The Wound and the Doctor

Glin Bennet, MA, MD, FRCS, FRCPsych, was born in 1927 and is a Senior Lecturer in the Department of Mental Health, University of Bristol, a psychotherapist and a consultant psychiatrist. Before taking up psychiatry he worked as a surgeon, and an earlier book, *Patients and their Doctors*, is about the reactions of people to illness, to hospitalization and to surgical operations. In *Beyond Endurance*, he described how people respond to extremes of physical and psychological stress.

By the same author

Patients and their Doctors: the Journey through Medical Care
Beyond Endurance: Survival at the Extremes

The Wound and the Doctor

Healing, Technology and Power
in Modern Medicine

Glin Bennet

Secker & Warburg · London

First published in England 1987 by
Martin Secker & Warburg Limited
54 Poland Street, London W1V 3DF
Re-issued in paperback 1988

Copyright © 1987 by Glin Bennet

British Library Cataloguing in Publication Data

Bennet, Glin, *1927–*
    The wound and the doctor.
    1. Medical technology
    I. Title
    610'.28

ISBN 0 436 04008 5

Typeset in 10½pt Linotron Bembo by
Hewer Text Composition Services, Edinburgh
Printed in England by Redwood Burn Ltd, Trowbridge

for James, Catherine,
Patrick and Julia

Contents

Contents

PART V – RE-VISIONING MEDICINE

Acknowledgements

I am grateful to the following publishers for permission to reproduce extracts from their works:

Allison and Busby (from *The Method* by P. Korovessis), Amnesty International (from *Professional Codes of Ethics* by A. Heijder and H. van Geuns), Atheneum Publishers (from *Married to Medicine* by Carla Fine), Blackwell (from *Barbers and Barber-Surgeons of London* by J. Dobson and R. Milnes Walker), The Bodley Head (from *Cancer Ward* by A. Solzhenitsyn), *British Medical Journal* (from 'Characteristics and prognosis of alcoholic doctors' by R. M. Murray, from 'I am an alcoholic' by G. Lloyd, and from 'Patient participation in a primary care unit' by A. T. M. Wilson), Cambridge University Press (from *Heraclitus* by G. S. Kirk, from *The Presocratic Philosophers* by G. S. Kirk *et al.*, from *Science and Civilisation in China*, Vol. 2 by J. Needham, and from *Joan-Baptista van Helmont* by W. Pagel), Clarendon Press (from *A History of the Royal College of Physicians of London* by G. Clark), Collins/Harvill (from *The Gulag Archepelago, 1, 1918–1956* by A. Solzhenitsyn), Constable (from *An Introduction to the Study of Experimental Medicine* by C. Bernard), Faber and Faber (from *Four Quartets* by T. S. Eliot), Victor Gollancz (from *Russia's Political Hospitals* by S. Bloch and P. Reddaway), Harper and Row (from *The Authoritarian Personality* by T. W. Adorno *et al.*), Her Majesty's Stationery Office (from *Cannabis*, and from *Committee of Inquiry into the Regulation of the Medical Profession*), Macmillan (from 'Newton the man' in *The Collected Writings of J. M. Keynes*), MIT Press (from *The Theoretical Foundations of Chinese Medicine* by M. Porkert), *New England Journal of Medicine* (from 'Compounding the ordeal of ALS' by D., P. L. and R. Rabin), Nuffield Provincial Hospitals Trust (from *High Technology Medicine* by B. Jennett), Open Court Publishing (from *Man a Machine* by J. O. de la Mettrie), Oxford University Press, New York (from *A History of Medicine*, Vol. 2 by H. E. Sigerist), Penguin Books (from *Discourse on Method* by R. Descartes, trans. by A. Wollaston, and from *Inequalities in Health* by P. Townsend and P. Davidson), Routledge and Kegan Paul (from *The Collected Works of C. G. Jung*, Vols 7 and 16, and from *Tao te Ching*), Tavistock (from *Married to their Careers* by Lane Gerber), University of California Press (from *East Asian Medicine in Urban Japan* by M. M. Lock), University of Pennsylvania Press (from *John Morgan: Continental Doctor* by W. J. Bell), Weidenfeld and Nicolson (from *Prisoner Without a Name, Cell Without a Number* by J. Timerman).

Preface

Why are so many doctors unhappy, despite their interesting work for which they are well rewarded; and why are their patients unhappy about the care they receive?

This book is devoted to understanding and, if possible, resolving that anomaly. Medical technology advances, yet the human problems remain. The more doctors can do to make life agreeable, and the more people know about their bodies and minds, the greater seems to be the dissatisfaction.

It is odd that a caring profession can be so accepting of the public's distress. Doctors hold the initiative and determine exactly how health care is delivered, and it has been difficult for me to accept that the medical profession (of which I am a part) does not at all times act as though it exists to help people in need. This is another anomaly: the doctors espouse high principles of caring, and have the power to implement those principles, but they do not implement them. Why not?

Anomaly and paradox pervade this subject, not only in the recognition of difficulties, but also in the daily work of a doctor, face to face with patients – hence the title which links 'wounds' and 'doctors'. I have tried to identify the essence of these contradictions, and then seek ways of resolving them. This book is the result of my explorations and endeavours.

The anomalies of the medical life are developed in the Introduction, and I explain my own relationship to them, as this is something of a personal book. Parts I and II are devoted to descriptions – given with a minimum of comment – of the troubles and vagaries of doctors: first at a personal and domestic level; and later at a professional level, when doctors are acting collectively as 'the medical profession' or in their individual public roles.

In Part III, there is an attempt to explain some of the peculiarities of doctors. Many of the difficulties doctors experience seem to be connected with the way they think about illness. Part IV, therefore, is devoted to ideas doctors have held about illness in ancient times, in medieval Europe and in the traditional medical systems of India and China; and a brief study of these reveals something of what we have lost as a result of the rise of technological medicine. In Part V, specific suggestions are made about how the quality of medical care can be improved. These involve: more realistic thinking about the nature of illness; better ways for doctors to manage their work and their personal lives; better ways of working in partnership with their medical colleagues, with other health professionals, and of course with their patients.

The book is written from the viewpoint of a doctor. It could have been written from a patient's viewpoint, or from both. It is placed 'within' the doctor, so to speak. I am not concentrating here on the deficiencies in medical care which derive from lack of resources, important as material resources are. The book concerns the person of the doctor and what goes on within, because I believe that the changes which will most improve the quality of medical care will come about through developments in the attitudes of doctors, rather than by providing more money and material resources; and so the emphasis is psychological rather than sociological.

The contemporary material is drawn from all over the English-speaking world. I have used the terms 'doctor' and 'physician' synonymously, and 'internal medicine' is used for 'medicine' as the term is understood in Britain. The hospital grades 'registrar' (UK) and 'resident' (USA) are also synonymous.

Most of the empirical work on doctors, until very recently, has been based on male doctors, and so there is a bias in my reporting. However, most of the serious difficulties in the medical profession are connected with men, as indeed are many of the difficulties experienced by women doctors. A book written in the future, with women doctors sharing the professional power equally with men, would be very different from this one.

I have made my career in medicine, and have experienced great variety in the quality of medical practice – from the excellent to the distinctly bad. The best is very good indeed, and I have an abiding respect for a great many doctors, famous and unknown. I also have a special regard for the present generation of junior doctors, and often feel, listening to criticisms of the medical profession, that people do not realize how fortunate they are to have so many able young doctors waiting to serve them.

Many people have contributed one way or another to the writing of this book – patients, medical colleagues and others; and to them I am most grateful. In particular I want to thank Liz Robinson for her valuable critical advice throughout the writing; Eveline Bennet for her detailed editing; Mark Bryant for guiding the book through publication, and Anthony Raven for his meticulous copy-editing; Susan Benn, Jeffrey Boss, Lucy Macaulay and Christopher Rowe for their specialized criticism; and Rosalind Bennet, who helped create the setting in which the book was written.

Introduction

Medicine Lost

Doctors seem to have the perfect answer to the dilemma of finding a life with meaning. They obviously do good for others, and while they may be criticized, everyone is glad to see them in a crisis.

Medical work is extremely interesting and varied. It may at times be demanding but it should never be boring. Doctors are privileged people. Allowances are made for them on the assumption that they live their lives poised in readiness to dash to the bedside of a sick person. They have high status, high incomes carrying complete security and a pension at the end, and it is exceptional to find one unwillingly out of work. There is no other group in society which is quite so well placed in terms of opportunities for a satisfying and well rewarded life.

The private lives of doctors contrast sharply with their professional style. Some difference between the outward image and private reality is to be expected, but not in an extreme degree, nor in those whose job it is to maintain the health of the population. They should know what makes for a good and healthy life, and how the hazards can be avoided. But doctors, taken collectively, compare badly with their patients when it comes to managing their private lives.

Doctors feature prominently in statistics for alcoholism, drug abuse and suicide.[1] They are not at the top of these tables but they are disturbingly high up in them.

Doctors can justly feel proud of the achievements of the medical profession over the past two hundred years or so. Technology may not increase our life span, but unquestionably it makes our lives more agreeable, so that the vast majority of people in the Western world can expect their lives to be free from chronic discomfort and disability, to an extent which would have been unthinkable early in the nineteenth century. Childbearing can be supervised so that it is mostly a joyful experience and the tragedies are rare; and dying no longer needs to be agonizing or endured in a state of stupor.

While doctors are respected for what they can do they are not always liked, and even actively disliked, being regarded as arrogant, unfeeling and condescending towards their patients.

Large modern hospitals house a huge range of diagnostic and therapeutic equipment so that their main function is technological. Patients can be assessed rapidly and safely, and there is seldom any complaint about the standard of professional expertise; but there are deep dissatisfactions at the human level. This is borne out by numerous surveys of the quality of communication between doctors and patients, and the feelings patients voice about the quality of the care they receive: overall, a good two-thirds of patients express dissatisfaction in this area.[2] They want to know more about what is wrong with them, what treatment is proposed, what effect certain treatments will have on their lives (notably on their sexual and reproductive functions), how they can participate in their own care, and whether there are any different approaches to their condition. Doctors would agree that these are reasonable requests, yet this level of communication between patients and doctors is rare. The lapses in the aspects of medical care which involve consideration for the patient are far too common, even in the best appointed medical centres, and I regularly hear stories which disturb and embarrass me – for I am part of the medical profession. What am I to say when people recount experiences such as the following?

A married woman of forty-eight was admitted for treatment of suspected breast cancer. The plan, as she understood it, was that she would have a biopsy examination under general anaesthetic, but when she woke her left breast was gone. She was told the growth was more extensive than had been anticipated. Next day, she complained to the surgeon that she should have had a chance to think things over once the biopsy report was available. She also resented having to sign a form allowing the surgeons to do whatever they judged necessary. The surgeon merely said, 'What's a breast, anyway? It's only the icing on the cake.'

A four-year-old child required drops in her eyes before having an eye examination. Her mother (who was familiar with ophthalmological procedures having had an eye removed for a malignant tumour) offered to put them in: the offer was refused. She then offered to hold her daughter while the staff put them in: this was also refused. Finally, the little girl was taken to another room by four nurses who had to hold her down. The diagnosis was duly made, and the subsequent treatment was entirely satisfactory, for this was a hospital with high standards, staffed by capable and committed people, and in which I would feel safe as a patient. Yet, at the human level – which is the level at which most people evaluate their medical care – there are frequent lapses.

Here, then, are two anomalies concerning the medical profession at the present time: the doctors, with high income and interesting work, who have such trouble in their personal lives; and the excellent medical services which yet allow so much personal dissatisfaction. The doctors are in difficulties with themselves and with their work.

These dilemmas encompass most of the problems facing doctors and the medical profession in general. They provide a point of departure for this book and a unifying theme throughout it. They are issues I have grappled with, and, recognizing their anomalous or paradoxical nature, I will not mistake them for questions which, generally speaking, have answers. Anomalies and paradoxes, in their nature, are less clear: they lead to resolution rather than to answers, and the succeeding pages will be an attempt at such a resolution.

It is unwise to try to explain human behaviour. In psychiatric practice people seek help for all kinds of reasons, and it is usually clear to those outside the immediate problem what has gone wrong and the various steps which have led to the person's breakdown. To say why the breakdown occurred is much more difficult, even when there are clear precipitating circumstances. Explanations can be offered in terms of simple causes and effects, and at first sight these can seem impressive, but in the long run they are not likely to be illuminating.

However, if this book is to achieve its objectives, which include making doctors more aware of what they are doing, I cannot avoid making some attempts at explanation for the habits and peculiarities of doctors; and for the misdemeanours and even actual crimes committed by them.

Much of the descriptive material and the discussion of the issues touches on questions of authority and power. Authority and power feature prominently in the book, and require to be set in some kind of context, otherwise Parts I and II will represent doctors in an unduly negative light.

Authority in medicine is not a simple matter. It is important at a time of crisis that a doctor can take charge: to be able to provide confident support and informed advice for someone stricken with serious illness which may involve major surgery; to guide a person towards the acceptance of fatal illness; or to sustain a bereaved family. Authority is needed in other settings, for example, after a major accident, to maintain a firm grip on the organization to prevent the medical services being overwhelmed; when dealing with colleagues and administrators to obtain the resources necessary for the discharge of one's clinical responsibilites, and then in utilizing these resources in a proper manner; when dealing with medical colleagues who are sick or in need of personal support. All clinical doctors need at times to be able to act decisively. They can do this because of their knowledge and the rights given to them by society – rights which are sanctioned by statute.

There is a negative side to authority. Most doctors respect the authority invested in them and they are not temperamentally disposed to abuse it. Sadly, some doctors do abuse their authority, causing great suffering to individuals and bringing the medical profession into disrepute. Other doctors unwittingly fall victim to the temptations of authority.

There is the benign authority of the doctor who uses power sparingly yet effectively, and the more malevolent authority of the authoritarian doctor.

Doctors have more immediate power over their fellow citizens than any other group in society, but when I started writing this book I had not anticipated just how pervasive the issues of authority and power would turn out to be. Authority and power seemed to crop up everywhere, and I wondered if perhaps I was projecting my own preoccupations, and highlighting these issues to an excessive degree. Objective reporting is naturally an illusion, and in a book like this there must be biases in the selection, yet I would be sorry if all I was doing was documenting my prejudices. I have been as vigilant as I could be about this, and at the same time take comfort from Aldous Huxley's words: 'having a beam in one's own eye may actually sharpen one's vision for beams in the eyes of others'.[3]

Partly because this is a personal book and partly because I want to make my biases as clear as I can, I will indicate briefly something of the influences to which I have been exposed. There was never any plan to my career, and at the major turning points I was guided by a vague sense of what was right and meaningful for me at the time.

I happened to start off in surgery because of a greater interest at the time in the practical over the theoretical, and indirectly through one of those formative experiences as a student which are small in themselves but have far-reaching consequences.[4] I had an opportunity to remove an appendix (under supervision), and that fired my enthusiasm for surgery and the technical challenges involved in performing operations.

There then followed busy surgical jobs in hospital, and later national service as a junior surgeon in the army in Cyprus at the time of the terrorist activity, in Egypt during the Suez crisis, and then in Libya which did not at that time have oil and so was still a poor country. It was instructive to encounter people who had great medical need yet did not appreciate what I regarded as the great benefits of Western medicine. I felt helpless and misunderstood in the face of the indigenous practitioners and sick people who had a totally different view of illness from my own. Lacking any understanding of their conceptual framework, and, I am ashamed to say, not even realizing then that they had any coherent way of thinking about illness, I tended to regard their attitudes at best as quaint, and at worst as wicked. I never could understand how a man given a tube of antibiotic cream for his trachoma could take it straight to the market and sell it for a few pence; or how a man would donate blood to help a sick son but not to help a sick daughter.

Immediately after the two years of national service, I was catapulted, so it felt, into the highly technological medicine of London, first in neurosurgery, and later in the currently spectacular medical occupation of cardio-thoracic surgery. With hindsight, I cannot now imagine what I was doing there, although it was exciting to feel that one was part of the vanguard of medicine. It was what I would now call a 'nineteenth-century' feeling, in which it seemed that all the ills of mankind could be cured by technological medicine.

The recollection of those years is mainly in terms of the very gifted and creative men for whom I worked. I came across other physicians and surgeons who were famous, pompous and incompetent; some who were simply rude to everybody; a few who were scholars; those who only became interested when a substantial fee was involved; and others still who were engrossed with the politics and ceremonial of medicine to the exclusion of practically everything else. Someone else looking back might recollect more of the actual work or the patients he looked after, but I think my attitudes were fairly typical of the junior doctors of those days. We did view the medical profession in hierarchical terms. These men were unquestionably at the top of the profession, and their position was a feature in their favour besides their outstanding abilities. Of course the two should go together, and often did, but not always by any means.

By 1962, I should have been in a senior registrar post but I had stayed longer than usual at a more junior level to gain broader experience. When the desirable senior registrar post came up, I found that I did not want it, and let it go. I had by then performed practically all the operations in the surgical repertoire, and the prospect of repeating them for the rest of my working life was not appealing. Learning operations and doing them for the first, second or third time, is one thing. Repeating them endlessly was not for me, so I took leave of surgery.

The decision to take up psychiatry came two and a half years later during an unexpected meeting with a friend while skiing. He told me he had recently begun a psychiatric job, and that must have activated a latent intention in myself because I knew in that instant that I, too, was going to 'take up psychiatry. The idea did not arise altogether out of the blue as I had long been interested in psychological ideas and already had part of the professional psychiatric qualification which I had taken at the same time as the surgical examinations, but the actual decision was immediate.

I started psychiatric work in Bristol where my switch of careers was regarded as an amusing eccentricity. I still found myself interested in surgical matters, and in medicine also, and enjoyed the company of the surgeons and physicians. This gradually led to my becoming involved in consultations about psychological and social problems affecting patients in the medical and surgical wards, and I found that having a surgical qualification rendered me somehow more credible to my medical and surgical colleagues.

My experiences in these wards, however, were not what I had anticipated. I was returning to a familiar environment but with different spectacles, and the images were quite disturbing. In the psychiatric department we talked about relationships, people's reactions to their difficulties, the significance and meaning of problems, how patients related to the staff, and other matters not connected with diagnosis or treatment in a medical sense. The medical and surgical departments were then, and to a great extent still are, primarily concerned with diagnosis and treatment at a physical level. Nothing else about the patient mattered to anything like the same degree.

An awareness of the patient's point of view is not necessarily an advantage for the doctor. It becomes harder to be concerned purely with the minutiae of pathology or the technical problems of an operation. It changes twenty or thirty 'cases' in the ward into as many people who are silently enduring great fear and distress. Open the doors a little, and the weight of emotion can be overwhelming. All the doctor's anxieties about mutilation, disability and death are brought to the surface and they are acted out by the patients.

It had been so much easier when I was a surgical junior, as matters such as these were simply never discussed. Our teachers got by with platitudes: 'treat the patient, not the disease', but nobody stopped to think what that meant in actual clinical practice.

Nowadays it is rather different. Much more is known about the function of large organizations. Researchers have taken a great interest in hospitals, how the staff impose their will upon patients,[2] and strip them of their identity in order to make them easier to manage,[5] and how even nurses condition patients to meet their expectations.[6]

Along with this, patients are much better informed than ever before about medical matters, and are more pressing in their demands to be treated as responsible, intelligent and sensitive beings. Nevertheless, they are still bound to feel a mixture of fear and awe on entering the seemingly monolithic institution of a hospital. The staff, for their part, far from responding positively to these aspirations, often take up a defensive position. But why should this group, which has all the power, be so suspicious of the other group, which effectively has none? It is yet another of the paradoxes which pervade medical practice, especially in hospitals.

This introduction began with the paradoxes of the outwardly confident doctor who is inwardly distressed, the excellent medical services which are unappreciated, and the high technology which fails to meet the needs of people. I have used a few autobiographical fragments to illustrate some of the sources of dissatisfaction, and also to make clear my ambiguous position in the story. If I have used examples of the actions of others, it is not because I think I am blameless – far from it – but because in those days I was quite unaware of what I was doing, and so my own misdemeanours were never recorded. I am writing, therefore, very much as an insider, with admiration for the expertise of many members of the medical profession, yet aware that things could be better.

Part I

Personal Strains

1

How Doctors Work

Many doctors lead contented and useful lives in which they achieve fulfilment in their work and personal relationships. Such life-styles have been portrayed as fact and in fiction,[1] and these accounts represent what the public and some doctors would like to believe. To what extent they conform with what a young doctor might reasonably expect from a career in medicine is quite another matter.

One thing is sure, that there is a niche for every doctor, as in this respect the medical profession is a club which can provide a congenial way of life somewhere in the world for people of every temperament. Doctors take on diverse responsibilities as they become established in the profession; they acquire a reputation in their hospital or community as being kind, conscientious, obliging, energetic, or perhaps the opposite of all these. In what seems a very short time, the young doctor becomes embroiled in the system. In Britain, this refers to the National Health Service, the medical organizations, and the delicate network of professional relationships with immediate colleagues and wider circles. In countries with different medical arrrangements there may be less involvement with the state, but then there will be private practice and its own rewards and worries.

In this chapter I want to describe something of the doctor's working life, and will do this, not by trying to cover the whole range of medical activity, but by concentrating on one issue which affects all clinical doctors, and one which has ramifications throughout the doctor's personal and professional life: that is the issue of being busy, with the consequences of excessive busyness which are inefficiency, and, in the longer term, burning out.

Professional busyness

I know a general practitioner who always used to break into a run on the path between the front door of his house and his car parked by the roadside. The message to neighbours was that he was on his way to urgent business. At times, doubtless he was, but not every day. Then he had his heart attack, and after that he walked.

It is very convenient to have it assumed that one is perpetually busy with humanitarian work. Allowances are made and life is smoothed in all kinds of ways, from flexibility with car parking to prompt attention to one's telephone. Medical prestige is not what it was but it is still advantageous, and all the more so when the doctor can create an impression of being in permanent demand. The process is a reciprocal one. The doctor probably is in demand, but the public also likes to invest the doctor with heroic qualities, since it needs heroes as much as they, in turn, need public adulation. The public also has an interest in exalting doctors in general, because people want to believe that their own doctor has superior skills. This leads all doctors to enjoy a vicarious prestige.

The medical profession makes a virtue out of busyness and working long hours, even though its spokesmen complain publicly about how hard doctors work. When I was a junior doctor, my seniors made it abundantly clear how much harder they used to work than we ever did. Nowadays, it seems to me that the juniors have an easier time than we did. And so the illusion endures.

From my surgical days, I can remember a misguided pride in staying up all night, having spent the whole of the previous day in the operating theatre, and then going on to assist at an operating list the next morning. I can clearly recall twenty-eight hours without getting out of theatre boots, and a good thirty-six hours of continuous surgical work in and out of theatre. It seemed at the time quite natural, and we really believed we were doing good work, in the best traditions of medicine: there was a job to be done and we got on with it. Workers in other departments and disciplines might go home at five, but if patients needed our care, we would be there to give it. We liked to think we worked longer hours than anyone else in the hospital, and that made us feel superior. We accepted without question the long days, often lasting until late in the evening, and busy emergency duty every other night. Without realizing it, we were adopting the ethos of the busy doctor, and equating it with quality; which was reasonable to the extent that, as trainee surgeons, we learned a great deal very quickly, but from the point of view of good doctoring, it was absurd.

Being unattached at the time, such extremely long hours did not really matter to me, except that no regular social life was possible. For those who were married it was much harder. A colleague at St Mark's Hospital in London, in the 1950s, used to stay in the hospital every weekday night and only saw his wife and children at occasional weekends, when he was not on duty. Sometimes he was away from his children for so long that

4

they resented his coming between them and their mother. At St Thomas's Hospital and the National Hospital for Nervous Diseases, Queen Square (and doubtless several other London hospitals as well), aspiring surgeons would virtually live in the hospital on indefinite tours of duty. These were prized jobs because they carried with them an implied promise of a consultant post at a good hospital; so to immure oneself in hospital for a year or so was judged a good investment.

The occupants of these posts in teaching hospitals were by then well conditioned to the supposed virtues of long hours of work, having already made many personal sacrifices to this end, and the more junior doctors and medical students regarded this virtual incarceration in hospital as an unavoidable step in the struggle to the top. The top, in those days, carried considerable prestige within the profession, positions in the Royal Colleges, honours, wealth from private practice – a kind of success more generally valued then than it is today. The average junior doctor might not have aspirations to become President of a Royal College, but he almost certainly did have a belief, albeit an implanted one, that working long hours was a good thing.

Doctors work hard, as do many other people in society. Clinicians probably experience more irregularity than other professionals and people in business, but they work against a background of financial security, and they have unusual scope for determining their working conditions. General practitioners and hospital consultants have great freedom in how they design and organize their lives. Not only can they choose the exact kind of medical activity which will suit them temperamentally, but the structure of contemporary society usually enables them to control the style of their personal life as well. Doctors have a fair choice of countries and climates in which they can work. They can choose an urban or a rural environment, and once there can usually construct their working conditions with considerable freedom, even though some will have committed themselves to deprived regions where the material resources and rewards are limited.

Many doctors say they are trapped in a treadmill, but many more have bent the system to suit themselves. General practitioners can acquire large lists spread over a wide area, they can take on clinics here and there, insurance examinations and other special assignments which keep them continually on the move. They can organize appointments at their surgeries (and most do) so that people do not have to wait, or they can have a free-for-all where people just turn up and are eventually seen. In the afternoons they can cultivate their gardens or run clinics where they can see people in longer consultations, and in the evenings they can see their families and friends, or hold surgeries and make house calls.

The specialists also have great choice, and here there is much more scope for quirks of personality. Anyone who comes to see himself as an embodiment of one of the grand physicians or surgeons of the past can act out this fantasy with ease, even in the framework of a nationalized health service. Thus, impressive ward rounds can be staged with the entire staff in attendance; out-patient clinics with large numbers of patients waiting to be seen, and the consultant seated at the centre of a large room with his assistants ranged around. These clinics in turn lead to the creation of long waiting lists of people for operations or other treatments. Such a specialist, needless to say, is going to be exceedingly busy, since the hospital style is merely one part of the realization of a self-image which will eventually dominate all his waking hours.

Most doctors take the path of busyness. This may also be the way to achievement but not always. Busyness is allowed to become a way of life, so that opportunities to fill up one's time are either positively sought or else accepted without demur. The doctor is in constant demand and his status rises accordingly, and so he becomes better able to structure his life as he chooses. It may seem contradictory to say that the busier the person the more he can mould his life to his choosing, but when the demands are professional they are ultimately in his control.

This contrasts with a life where there are substantial family demands with continuing domestic and personal relationships. These cannot be controlled in the way that professional relationships can, neither can they be abandoned at the end of the day, and some doctors come to find the professional relationships altogether more congenial for this reason.

Inefficiency and errors

It would be unfair on the thousands of junior hospital doctors to suggest that they work dangerously long hours because they choose to. These conditions are imposed upon them by their seniors who are now making the present juniors do what they had to do when they were at that stage. The seniors often act as though they believe it is good for them to work through the night or at any rate that it is the only way to learn. However, the attitude is not rational, at least it is not quite what it appears to be. It is rather that these long hours of duty constitute some kind of initiation rite to the medical profession proper. Anyway, no change in this practice is likely, since more doctors would have to be employed who would then not find a permanent place in the medical pyramid.

A few years ago I studied the effects of physical and psychological pressure on the quality of decision-making and performance.[2] The main research was on sailors in isolation in small boats on the ocean: people

6

who had to function at a high level of efficiency if they were to survive and reach their destination, despite lack of sleep and proper nourishment, and moments of anxiety and fear. The work also involved studying the experiences of adventurers in other extreme conditions; and also those of airline pilots, train drivers, and others who worked in comfortable physical surroundings yet had to function effectively for long periods of time. Frequently in these studies I was reminded of events I had experienced or witnessed in hospital work, and it was disturbing to realize how often the junior doctors in hospital were working in circumstances almost certain to lead to impairment of function.

The present generation of junior hospital doctors is still working excessive hours; and according to recent surveys,[3,4] the average junior hospital doctor in Britain works about a 90-hour week, of which 84 are spent actually on duty. 32 per cent are on duty for more than 100 hours and 8 per cent for more than 130 hours. The average for juniors in trauma and orthopedic surgery is 101 hours, while for psychiatry it is 62 hours. The work of these doctors is relatively easy to measure because they have essentially one job in one place. The working hours of specialists are less easily measured as their lives are more complicated, although an average of 49 hours has been quoted for whole-time consultants in Britain. General practitioners also lead complicated lives and their working patterns have so far eluded study,[4] a conclusion which suggests that there is great variation in the hours worked.

A peculiar aspect of the present position of junior hospital doctors (whose situation best highlights the issues under discussion) is that they are overworked despite abundant knowledge about the deterioration in the quality of performance after long hours of work. Elsewhere precautions are taken to prevent fatigue from excessive hours of work wherever a sustained high level of performance is required, such as piloting aircraft, driving trains or heavy road vehicles. But the need for such precautions is totally disregarded in the medical profession, mainly, I think, because it conflicts with the collective medical fantasy of the doctor as a person who is above human frailties, and who has to survive the hospital years as a kind of *rite de passage*.

Out of the great variety of reactions to fatigue – extending to hallucinations and complete psychological disorganization – three appear conspicuously in medical practice: simple errors, poor concentration and forgetfulness; false expectations; and preoccupation and distraction.[5]

Simple errors, poor concentration and forgetfulness. At any given moment in the day or night, large numbers of people are bringing serious problems to doctors who they assume will be in a position to make accurate observations and judgements. Every doctor knows that this is by no

7

means the case, especially at night – just consider all those appendixes removed in error.[6] Any observer in a hospital at night can identify the people who have been working all the previous day. These doctors have a ponderous manner, everything is done laboriously and takes far longer than it would have done sixteen hours earlier. During such long spells of duty one can become almost like an automaton, devoid of emotion, and dehumanizing patients by pointedly disregarding everything except the diseased organ. With hindsight, I find it hard to believe that, on several occasions, at the beginning of yet another abdominal emergency late at night, I could earnestly hope that the case would prove inoperable so that I could get some sleep, because a bowel resection might have us there another hour and a half.

When subjects are tested in a psychological laboratory, a deterioration in performance can be demonstrated reliably after one night with only two hours' sleep, or after two consecutive nights with only five hours' sleep on each. Where one whole night has been spent without sleep, performance is much more seriously impaired, and even one good night's sleep is insufficient to restore the subject to full efficiency.[7]

Now these are results from inevitably dull tests, so how relevant are they to the activities of highly motivated young doctors doing work which interests them and which they regard as important? The short answer is, not very relevant, except after prolonged sleep loss when no amount of motivation can keep a person functioning effectively.

At the Presbyterian Hospital in New York City, a group of thirteen interns were given electrocardiograms to read for arrhythmic episodes, first, when they were rested, and again after an average of 1.8 hours' sleep (range 0–3.8 hours). They worked more slowly and made significantly more errors in their sleep-deprived state. 'Difficulties thinking' were described by twelve out of the thirteen, 'depression' by ten, 'irritability' by nine, 'referential feelings with extreme sensitivity to criticism' by six, 'depersonalization and derealization' by six, 'inappropriate affect usually associated with black humor' by five, and 'recent memory deficit' by five.[8,9]

In a more detailed study from Cambridge,[10] junior doctors were given tests of grammatical reasoning, and also had to pick out the abnormal results from a batch of twenty-four laboratory reports dealing with haematology, blood electrolytes, enzymes, blood gases, etc. With a sleep debt (the number of hours less than their average sleep) of three hours or more, 'there was a reliable increase in the variability in the rate of work'. If the same doctors knew that an extra effort was needed they could perform as accurately in these short tests as when they were rested, if not better. It would have required a test lasting twenty minutes or more to demonstrate any reliable deterioration, but no tired doctors would willingly submit to this at the end of a night's work. After a cumulative sleep debt (the sum of the sleep debt for up to the three preceding nights) of between three and five hours there was a deterioration in efficiency, but it could be compensated for by extra effort. However, no such compensation could be made once the cumulative debt reached eight hours.

Tiredness may occur by itself, although in clinical work it is more likely to be associated with a measure of anxiety. Doctors become anxious if they doubt their ability to cope with their work – because there is too much of it or because they doubt if they possess the necessary knowledge and skills. They can also become anxious about more remote matters relating to their employment, money and personal relationships; and there is a great deal of field work and experimental research which shows how anxiety can affect the quality of observation, reasoning and performance.[11,12] For practical purposes, tiredness and anxiety can be taken together, each augmenting the effects of the other.

False expectations means seeing what you want to see as opposed to what is actually there. At night this means diagnosing gastroenteritis (which allows you to go back to bed) as opposed to acute appendicitis (which means you must operate). It is one of the commonest reactions to fatigue for a doctor to narrow his perception and distort his interpretations to meet his reduced capacity. When fresh and relaxed, there is a fair chance that he will take in all the available clinical information and process it accurately; when fatigued, a dangerous tendency to select often appears. Surgeons are especially at risk. At the end of a difficult dissection in the region of the gall bladder, the surgeon finds a bile duct. He earnestly wants it to be the cystic duct, and not the common bile duct. If he is tired and troubled about professional and personal matters – perhaps far away from the operating theatre – he is in danger of believing that the hollow structure he is holding in the clamp is the duct he has been searching for.

The other reaction, which is partly a variation on the foregoing, is *preoccupation and distraction*; and it means that the doctor concentrates on a detail at the expense of the whole. The tired house officer concentrates so hard on the blood pressure, pulse rate and pupil reactions of a patient with a head injury, that he fails to notice that the patient has become unconscious.

The same doctor examining a boy with abdominal pain finds he is tender on the right side of his abdomen, low down, and he decides the boy has acute appendicitis. That observation is accurate but he fails to take proper account of the history of diarrhoea and vomiting, gurgling in the

9

gut and a temperature of thirty-nine degrees Celsius. This doctor is eliciting a basic clinical sign and making assumptions about it which are not then subjected to critical analysis or modified in the light of other information. If the same doctor had been fresh and relaxed, he would have considered acute appendicitis, but also other possible diagnoses such as gastroenteritis or some fever, and then would have made further observations to reduce the diagnostic possibilities.

The fatigued doctor will often narrow the range of his clinical observation. He may also become inflexible in his reasoning, and refuse to revise his initial hypothesis in the light of subsequent information, because at that time he is incapable of the mental effort needed to handle all the variables. On the basis of limited observation, he seizes on one diagnosis and sticks to it, regardless of other clinical information which he simply fails to register. This can have grotesque consequences, as when I saw a junior doctor so unnerved by a cardiac arrest that he threw himself into the business of getting a blood transfusion going, which he insisted was an essential preliminary to cardiac massage, despite the uselessness of such a course and the objections of the rest of us. He was preoccupying himself not only with a detail to the neglect of the whole, but with an irrelevant detail at that. Faced with a problem which was beyond him, he was concentrating on an activity which he could understand, but, more importantly and dangerously, he had reinterpreted the problem of cardiac arrest to suit his limitations, and nothing anyone could do at the time could shift his beliefs.

A variation on this pattern occurs when the fatigued doctor is unable to settle on any single diagnosis, and instead flits from one possibility to another. He is responding to every bit of clinical information as it appears, and becomes overwhelmed by it all since he cannot integrate his observations into a coherent hypothesis or diagnosis that will not be blown away completely by the next new item of information. It is a phenomenon particularly connected with a high level of anxiety. [13,14]

This kind of grasshopper indecisiveness is especially serious in a surgeon, who should be able to make up his mind positively on all occasions (even when the positive decision is that no firm decision is possible at the time) and not have to look to a supportive assistant, anaesthetist or theatre nurse to help him make up his mind.

Those in surgical specialties are most prone to the effects of fatigue because of the irregular nature of their work, the need to be decisive, and the prevailing background of disaster which maintains their anxiety at a high level, however relaxed they may say they feel when operating. Despite these considerations, I have not found that surgeons (or any other doctors for that matter) are interested in studying the quality of their work at different times of the day or night, even though quite simple methods of study have been proposed.[15]

Running down and burning out

Fatigue, with its attendant errors and behavioural disturbances, is in the nature of a short-term or 'acute' phenomenon. There is also the chronic deterioration in performance spread over years, and it goes under the currently fashionable name of burn-out.

The term 'burn-out' was introduced by a New York psychoanalyst in 1974[16] to describe the emotional and physical exhaustion that overtakes many dedicated front-line community and mental health workers trying to grapple directly with people who have difficult and intractable problems. Examples would be crisis intervention workers, alcohol and drug counsellors, psychiatric nurses, health visitors, social workers, child care workers, teachers, probation officers. The concept of burn-out caught on at once as it described an all-too-familiar set of responses in the caring professions, and it has given rise to a large literature.[17-22] It is a somewhat vague term, like 'stress', which has no agreed meaning, but the concept is a useful one for all that.

The path to burn-out is described with regard to people whose conditions of work are very different from those of doctors. These community workers are more directly exposed to their clients, and they do not have the status, the professional autonomy or the income which serve to protect doctors. Nevertheless, the sequence of deterioration for doctors is much the same.

In the course of several years of effective and satisfying medical practice, an equation is operating, so to speak, in which the physical drive and emotional energy put into the work is balanced by satisfaction gained from the work, as well as the individual's own recuperative capacity. If a great deal of physical and emotional effort is being put into the work and the level of satisfaction is low, then the doctor's resources are being depleted, and in time the consequences of this will appear. The compulsive busyness and the denial of human limitations, mentioned earlier, are examples of behaviour which will eventually deplete a doctor's resources, unless he has somehow managed to develop recuperative activities which will balance the equation. A few doctors manage to work compulsively and yet remain in balance; the majority are liable to run down slowly over the years.

A series of downward steps has been described[23] which matches the experience of many doctors. There is an *initial enthusiasm* for the work:

11

this is a feature of all burn-out, which is, by definition, a phenomenon affecting people who are strongly committed to their work and believe in its importance. In other words, 'you have to be on fire before you can burn out'.[24] In the early years of medical practice, there are high hopes, high energy and high expectations. The work is everything: a powerful identification with the profession, an impressive commitment to the patients, and even a feeling that nothing outside the work really matters all that much.

After a number of years, a sense of *stagnation* develops as the work ceases to be sufficient sustenance on its own. There is a desire for time away from work, time with family, a desire for more material comforts and benefits, and a rewarding career to look forward to. This phase introduces an element of reality and a sense of balance in life, so it may herald only the end of unrealistic enthusiasm, not necessarily the beginning of a decline.

A true decline is apparent once feelings of *frustration* begin to predominate. There can be frustration and irritability about the inconsiderate habits of patients, colleagues and the administrative machine. The early idealism and the over-riding commitment to patients have given way to a mild cynicism, and the feeling that nothing one does really makes any difference. The doctor may also begin to doubt his own competence.

A common symptom is resentment at the trivial nature of the demands made by patients; and this suggests that the doctor is dismissing from his mind the human aspects of the problem, such as the patient's anxieties: something doctors commonly do when under pressure of any kind. Such a call will be felt as yet another unreasonable demand on his time, although if he reflects, he will remember how in the past he met such calls as a challenge.

Gradually conditions deteriorate into a state of *apathy* in which only minimum energy goes into the work that was once so stimulating and rewarding. The apathetic position is regrettably stable, unlike enthusiasm which is ephemeral. Apathy also has a good deal of realism about it as it is almost impossible to bring about many of the changes hoped for in one's youth. The problems facing all members of the helping professions are to do with people, their ailments and their wayward behaviour; and these are notoriously resistant to change. Apathy also occurs when the doctor stops learning, when he admits to himself that he does not really want anything to change, and when job security becomes the primary consideration. By this stage, the quality of his work is probably below what is acceptable. He may have found, or created, a niche for himself in which he can eke out his time.

The concept of burn-out is formulated in terms of the pressures of a particular kind of work, and that leads on to the question of what sort of person chooses such work in the first place. This interplay of the doctor's personality and the style of medical life runs throughout the book, and I take the broad line that the personality comes first, and that it determines how the doctor will live and work.

2
How Doctors Live and Die

In England and Wales the life expectancy of male doctors is better than that of the population as a whole but worse than that of the professional classes (Registrar General's social class I). This can be expressed in numerical terms by use of the Standardized Mortality Ratio (SMR) which is the annual number of observed deaths for a given population (in this instance, male doctors), expressed as a percentage of the deaths expected for the whole population, standardized for age and sex. The average likelihood of dying is then, by definition, 100. Doctors score 81, the clergy 76, the legal profession 93, and primary and secondary school teachers 66; and the professional classes altogether score 75.[1]

United States doctors seem to be equally favoured. Three groups of male medical graduates from Harvard (which contained fewer than one per cent non-whites and were judged comparable with American doctors in general) were followed for up to forty-five years from graduation, and showed a significantly lower mortality as compared with US white males in general.[2]

A hundred years ago the position of doctors was worse. In terms of death rates per thousand for males aged 25–65 for the years 1880–82, doctors scored 17.3 compared with 'all occupations' scoring 15.4. By comparison, the rate for the clergy was 8.6, for the legal profession 13, for schoolmasters 11.1. At the top end were 'earthenware manufacturers' at 26.8. The death rates for doctors had been rising steadily between 1860 and 1880. Out of twenty-seven different causes of death, the doctors had lower rates than the general male population for only seven. Notable amongst these were the deaths of doctors from pulmonary tuberculosis ('phthisis') which were only about half the rate for the general population – a consequence of their good living conditions despite exposure to the disease. Deaths of doctors from smallpox were about one-sixth of the average – the result presumably of vaccination, because the doctors' death rates from diphtheria, scarlet fever and typhus, for which there was then no immunization or treatment, were well above the average.

14

The death rate from hernia for doctors was only one-seventh of the average.[3]

In the 1930s doctors were still at extra risk, with an SMR of 106 (i.e. worse than the average male), compared with an SMR for professional men of 83; but by 1951 the SMR for doctors had come down to 89 and the SMR for all 'professional and technical' men had fallen to 80.[4]

In the second half of the twentieth century there are still risks associated with particular medical occupations, such as radiologists and the effects of ionizing radiations, pathologists and tuberculosis, workers in renal dialysis units and hepatitis, paediatricians and minor infections.[5] The medical profession in England and Wales does not, overall, have a significantly raised mortality from cancer, but studies from various parts of the Western world suggest that certain groups of doctors show an increased incidence of lymphoma and brain tumour.[6]

The spectacular change in recent times has been the fall in the number of deaths among doctors from lung cancer and other smoking-related diseases.[7-9] Differential mortalities within the medical profession have also become apparent, although the meaning of these is not clear.

In a survey of over 20,000 male doctors in Britain over a twenty-year period up to 1971, the overall death rate among general practitioners was about 23 per cent higher than that for hospital physicians and surgeons of similar ages. The GPs smoked 37 per cent more cigarettes, and their higher death rate could be accounted for by the 38 per cent excess mortality (over the expected death rate for all male doctors) from smoking-related diseases such as lung cancer, chronic bronchitis, and ischaemic and pulmonary heart disease.[9] This survey was not designed to investigate the reasons why the GPs smoked more than their hospital colleagues, but it was noted that over half of the GPs in the survey were in singlehanded practice (compared with about 11 per cent in the 1980s). General practice in the early years of the National Health Service was a pretty depressed occupation. GPs were given inadequate resources compared with the hospital doctors, their status was reduced and they were a demoralized group.[10] Nowadays their position is quite different: they smoke less and they work under much better conditions. Over the period of the survey, the SMR for all doctors fell from 89 to 81, and the SMR for professional men fell from 80 to 75.

The only current mortality statistics in which male doctors figure prominently are those for cirrhosis of the liver (SMR 311, based on 14 deaths), suicide (SMR 335, on 55 deaths) and accidental poisoning (SMR 818, on 15 deaths).[1] These are all causes of death which have a relationship to the doctor's attitudes, state of mind and style of living. Put the other way round, the doctor's attitudes, mental state and life-style have a definite connection with how long the doctor lives, and also how much distress is endured.

Quality of life

The contemporary question, then, is not about the doctor's physical health, which is better than average, but about 'psychological' health; or, more precisely, about personal distress, emotional disturbances and frank psychological disorders.

Characteristically the male doctor's difficulties develop in the late thirties when he is established and has achieved the objectives which have occupied him so intensely over the preceding twenty years. The doctor not only has his partnership in general practice or his specialist appointment but has found his place in the system. He has also begun to accept, or at least to become aware of, his personal and professional limitations; and of some of the intractable problems of medical practice, which vary from country to country. For example, in Britain the bureaucracy of the National Health Service is commonly seen as the barrier to a fulfilling professional life; and in the United States it may be the threat of malpractice suits, physical violence or peer review.[11] While not denying the reality of these difficulties, they can also become focal points for a more general realization of how little can be changed in life and how few of one's early aspirations will ever be fulfilled.

The doctor also – probably – has his wife and children, his own home, a nice car and perhaps a boat as well; even a place in the country. He has all the material trappings, in the traditional sense, that a professional person can reasonably expect. Through enormous effort and sacrifice he has made it, personally and professionally, yet what awaits him may not be contentment but disillusionment. He is at the classic 'mid-point' in life where he can look not only backwards in time to find some boundary to his existence, but forwards as well. The endless striving upward towards a limitless future, in which all kinds of discomfort and inconvenience are tolerated on account of what lies ahead, is now tempered with the new realization that life is actually finite, and that he will not be advancing uphill for ever. Rather, in the thirties, forties and fifties the average professional man is on a plateau, after which there is a tendency to run downhill. In a social system based on endless achievement, problems can be expected if this success does not occur; and there can be difficulties even when the success is considerable, because for many men the essential element is the striving or yearning for what they have not got.

There are no statistics about the quality of doctors' marriages or divorce rates but some pointers emerge in the course of more general studies of the mental health of doctors.[12-15] Doctors seem to experience considerably more marital discord and higher rates for divorce than other professionals. Studies of the health and the problems experienced by their wives indicate a good deal of unhappiness, and that bears on the quality of marital life.[16] These and other matters surrounding doctors' marriages and families will be discussed later.

It is difficult to investigate the quality of life in a quantitative way, and I know of only one study that has managed to do this. It is particularly interesting as not only is it a controlled study but the subjects were followed up for a total of thirty years. It is the well-known work of George Vaillant and his colleagues at Cambridge, Massachusetts.[13] They began by investigating 268 male students selected on the grounds of good health and satisfactory academic performance. Details of the subjects' early lives were obtained by interview and home visit, and the subjects were contacted thereafter at two-yearly intervals. Forty-seven of the original group of 268 attended medical school. Two-thirds of them were at Columbia, Harvard, Johns Hopkins, Pennsylvania and Rochester; and all but one graduated. They were compared with 79 'socio-economically matched controls' also from the original 268.

Over three-quarters of the doctors had passed their specialty-board examinations, and all were currently 'gainfully employed'. At the time of the investigation, when the subjects must have been approaching fifty, the authors felt that the doctors were in better than average general health, yet 47 per cent of them had 'poor marriages' or had been divorced (compared with 32 per cent of the controls), and 20 per cent had actually been divorced (controls 14 per cent). 36 per cent reported 'trouble with control' of alcohol, 'often' used sleeping pills, or had taken amphetamines or tranquillizers daily for more than one month (controls 22 per cent).[17] Thirty-four per cent of the doctors had paid ten or more visits to a psychiatrist (controls 19 per cent). These differences were all statistically significant.[18]

In a more medical framework, there is another quantitative study, made by Robin Murray,[19] who took advantage of the very detailed records of hospital admissions and discharges which are kept in Scotland; and he followed all the psychiatric admissions there between 1963 and 1972. Altogether 110 male doctors were admitted during that period, and, as a control group, 379 non-medical professional men (Registrar General's social class I). Murray selected the age group 25–64 years and found that the discharge rate[20] for doctors was greater than that for other social class I men for 'all psychotic illness' (1.8 times social class I), 'all non-psychotic illness' (3.1 times), 'alcoholism' (3.3 times), and 'drug dependence' (10.8 times).

So far all the surveys have been about male doctors, and that is a historical phenomenon. There were relatively more male doctors when many of these surveys were started; and the standing of women doctors was lower than it is today, and so perhaps of less interest in research.

A group of 111 women doctors in St Louis had significantly more psychological disorders than a matched group of 103 women with PhDs: 57 per cent to 42 per cent.[21] The great majority of both groups were classified as being depressed. Among the depressed women doctors, 28 per cent gave a history of depression before entering medical school (and all had subsequent depressions), 33 per cent were depressed during medical school or residency, and 39 per cent had their first depression after their training was completed. Sixteen of the twenty-two psychiatrists and child psychiatrists (73 per cent) in the survey were depressed, compared with forty-one of the remaining doctors (46 per cent); and this statistically significant loading by the psychiatrists accounts for most of the differences in the prevalence of depression between the women doctors and the PhDs.[22]

While there is disagreement about the precise meaning of certain labels used to describe many varieties of mental disorders, it is fairly clear what is meant by the term 'depression', even if it does cover a wide range of appearances – from a sense of meaninglessness about life and work to an incapacitating condition requiring institutional care. The former state usually represents, I believe, the beginning of the downward slide currently encompassed in the literature about burn-out.

The early stage characterized by apathy and a sense of meaninglessness can proceed, if no remedial action is taken by the doctor, family or colleagues, to the more severe forms of mental disorder, alcoholism, drug abuse and finally suicide.

The concept of burn-out coincides in the medical profession with a concern for what is called in the United States the 'impaired physician'. The 'impaired physician' requires personal help, although there is also a commendable interest in protecting the public from dangerous or incompetent doctors. A large literature has grown up on the emotional problems experienced by doctors, and on figures for their admission to psychiatric units.[12,15,23-37] These describe the different presentations of the sick doctors, what was done for them, and how they progressed back towards work or on to retirement from practice; and they all confirm the high proportion who are dependent on alcohol and drugs. There are also some longitudinal studies of the progress of medical students after they graduate.[11,38]

Severe mental disorder

Bizarre behaviour and disorders of thinking processes may erupt suddenly in vulnerable personalities. More usually they represent the end point of a steady decline through inability to cope with external circumstances and the vagaries of temperament. Before any specific symptoms appear, it is quite possible for a doctor (or indeed anyone else so afflicted) to work inconspicuously while harbouring dangerous delusional ideas, yet maintaining sufficient insight to realize the consequences of acting them out. Such a condition is always liable, at a time of crisis, to decompensate into florid psychosis. For example, 'a junior hospital psychiatrist' had become 'increasingly capricious, prickly and withdrawn . . . and . . . on one occasion he sprinkled a patient with water while chanting from the Koran, explaining to an attendant nurse that "the patient's being would be made pure". This was followed by him writing a long, untrue and defamatory account about another doctor in the patient's case notes.'

It transpired that this doctor had only recently arrived in Britain 'from the Middle East, had no family or friends, and was resident in the hospital'. He was 'an extremely lonely man who spent his off-duty time either studying or impassively watching television in the Doctors' Mess'. The author of this case-history reported his fellow junior doctor's plight to the senior consultant. The senior's response was 'authoritarian, defensive and dismissive', making the reporting doctor feel he had behaved in an 'inept, impudent and unethical way'. Soon after the sick doctor 'died from a suicidal overdose while still an employee of the hospital'.[39]

Three New York and New Jersey psychiatrists reported details of thirteen doctors who had come under their care.[40] Here are some extracts from their account.

A surgeon . . . rewrote house-staff orders because he believed that the orders had been written to embarrass him.

A physician tormented his patients with unnecessary diagnostic tests, always doubting that he had done enough. As a house officer, he had spent long hours attempting to revive deceased patients.

[Another physician was proved to have] consistently falsified medical data. For example, when instructed to watch a bleeding patient throughout the night, he did not do so, entering bogus hematocrit data in the chart at a convenient time the next day. He never showed any remorse when confronted with evidence of fraudulent activity.

19

A profoundly depressed internist flattered his patients by confiding in them, but some admitted that they could not tell him about their troubles since *his* troubles occupied so much of the consulting time.

[A young physician's comments at meetings] were often incomprehensible to others, but they assumed that they simply failed to grasp his humour or imagination, and that he practiced good medicine, since he was well read and well informed. His strange comments were an illustration of a schizophrenic thought disorder, reflecting unusual associations, autism, and idiosyncratic thinking.

A physician who appeared to have had a successful result from cancer surgery dealt with fears of recurrence by the defence of denial. . . He minimised his patients' complaints and failed to investigate potentially dangerous symptoms.

A surgeon said that he believed in telling the truth to his patients. He gratified his sadistic impulses by emphasizing the least likely and gravest possible outcome of the patients' illnesses.

Two Boston psychoanalysts have published detailed accounts of the breakdowns of the two doctors mentioned below.[41]

After a week of debilitating depression, Dr. F, a hematologist in midlife, tried to get out of bed and return to work. Unable to mobilize himself and resume his professional duties, he became acutely suicidal. He began to plan the details of his demise, from thoughts of obtaining a specific lethal chemical from his laboratory to telephone inquiries of a local mortuary regarding the ultimate disposal of his corpse.

Dr. L was a senior resident in a surgery program. . . During the few days preceding his admission, he had been attending a conference in medical hypnosis, a special research interest of his. In his delusions he had begun to think that as a member of [an extra-terrestrial race of superhuman beings] he could become anyone he wished just by willing it. He had felt he could become chief resident just by deciding that was what he wanted to be. Or he could become the famous psychiatrist who was conducting the hypnosis conference if he wanted. At times he had thought he was this psychiatrist, while at other times he had thought he was having a homosexual relationship with this man. It was only when he had walked on the stage, introduced himself as the psychiatrist, and started to address the group in incoherent and delusional terms, that his decompensation had become evident.

In Britain, members of the Committee of Inquiry into the Regulation of the Medical Profession[42] were very concerned about what they called 'the sick doctor'. They wrote:

> Nobody who had seen the detailed evidence presented to us would underestimate the nature and scale of the problem of the sick doctor.
>
> [They referred to a] doctor whose appearance at the locum bureau always frightened the clerical staff; [a] doctor who believed that his practice of a sexual perversion on patients was beneficial to their particular condition; and [a] doctor who was sure that the electricity supply was being systematically contaminated. A particularly horrifying feature of the evidence was the length of time such doctors continued in practice: we received details of chronic alcoholics who had been known to be such for 20 years or more.

They gave some more detailed accounts of a few cases, including that of the unorthodox Dr C.

> Dr C. was a locum who piled all the drugs in the surgery into a bucket which he then put in the surgery waiting room, with a label requesting patients to help themselves and not bother him. When taxed with this by the General Medical Council, Dr C. said his method of treatment was no more random than that of other doctors.

These examples are clearly extreme, and represent but a small proportion of the doctors who become depressed or otherwise temporarily incapacitated, but who will in due course resume professional work. More again will experience the profound disillusionment already described which has a lowering effect on their personal and professional life.

Alcoholism

Drinking is a huge and enduring problem for doctors. In a survey published in 1976 it was estimated that in the United States there were between 13,600 and 22,000 alcoholics among the 324,000 doctors there, and about five million alcoholics overall.[43] On the assumption that doctors in the United States have the same drinking habits as the general population, it was estimated in about 1983 that 384,000 out of the 483,701 physicians there would be drinkers, and therefore it was expected that between 20,000 and 25,000 would be, or would become, alcoholics.[44] For England and Wales there are no figures of prevalence, and the published reports are from prestigious centres which are not representative of the country as a whole. The most useful information comes from Scotland where the rate of first admissions for alcoholism is 2.7 times that for other men in social class I,[19] and the SMR for cirrhosis of the liver in England and Wales is over three times the expected.[1]

William Ogle's figures of a hundred years earlier[3] record well over twice the rate of deaths from 'cirrhosis and other diseases of the liver' among doctors, as compared with the general male population aged over twenty, and an excess of deaths among doctors from 'alcoholism', but these figures cannot be used to say anything more than that alcohol has been a problem for the medical profession for a very long time.

At a more direct and personal level, Murray's study of forty-one doctors (including five women) treated in the Maudsley and Bethlem Hospitals in London is interesting.[45,46] Five had started drinking as students, three as house officers, five while in the armed forces, and for thirteen the onset was 'insidious'.

> Twenty-five thought that drinking had seriously affected their careers. Most admitted that alcohol had at times impaired their care of patients; this ranged from inability to do house calls or ward rounds when drunk to causing the death of a patient through negligence.
>
> Seventeen doctors had been in trouble with the law, the offences ranging from drunken driving to forging prescriptions and attempted murder. Several others had escaped prosecution only through the indulgence of the local police. Twelve doctors had attempted suicide.
>
> Only six sought psychiatric help entirely of their own accord. Sixteen came on the advice of colleagues, seven on account of their families or friends, and four on instruction from their employers.
>
> Invariably the cause for concern was not the alcohol consumption itself but the adverse consequences of that consumption. Patients were often amazingly tolerant of behaviour that included falling asleep during a surgery. Colleagues acted mainly because of obvious danger to patients. One referral came after an anaesthetist had refused to start an operating session because the surgeon was so dysarthric and ataxic.[45]

Gareth Lloyd has told his own story simply and impressively in the *British Medical Journal*.[47] He begins by saying, 'I am a doctor and an alcoholic', and then goes on to explain how the process began and developed.

> The drunken weekend antics of fellow students were incomprehensible to me. I just could not understand the point of getting drunk . . .
> Aboard the troopship *Asturias*, bound for Korea at the age of 25, my

relationship with alcohol suddenly and irrevocably changed. . . . The magic came, not from the taste or the scent or the texture but from the effect – a relaxing, uninhibiting, magic glow. In that moment the ingrained childhood distrust of alcohol evaporated.

At the outset I came to know that I could drink large amounts of alcohol without becoming drunk or sick . . . Drinking alcohol became a daily routine . . . Two years later I became dependent on alcohol but did not know it.

Returning to civilian practice and a career in obstetrics and gynaecology, I began to find additional reasons for drinking. The working hours were long . . . [and] studying for higher examinations demanded extra effort.

Within a few years minor symptoms of withdrawal – morning shakes, early awakening, and mild depression – emerged to confound the problem. I began to drink alcohol for symptomatic relief and to drink earlier in the day . . .

Each clinic or operating session became an increasing burden to dovetail into a demanding drinking pattern. That I was able to present a semblance of normality is a tribute to alcoholic cunning or a condemnation of my colleagues' sense of observation. Drinking now made me drunk and amnesic, but these excesses were always at home and consequently uncommon. On these occasions I would wake very early in a trembling, retching lather of sweat, craving for the alcohol I had carefully hidden. Sometimes I would forget the hiding place and become terrified of worsening symptoms of withdrawal.

The more common daily ritual included an intermittent and carefully titrated feed of alcohol, coupled with many mint or cough sweets. Some work suffered, particularly record-keeping and letter writing. The more tedious work became neglected. By some miracle of effort I maintained good clinical standards and obtained the MRCOG.[48]

Dr Lloyd sought help for himself before any disasters occurred, and in due course put his experiences to good use.[49] All too often, the doctor denies the seriousness of what is happening, and, worse still, fellow doctors connive by covering up. In my own junior days in hospital, it seemed only natural to 'help out' a colleague who had drunk too much. After all, heavy drinking was part of the robust medical ethos, and likely to be more acceptable in a junior doctor than an interest in left-wing politics, ballet or modern poetry. I did not connect regular heavy drinking by a junior doctor with alcoholism later on. That realization came later in the army where, at any one time, various stages of the

23

process would be on view in the Officers' Mess. Perhaps such covering-up is a habit of the past, and junior doctors will no longer feel obliged to use subterfuges to keep a drunken consultant from coming face-to-face with seriously ill patients whom he might be in danger of killing. The bizarre experiences of 'Mark Strega'[50] are familiar in their essence, although, I hope, merely reminiscent of an era when the power of seniors was such that they could not be gainsaid, however perverse their clinical judgement or tremulous their hand in the operating theatre.

Drug dependence and self-medication

All the accounts of alcholism among doctors indicate that a large proportion of these doctors were abusing drugs, either before becoming addicted to alcohol[45,51] or as a complication of established alcoholism.[46] The only comparative data I know of concerning these two habits come from the study of doctors in Scotland[19] which showed that while the discharge rate of alcoholic doctors was 3.3 times that of other men in social class I, the rate for drug-dependent doctors was almost eleven times that of other men in social class I.

Before the drug explosion of the 1960s, it was estimated that about 15 per cent of all addicts were doctors, with nurses and pharmacists accounting for another 15 per cent.[52,53] These were a different group from the present-day addicts, being older and capable, in many cases, of functioning effectively as professional people, despite their addiction.

Doctors nowadays start their downward slide from a different position to that of the great mass of addicts but the end point can be much the same. The physical surroundings will be better and the clothes more expensive, so that a colleague with slurred speech, or one lying stuporose on the sofa, conflicts with our stereotype of the junkie's pad and throws one off the trail. Upstairs, the picture can be more explicit: uncapped bottles of drugs in the bathroom with no effort made to conceal the traces. On one occasion during a visit to a colleague's home, the bedroom might have been deliberately arranged to illustrate the plight of the doctor-addict. There were the broken ampoules, a blood-stained syringe, blood-stained sheets, and, to complete the picture, white coat, stethoscope and medical textbooks.

Many doctors nowadays, particularly general practitioners, are in a very difficult position when they experience crises in their own lives. They have a mass of patients demanding relief from all kinds of emotional distress, and an aggressive pharmaceutical industry smothering them with agents promising to relieve this very distress. There are sufficient free samples of stupefying drugs on many GPs' desks to send a score of doctors into oblivion. They are handed out with an assurance that they will allay the patient's distress, but the equally unhappy doctor is not supposed to touch them at all.

A long way from the end of the line, yet a fair distance along it, is the bright-eyed, relaxed and slightly unsteady doctor who denies the existence of any problems. A well-meaning colleague may wonder about lateness in the morning, a new habit of getting someone else to do the driving on house calls, or the empty ampoules in the waste bin. These are danger signs: such a person has crossed the threshold and is heading for addiction, if not there already.

How, then, does this process begin, and where is the dividing-line between self-medication and drug abuse? All doctors are liable to take drugs on their own initiative or to obtain them for their families, but the extent of this perfectly reasonable practice is unknown. In one survey of the medical care received by 932 doctors, 39 per cent of the general practitioners and 29 per cent of the 'hospital' and 'other' doctors had 'self-treated illness within the last three years'. In only twelve cases the authors felt that self-treatment had been contra-indicated, and these were eleven doctors who reported 'mental illness' and one doctor who reported 'alcoholism'. Altogether, of the 321 'significant illnesses' reported, 135 (42 per cent) were initially self-treated.[54] There was a 66 per cent response rate to this postal survey, which was not completely anonymous,[55] and I think it is reasonable to assume that doctors who were misusing drugs might not reply, or at least not reply accurately.

The first time a junior doctor has to deal with an experienced doctor who has taken an overdose of drugs can be quite disturbing, even disorientating in a way. It shatters the fantasy that doctors are healthy and in control of everything, and only patients are ill; because here comes a doctor who is not only ill but has personally contrived the incapacity, or so it seems to the newcomer.

Suicide

Taking one's own life is the ultimate indicator of personal distress. It can be the end point of disillusionment, depression, alcoholism and drug abuse, all of which are common among doctors, who figure prominently in the suicide statistics, having well over three times the expected rate in England and Wales (Standardized Mortality Ratio 335, based on 55 deaths). They come fourth in the suicide tables, being exceeded by 'pharmacists' (SMR 464, based on 22 deaths), 'chiropodists' (SMR 374, based on 4 deaths), and 'labourers and unskilled workers not elsewhere classified' (370, based on 483 deaths). Nurses came eighth (SMR 297, based on 34 deaths) and dentists sixteenth (SMR of 206, based on 8 deaths), but the clergy, lawyers and teachers do not feature in the top twenty occupations with regard to the frequency of suicide.[1]

Turning again to the statistics for the years 1873 to 1882, the suicide rate for male doctors was 363 per million, compared with 238 for the 'general male population of corresponding ages', showing an excess of 52 per cent.[3] Using a slightly different population of doctors over the years 1878 to 1883, Ogle found that the medical suicide rate was 464 per million, compared with 123 for 'clergymen, priests, and ministers' and 354 for 'barristers and solicitors' of the same age-distribution (figures for the general male population were not given).[3,56] The considerable excess of definite suicides among doctors, as compared with the clergy and lawyers, seems to persist.

Because of the reluctance of courts to return a verdict of suicide if there is any doubt in the matter (and this was especially true before 1961 in Britain when suicide was a felony), the figures for accidental death, in particular death by poisoning, need to be scrutinized as well. The SMR for doctors dying of accidental poisoning is an alarming 818, compared with the clergy and lawyers, who are not listed separately at all. In 1881 to 1883 doctors were high up on the returns for accidental deaths, ahead of carpenters, joiners, butchers, farmers and agricultural labourers. There was no mention of lawyers and the clergy, presumably because they were well down on the list. Out of the 120 accidental deaths between 1873 and 1882, 48 were due to poisoning, including 18 from laudanum or morphia.[3]

In the United States, the *Journal of the American Medical Association*, since 1965, has published in its obituary columns the cause of death of all graduates of American medical schools and of doctors practising in the United States. These figures have formed the basis of a number of studies of the suicide rate in the medical profession. For male doctors, the rate is found to be very close to that for white males over the age of twenty-five, but the suicide rate for women doctors is between three and four times the rate for white women over twenty-five.[57-59]

Most of the surveys of suicide in the medical profession,[60-63] especially those which show high rates for doctors, are open to criticism on methodological grounds.[64] Doctors are more likely than others to succeed at killing themselves if suicide is their intention, as they have not only access to the agents but knowledge of how to use them (chemical methods being the most popular at present). The reports are based upon what, in statistical terms, are relatively small numbers: it is estimated that about one hundred physicians in the United States kill themselves each year – about one whole class of a medical school – and in England

and Wales the SMR is based on fifty-five deaths. This weakens the authority of statements about high rates of suicide in particular medical specialties or sub-specialties; although psychiatry seems to be over-represented, at least in the United States.[65] The rates are insufficiently standardized for age, place of residence, alcoholism or pre-existing drug abuse. Furthermore, the verdicts of suicide as given in the obituary columns of the *Journal of the American Medical Association*, on which several studies has been based, evidently can appear only with the approval of relatives of the deceased.

The most satisfactory study I know of is based on 'a computerized review of all death certificates filed in the State of California' for 1959, 1960 and 1961.[66] Here the suicide rate for doctors was more than twice that for men of similar social class standing, or for the population of the state as a whole. However, doctors still had only the fifth highest rate, being exceeded by 'chemists, dentists, pharmacists, and non-medical technicians'. When 'health-care' workers of all kinds (except psychologists) were taken together the suicide rate for men was more than double that of other 'professional-technical' workers, and for the women slightly less than double. There were no differences in the suicide rate between different medical specialties, although the numbers were small in each group, but there was a sudden rise in the suicide rate for all doctors after the age of sixty-five.

Nearly all clinical doctors have a plentiful supply of lethal drugs close at hand, and a knowledge of their effects. Pharmacists and nurses have the same access and knowledge, and they also have high rates for suicide.

There is a certain amount of evidence that adverse experiences early in the lives of doctors might predispose them to difficulties in their mature years.[13,17,35] This is a special instance of a fairly generally accepted proposition, and it prompted some investigators to try to predict which medical students would eventually commit suicide.[67] In a longitudinal survey of 1,198 students at Johns Hopkins Medical School, set up to investigate the 'precursors of hypertension and coronary disease', it was found that between one and eighteen years after graduating, nine had committed suicide. For the purpose of their 'retrospective-prospective' inquiry the investigators matched each of these nine with two controls from the larger survey, plus six 'distractors' who included two who had died 'under ambiguous circumstances'. Information which had been available during the student years (early medical and family history, academic record, smoking and drinking habits, results of various psychological tests) relating to these thirty-three subjects was then shown blind to an investigator who had no knowledge of their progress since qualification, and who was asked to arrange them in order for what was called their 'suicide potential'. The first nine places in the rank were occupied by the nine who had committed suicide.

This has been a rather melancholy catalogue of woes within the medical profession, but it is clear that these are end points. Rates and percentages are given because they are ways in which personal distress can be measured and then compared with prevalence for other groups in society, even though they take no account of the quality of the subjective experience.

3

Doctors' Marriages and Families

When doctors' marriages were first noticed by medical writers, it was in terms of the attributes of the doctor's wife. The (male) doctor was seen as the constant, and his wife a variable who conformed to his ideal with greater or lesser success. Gradually, the emphasis changed from the wife to the marriage, from the qualities of the wife to the quality of the relationship; and these general social changes are reflected in medical writings over the past hundred years.

Towards the end of the last century, a woman marrying into the medical profession might well find that her husband would expect to follow the advice of Sir William Osler, writing to a young doctor about to marry.

> There must be trust, gentleness and consideration. A doctor needs a woman who will look after his house and rear his children, a Martha whose first care will be for the home. Make her feel she is your partner arranging a side of the business in which she should have her sway and her way . . . console her and take her advice about the house and children and keep to yourself as far as possible the outside affairs relating to practice.[1]

Osler made the same point even more forcibly in an address to Canadian medical students.

> What about the wife and babies, if you have them? Leave them! Heavy as are your responsibilities to those nearest and dearest, they are outweighed by the responsibilities to yourself, to the profession, and to the public . . . Your wife will be glad to bear her share in the sacrifice you make.[2]

No one exemplified better than Osler the ideal of the physician of great erudition, medical wisdom and energy, with an inexhaustible concern for

29

his patients. Osler's views matched the social attitudes of the day, and in particular what society expected of a woman who had the privilege to be married to a doctor. They also conformed with the 'Protestant ethic' which was propounded formally by Max Weber around this time,[3] and it was an attitude which suited most men very well indeed.

Mrs Mayo clearly understood what was wanted. When her husband, Dr William Mayo, wanted to buy a new microscope costing $600, he realized he could only find the money if he mortgaged his house.

'Well, William,' said Mrs Mayo, 'if you could do better by the people with this new microscope and you really think you need it, we'll do it.'[4] In due course her husband went on to found the Mayo Clinic, but she was not to know that at the time.

A microscope also features in the private life of Robert Koch (1843–1910), as his wife saved enough from the housekeeping money to buy him one for his twenty-eighth birthday. She had her own talents and helped him considerably in his work, showing him how to obtain pure cultures of bacteria by using solid media instead of the liquid media which were in more general use at the time – and which led eventually to Koch's identification of the tubercle bacillus.[5]

Sir David Bruce (1855–1931) and his wife Mary provide another example of partnership and dedication on the part of the wife. They worked together in Africa on the part played by the tsetse fly in the spread of trypanosomiasis, and on his deathbed Bruce could say: 'If any notice is taken of my scientific work when I am gone, I should like it to be known that Mary is entitled to as much credit as I am.'[2,5]

The wife's role was to support her husband and to be a credit to him at all times. Many medical wives may have felt like Emma Bovary, but the great majority did what was expected of them and reaped the material and social benefits in the process.

The next phase in the history of the doctor's wife began when she came to be presented as a problem. These comfortably placed women were becoming depressed, developing anxiety symptoms, drinking excessively, and abusing drugs – which might have been prescribed by the husband (even at times injected by him) or removed from his supplies, with or without his knowledge. When admitted to psychiatric units the doctor's wives could present management problems, and, more often than other women, took their discharge against medical advice. They attracted a modest literature around themselves in the 1960s and 1970s.[6–8] Here is a typical story of the time:

Frequently [the doctor's wife] is bewildered as to why she is experiencing such feelings. Materially comfortable, with secure social status, usually a financially generous husband, and often envied, her unhappiness and anger may seem inappropriate to her. The husband seems no less bewildered. He has 'followed the rules' – worked hard, provided amply and wished the best for his family and is baffled by the turn of events which finds him with a depressed and suicidal wife and problem children. These men tend to be professionally competent and successful, but present as rigid, interpersonally distant and covertly or overtly controlling.[8]

The wife of an affluent New York City neurologist, participating in an inquiry about the attitudes of doctors' wives, had this to say about her drug addiction:

I was the perfect doctor's wife who just happened to be an out-and-out junkie on the side. My problems started innocently enough. I would complain about a headache, and my husband would give me whatever pill happened to be in his bag. . . Any drug I wanted was easily accessible. My husband would just give me pills to treat my symptoms – we never discussed their possible causes. I understand now that I used my various complaints to get his attention, but at that time I thought my behavior was the most natural thing in the world. My husband was usually so detached, so noncommunicative, but I always knew I could count on some interesting physical ailment to engage his curiosity. He especially liked to give me new drugs which weren't even on the market yet. Amazingly, instead of feeling like a laboratory animal in some experiment, I considered myself privileged to be able to take a pill that no one else could. It was like seeing a movie before it's officially released; I felt special.

My best friend's father had been a physician, and she was the only person who kept telling me that I was acting stoned out of my mind all the time. . . Not only did my husband not say a word about me acting like any Forty-Second Street junkie, but he also continued to give me my pills and injections on a regular basis.

Eventually this woman was admitted to a psychiatric clinic, and had convulsions when her medications were stopped.

I directed all my anger at my husband, who, by the way, was absolutely wonderful to me while I was at the clinic. But at the same time he was being so kind and caring, he was denying any responsibility for the condition I was in. He never stopped acting like the dignified doctor, and all the psychiatrists, except one, generally bought his

31

story. To them, I was the typical pill-popping, boozed-up doctor's wife. The one psychiatrist who was different helped me understand my physical and emotional dependence on my husband, and he literally saved my life. I came to see my husband as a man who, although he appeared completely disciplined and controlled, was unable to show any emotions unrelated to his professional role as a physician. I don't think he consciously wanted me to become dependent on drugs, but putting pills in my mouth was his way of meeting my demands for affection and recognition.[9]

It is abundantly clear from the various published reports that the women concerned were unhappy, and the symptoms offered were a reflection of the difficulties they were having in their relationships with their husbands, even though many of the husbands did not realize that these symptoms had anything much to do with them.

The third phase in the medical profession's awareness of the circumstances of the medical wife began in the 1970s when it was becoming more usual to think about couples and relationships rather than individual married people who happened to have symptoms, and more and more therapists were working with whole families. Thus the doctor's family relationships became the focus, rather than the sick wife.

The first image is of the overworked junior hospital doctor with a wife living in a home which he seldom sees. When he does get home, he wants a meal and then to sit in front of the television set until, in a very short time, he goes to bed and straight into a deep sleep. Alternatively, if he is working for higher qualifications, he disappears into his study after his meal, or, if there is no separate study, has the television turned off while he works on his books in the living room.

The wife becomes virtually a single parent, having to cope on her own with paying bills, decorating, gardening, as well as all the traditional women's duties, possibly with her husband, on top of everything, feeling guilty about not being involved in them. Then there is the impossibility of the wife planning a social life, even for herself, because of the irregularity of his night duties. And when he is at home he is often too tired to spend time with the children, or to bother much about maintaining and developing his relationship with her.

The difficulties are in no way evenly distributed. True, the doctor has many pressures on him at work from long hours on duty, having to take clinical responsibilities and make decisions for which he feels inadequately equipped, but he has the rewards of interesting work and almost unlimited opportunities for supportive relationships within the hospital. These relationships easily become sexual, intensifying the wife's sense of isolation even if she is unaware of what is actually going on.

A comparison was made in Edinburgh between junior hospital doctors and dentists at comparable stages in their careers, both being middle-class professional people; but the dentists contrasted with the doctors, as they worked more regular hours in a less hierarchical and competitive environment.

Both groups comprised married men, thirty-eight years of age or less, who had one or more children. Eighty-two per cent of the doctors worked over fifty hours in the week (compared with 12 per cent of the dentists), while 88 per cent of the dentists worked up to fifty hours per week (compared with 18 per cent of the doctors). As a result of this, the doctors spent much less time in family activities than the dentists, although they managed to spend proportionately more of it with their children. The doctors' wives were much less likely than the dentists' wives to talk in the evening to their husbands about events of the day, or to look to their husbands for emotional support; and it was not clear whether this was because the medical husbands were too tired or the wives felt they should not bother their husbands with such things, or because the medical wives lived more separate lives anyway.[10–13]

Most of the doctors' wives regretted the limited interaction with their husbands and the restriction of their social lives, but only a minority of the doctors saw these constraints as problems; the only lack regularly commented upon by the junior doctors was the brief time they had with their children.

A study from Australia about the pressures on junior hospital doctors referred to a similar differential perception. Thirty per cent of hospital registrars said they 'frequently' felt 'emotionally drained' when they came home, but 75 per cent of these registrars' wives said their husbands were frequently emotionally drained. The doctors tended to regard themselves as simply physically tired; and GPs and specialists in the same study showed a similar marked difference in perception of tiredness between doctor and wife.[14]

A particularly interesting investigation into the marriages of young doctors comes from Lane Gerber in Seattle.[15] It was to a great extent prompted by his experience of his father who was a doctor of the type who felt he had always to be professionally available, who seldom completed a meal with his family without a clinical interruption, who lavished love on his patients, leaving his children feeling neglected, and so on. Professor Gerber did not wish to replicate that way of life so he avoided a career in medicine, but he has taken an interest in medical students and young doctors, and in his book he followed the fortunes of forty male (fifteen married) and twenty female (eleven married) medical students for between two and ten years through their medical training and hospital posts. He also interviewed thirty physicians who were full-time or part-time faculty members. The result is a book that every junior hospital doctor and every junior doctor's partner should read, and then discuss the issues together one by one.

Here are two extracts which capture some of the flavour of the young doctors' problems.

I'm so tired all the time. I can't even be by myself, let alone with anybody else. At first, going home to Nancy was like a haven, a refuge from all this. But it's hard to go home, get used to that and then re-enter this world at the hospital. You have to keep readjusting and you get to the point where you just don't want to or can't anymore. It's easier just to be here so you're not torn by things at home . . . It's easier to be with the nurses, they know what it's like . . . There don't have to be any attachments. You don't have to give in the same way. Easier just not to think about home.[16]

You know I guess I had the typical woman's reaction when he talked about where he wanted to go for a residency program. You go where it's best for him. I'm supposed to understand and give. He gets all the credit. I can't complain about being lonely or his being really unavailable to me when he is at home because he works so hard helping others. You know mostly we don't complain about all this. What can you do? You don't want to be known as a complaining wife. So we put up with this bullshit even though it wrecks our relationship and makes us depressed.[17]

The American experience may be more intense than that of young married doctors in other parts of the English-speaking world, perhaps because the length of training means that the junior doctor will be relatively older when doing the hospital jobs; but overall the pattern is depressingly similar,[18] and the wives everywhere maintain an attitude of 'disgruntled forbearance'.[19]

The circumstances of young doctors and their partners are peculiar, and are best seen as an extension of the socializing process which is applied to medical students from the beginning of their studies. Hospitals are generally run as though there was a shortage of doctors, but there is never any real effort to rearrange schedules and the working habits of senior doctors to mitigate their arduous conditions, as might be expected if shortage of staff was the real problem. Junior doctors and their partners can be reassured that their difficulties are merely part of the price to be paid for entering a great profession.

The domestic life of the established male doctor continues to be dominated by his clinical commitments. The irregularity of clinical medicine causes families to adapt in different ways, with the wife and children developing their own routines, incorporating father when he is around but managing perfectly well when he is not. Sometimes they manage better when he is not there, especially if he expects the family to revolve around him when he is at home, however tired he may be.

The inevitable emergency hangs over doctors' families – these sick or needy people requiring his urgent and confidential attention. The word 'emergency' is supposed to be enough. It forces him, or enables him, to miss his daughter's birthday party or prize-giving, to neglect his wife's needs for time alone by herself or alone with him. It also enables him to do what he likes without having to account for his time. You cannot ask him not to deliver that baby, or not to go to someone in severe pain.

Another intruder is the telephone. Wives and children have to contend with distraught people on the line, pleading for attention. The children cannot make sense of the complicated messages and feel guilty that they may mistake some vital detail; or they may be asked to lie to someone about the whereabouts of their father, the doctor. The telephone becomes a symbol of disruption which brings only trouble, day and night. Then there is the bleep (or beeper), which is a blessing in that it allows the doctor to be mobile, and a curse because it follows him everywhere. On the other hand, its presence on the doctor's belt confers a certain extra kudos; and it has proved to be a great help when the doctor wants to be immediately available yet without anyone knowing exactly where he is.

One way to get the doctor's attention is to be ill, at least in the child's view, since father is always going to see sick people and apparently spending time with them and so is never at home. Yet, when the doctor's child falls ill, the sympathy supposedly lavished on ordinary patients is often missing, and the child is bundled off to school unless totally prostrate. The gentle fussing and coddling, from which everybody can benefit now and again, is often denied the children of medical parents, especially when the mother is a nurse; and a really substantial symptom and sign is needed to earn a day away from school. Then, if a medical opinion is required, the doctor/father – from the standpoint of the child – is not prepared to give the treatment himself but calls in a colleague. It can almost look as if father does not care. Wives do not fare much better either, and it has been said of doctors treating their wives: 'If he loves her he's afraid to. If he doesn't she's afraid to let him. No other doctor wants to, for there is neither fee nor praise.'[20]

Wives can so easily feel undervalued. They may have sustained their husbands, financially and emotionally, during the hard early years – especially in the United States – but once the doctors have arrived professionally their wives find themselves expected to be a credit to their husbands and help still further in promoting their careers, rather as though they were married to politicians.

The issues relating to medical marriages and family life are vividly displayed in entrepreneurial private practice in the United States, where it is desirable to appear prosperous, with a beautiful home in the right part of town and a capable wife – even if she does drink too much and abuse drugs. The lot of the American doctor's wife has been recorded by Carla Fine,[21] who is one herself. She interviewed one hundred wives of doctors and allowed them to tell their stories. Even though they emanate mostly from a background of demanding private practice, these stories make absorbing reading – and embarrassing reading for most male doctors. The pressures are less in the United States in academic medicine or federal health programmes, and also in Britain in the National Health Service, but the compulsion that drives doctors everywhere into excessive busyness has the same effect on personal and domestic life all over the world.

Throughout Mrs Fine's book, there is the cry about the conflict between their material affluence and the sense of emotional emptiness.

I'm always conscious that if I criticize my husband's compulsive dedication to his work, I will be regarded as a spoiled princess. When I have to attend a family gathering or a friend's cocktail party by myself – which is quite often – people will just ooh and aah after they learn my husband's absence is due to the fact that he had to deliver a baby. 'How terrific,' they'll say, 'You must be so proud.' Yet if I were married to a lawyer who had stayed home to finish some briefs, their reaction would probably be: 'Your husband is really a workaholic. You should get him to relax.' I'm in the position of having to smile appreciatively about his accomplishments when deep down I'm really resenting the closeness between my husband and that other woman giving birth.[22]

One of Mrs Fine's interviewees was consoled by her mother with the statement that most women are unhappy in their marriages but that doctors' wives are fortunate because they are at least *rich* and unhappy.[23] The men, whose prime preoccupation is their work, tend to be less unhappy about their personal lives; and the disparate views about the quality of the marriages noted among male junior doctors and their wives persist into the mature years.[24]

Wives who are doctors

A significant variation on the very traditional pattern might be supposed to occur when the wife in question is medically qualified. However, it seems that medical women work as hard as the men, and in the groups studied, at any rate, they attend to most of the cooking, cleaning, shopping and child care as well.

Several surveys in the United States over the years 1957 and 1976 have shown that between 84 and 91 per cent of the women doctors were working, compared with between 94 and 99.4 per cent of the male doctors.[25,26] The proportion of women working has increased over this period, especially where primary care is concerned (defined as family practice, general practice, obstetrics-gynaecology, internal medicine, paediatrics); and 51 per cent of the women doctors were in primary care practice compared with 39 per cent of the men. Part of this study focused on a random sample of eighty-seven women doctors in Detroit with substantial domestic responsibilities.[27] It was found that considerably more women (median age 46) than men (median age 51) had undergone additional training after graduation; and that throughout their professional lives women work about 90 per cent of the time that men do.[25] This last statistic may surprise some, and it needs a little amplification. The authors of this paper are aware of the claim made two years before, based on composite data from the 1960s onwards, that women doctors work only 60 per cent of the time that male doctors work.[28] The authors of the Detroit study used medians rather than means (this is a statistical device to prevent the overall picture being distorted by a few extreme values, as it can be when 'means' – i.e. averages – are used); and they calculated a ratio of the number of months worked full-time since graduation, divided by the total months since graduation. The ratio was 0.88 for the women, and 0.99 for the men. The ratio of the ratios was 0.89, hence the 90 per cent. This difference, the authors claim, was due to time taken out for 'childbearing and childrearing'.

In Britain, it is estimated that women doctors with children will work about 60 per cent of the possible time they could work.[29] If a woman doctor has completed her postgraduate training by the age of twenty-eight, then she will have thirty-two years of professional work before the current retirement age of sixty. If she has two children, she might miss up to twelve years of working time, according to how long she spends in full-time or part-time care of the children before they are fifteen. In that

37

case, the twelve years out of a working career of thirty-two years would mean she worked 63 per cent of the time that a man could work.[30]

Whatever the actual figures, it is clear from all the surveys that the woman has to cope with the domestic planning and organization. Even if the men help willingly and do whatever tasks are assigned to them, the woman has the main responsibility. In many cases this evokes a 'superwoman' response from the obviously able women who complete the medical training, such as one of Mrs Fine's interviewees.

> I want to be a superwife, supermom, and superdoc [said a forty-year-old internist]. I've been pushing myself since high school, and I'm just beginning to realize that if I don't tone down some of my expectations, I'll start to fragment into little pieces. When my daughter was born five years ago, I took only two weeks off from work. I was doing my fellowship at the time and didn't want any of my male colleagues at the hospital to think that a 'little thing' like a birth would slow me down. Of course, it was too short a time, for both me and the baby. But a woman doctor is constantly forced to prove that she can do anything, that she's as strong as an ox. There's a terrible price to pay for this attitude. Your children suffer, your career suffers, and your marriage suffers. Even though Wayne [her dermatologist husband] is supportive of my work, he just takes it for granted that Nicki is my responsibility. In other words, in his mind I have two careers – physician *and* mother. I'm also expected to supervise our full-time housekeeper and make sure that the household runs evenly. The result is that my husband's practice is flourishing while mine is barely limping along. I sometimes think that in Wayne's heart of hearts he wishes he had a full-time wife, a woman who would look after his needs. Well, I'm right there with him. There's nothing I would like better than the luxury of having a full-time wife around the house who would also take care of me![31]

The Detroit survey basically supported this woman's comments, since 'thirty per cent of the women physicians have no domestic help at all, while two thirds have help only one or two days a week. Except for cleaning and laundry, in which case hired help may do the actual work, 76% of the respondents do *all* of the cooking, shopping, child care, and money management in the household.'[27]

Other writers have painted a less grim picture of the woman doctor's life,[32] but even though, in the mid-1980s, one quarter to one half of medical graduates in Britain and the United States are women, there is little preparation for the dual role which will probably be expected of them, few models from women who have coped well, and not much understanding and support from medical institutions. There are now examples of medically qualified couples who are really trying to share the domestic work, with the father wanting to participate actively in the child-rearing, accepting that the wife's career is as important as his own, and prepared to move house in accordance with her appointments; but there is little encouragement in this from the top of the profession. Little effort is made to develop part-time specialist training or permanent part-time posts, which more and more men as well as most women would like.

I suspect there are still a majority of male junior doctors who have no desire to share domestic duties, and no interest in the concept of a dual-career family.[33-36] Bearing in mind the competitive nature of the medical profession, these are the ones likely to end up in the most influential jobs, and so help perpetuate the present system. Some of the general aspects of the relationship of women doctors to the medical profession as a whole will be taken up in Chapter 5.

Divorce

Statistics tell only part of the story. In private medical practice, appearance is all-important, and to some extent this applies throughout the medical profession. The marriage as an intimate and supportive relationship may long since have rotted away, members of the family may be leading aimless lives propped up with drugs and alcohol, yet they can all turn out together to church now and again, and chat amicably in public, giving an impression of warmth and unity. 'Marital dry-rot'[37] is prevalent in the medical profession, and it describes the intact external structure concealing atrophy and incipient crumbling within.

Although it is the quality of marriage which matters rather than the quantity of apparently intact marriages, divorce statistics are worth looking at if only to provide a basis for comparison between groups.

George Vaillant and his colleagues in Cambridge, Massachusetts, who followed up the group of male doctors and controls for thirty years (up to 1967), found that 47 per cent of the doctors had 'poor marriages' or had been divorced, compared with 32 per cent of the controls; and that 20 per cent had actually been divorced, compared with 14 per cent of the controls.[38] In other words, in that sample, male doctors were more likely than other professional men to have had 'poor marriages' and to be divorced.

The only other controlled survey I know of concerning medical divorce reached a different conclusion. It was based on an analysis of 'all the complaints for divorce and annulment filed in California for the first six months of 1968', with the knowledge that 90 per cent of these 'complaints' end in divorce.[39] California had a divorce rate 50 per cent higher than the US national average in the late 1960s, which was also the time of the burgeoning of the growth movement there, but doctors seemed to have divorced less frequently than others. The annual 'complaint rate' for all men over twenty-five in California was 22.6 per thousand population, 19 per thousand for professionals (dentists, lawyers, architects, engineers, etc.) and 16 per thousand for male doctors. Out of twelve professions listed, the doctors came eleventh in the complaint rate, even though they ranked first in the list in terms of professional prestige.

Of the women doctors, 56 per cent were married, compared with 90 per cent of the male doctors; and their complaint rate was twenty-four per thousand, as opposed to sixteen per thousand for the male doctors. The reasons for their higher rate were the same as those already mentioned for all married women doctors – having to cope with a demanding job and in the evenings to run the house and family as well, with or without emotional support from the (usually medical) husband.

Overall, the doctors (men and women) married later, stayed married slightly longer, and divorced later than other men and professionals;[40] and the peak period for 'complaints' was between the ages of 35 and 54 when the doctors were clear of their training and generally well established.

Lane Gerber was studying medical students and residents (in Seattle), and among his group a quarter were married or engaged by the end of the medical course, and half of those who were 'married at some time during medical school were divorced by the end of the first year in residency'. He seemed to think that divorces were commoner at times of transition from medical school to residency, and then from residency to practice, and then again after about ten years in practice.[41]

Whether or not doctors have more difficulties in their marriages than other professionals remains an open question, but they certainly have plenty, and their painful conflicts are liable to be acted out behind a front of respectability, which in the end merely intensifies the distress. The doctor can be struggling with intractable personal problems at home, and then, next morning, advising patients about the very same problems. According to how you look at it, it is a paradox, an aberration, or merely a sign that we are all human.

Part II

Medical Maladies

4

Centuries of Medical Power

Professional people display their greatest eagerness and anxiety when discussing questions of power and control. No academic or technical topic is ever charged with the same urgency; and no new medical advance will draw the same passionately interested audience as a meeting devoted, say, to reducing the clinical freedom of doctors. Although there are moves to liberalize the medical profession, there is a basic structure that it is not in any doctor's material interest to alter.

A great deal of Part II of this book is about power because it affects all aspects of medical work. This chapter will be devoted to the collective power of the medical profession, with special reference to its history and whatever lessons may be learned from the past; and the next chapter to how individual doctors conduct themselves in relation to their patients in order to maintain their position of authority. In later chapters in Part II, particular topics will be explored: the training and socializing of doctors; high-technology medicine detached from the real needs of people; the irrational in medical practice; and the relationship of doctors with the state.

The ancient scene

There is no date at which medical expertise can be said actually to have begun, since there is a steady development in skills, from animals taking care of themselves and one another by licking wounds and sores, and, in the case of primates, removing thorns and parasites. The most basic care that humans or their forebears rendered for each other was probably assistance at childbirth; and evidence from round holes in skulls and long bones with clean cuts suggests that very soon after primitive man had learned how to make tools, he was performing surgical operations on his fellows.[1] The Cro-Magnons of 20,000 years ago made definite efforts to care for their sick and injured.[2] How primitive people conceptualized disease and injury is another matter.

43

At some remote stage in human development, questions must have been asked about how and why. In primitive times these questions were answered in animistic terms, concerning the intervention of spirits, good and evil. That was the moment when a need developed for someone who could intercede with these spirits, and so the first medical practitioners came into existence. These primordial practitioners, then, were priestly figures since they knew about the spirit world and what the spirits required of mortals. They were both priests and healers, and so of considerable importance in their communities, as they still are today in many tribal societies.

Organized medical practice carried on by a medical profession of a type recognizable to us today goes back in Egypt at least to the third millennium BC. Henry Sigerist[3] describes an inscription commemorating a physician by name of Irj who lived around 2500 BC which would do justice to any eminent medical man of later ages. Irj was Superintendent of Court Physicians, 'palace eye physician', 'palace physician of the belly', 'one understanding the internal fluids' and 'a guardian of the anus'.

Medicine seems to have been strictly hierarchical, like the priesthood, for most of the span of ancient Egyptian history. The four major ranks were: Physician without special attribute, Chief of Physicians, Inspector of Physicians, and Superintendent of Physicians. In addition there was a corps of palace doctors headed by a man bearing the title, Greatest Physician of Lower and Upper Egypt; and at the top of this tree was a kind of minister of health called Administrator of the House of Health and Chief of the Secret of Health in the House of Thoth.[3]

When Herodotus was visiting Egypt in about 450 BC, he noted that 'Medicine is practised among them on a plan of separation; each physician treats a single disorder, and no more: thus the country swarms with medical practitioners, some undertaking to cure diseases of the eye, others of the head, others again of the teeth, others of the intestines, and some those which are not local.'[4]

Mesopotamian medicine had an approximately similar span to ancient Egyptian, from the third to the first millennium BC, but little of it is relevant to us today except the Code of Hammurabi (1792–1750 BC) which was the first attempt to regulate medical practice by law. A scale of fees was laid down for different surgical procedures, which varied with the social standing of the patient. In the event of an operation ending fatally or the patient losing an eye, then the doctor's hands were cut off. If the patient who died was a slave, the doctor merely had to replace the slave, or half the price of a slave in the case of an eye lost. It is unlikely that these penalties were actually carried out as that would not really have been in the interest of the society, but they remained on the statutes as a warning.

Ancient Greek medicine was vastly important but its practitioners mostly showed little interest in forming an exclusive company, and anyway the principal figures were widely spread across the ancient world. For example, Pythagoras worked in southern Italy, and, some time later, Hippocrates in the eastern Aegean.[5]

After the Hippocratic period (around the third century BC) until the appearance of Galen some five hundred years later, a number of medical sects flourished. There were, amongst others, the empirics, the sceptics, the methodists and the pneumatists.[6,7] The details are not important here; they are interesting as they offer us a prototype of medical ideological conflicts which have existed on and off ever since.

After the collapse of the Roman Empire, the medical knowledge of the ancient world was to a great extent kept alive in the Near East, mainly in Arabic translation. It was then to come back to Europe in the Middle Ages, along with most of the Greek classics, and there to be preserved and fostered in the Christian monasteries of northern Europe.

Medieval medical politics

The monasteries were about the only stable institutions in early medieval Europe, which was continually being raved by wars and disease. The ecclesiastics also provided a reasonable standard of medical care, although they felt that their prime task was to assist the soul rather than the body. Nevertheless the demands on the monks' services increased so that they would go on consultations outside the monasteries, with consequent neglect of their religious duties. Therefore, in the twelfth century, various church councils placed a ban on these excursions and later restricted the monks' medical activities altogether.[8] The decline of monastic medicine led medical teaching and practice into the hands of the laity, and to the foundation of secular medical schools and the beginnings of a medical profession in modern times which was separate from the church.

Notable amongst these was the medical school at Salerno. It began in the ninth century in a healthy and agreeable setting in southern Italy, and teachers and students gathered there from all around the Mediterranean. The classical texts were the basis of the teaching for the numerous students who included Arabs, Jews and Orientals, as well as monks from northern Europe. The school reached its zenith between the twelfth and fourteenth centuries and thereafter declined.

It is easy to imagine the collection of medical scholars at Salerno in rather idealistic terms, but medical historians agree that it was a very good period in the history of secular medicine. There was active study and interchange of ideas without the encumbrance of a profession as we know it today: perhaps these early physicians conducted themselves like the early Christians before the foundation of the church.

In Britain at around the same time the monasteries were active, although secular medicine was rising fast with the development of the City of London guilds. These were essentially protectionist organizations to control competition in trade; and much of medical practice, such as it then was, was seen in terms of commerce.

There were the apothecaries who were part of the Company of Grocers, and this was a natural association since they dealt with plants, herbs and spices. The apothecaries also dealt in the corpses of animals, birds and fishes, and in imported drugs and fragments of human mummies, insofar as these were judged to have medicinal properties. They must also have given medical advice at least on how to take the medicaments supplied, and so were acting beyond the role of pure tradesmen, as indeed they had been for a long time past.[9]

Another group comprised the barber-surgeons, as barbering and medieval surgery seemed to go quite well together. In different parts of England the surgeons were linked with other trades, such as scriveners, skinners, parchment-makers, and wax-chandlers. In Amsterdam they were linked mainly with the wooden-shoe makers.[10] The Barber-Surgeons Company was a well-established City of London guild, and there is a record from 1308 concerning 'supervision over the trade of Barbers etc.' in the City of London.[11] Throughout the fourteenth century there is abundant evidence of a well-organized group who were regulating their affairs, maintaining standards and supervising training. At the same time, of course, they were dealing with the competition, and very effectively too, it would seem. They managed to have laws enacted which enabled them to prosecute, or have prosecuted, 'unqualified' surgeons, some of whom were doubtless charlatans, but not all of them.

There was also a small group called the Fellowship of Surgeons, who considered themselves of superior standing to the barber-surgeons. They were full-time surgeons, which may have given them higher status but inevitably less trade. The rivalry was intense, and the barber-surgeons won, as, in 1462, they prevailed upon Edward IV to grant them a Charter of Incorporation. It gave them control over the practice of surgery in the City of London and the suburbs, and was a powerful blow against the Fellowship of Surgeons.[12] It also reduced the religious element in the Barber-Surgeons Company. Nothing more was heard of the rivalry for almost a century, when the two groups amalgamated for their mutual benefit.[13] I think this must have been the first example of intra-specialist rivalry where legal sanctions were invoked to quell the opposition, and it provided a fine model for medico-political dealings. The golden rules exemplified here are: keep close to royalty and involve the monarch (or the ruler) in your organizations; identify with the ruling group and the organized church; consolidate your position with legal sanctions.

The physicians had not been silent all this time, but the guild structure, which dominated so much gainful activity in the Middle Ages, was uncongenial to them since they regarded themselves as educated men who should not have to demean themselves by drawing blood or compounding medicaments. They identified with the senior secular profession, the law, which was above City guilds and that sort of thing, but they still charged fees for advice. The lawyers, however, would take on apprentices (and do to this day), and that proved unacceptable to the physicians, perhaps as it conflicted with the academic image they had of themselves.

Oxford University had been conducting some kind of medical teaching since the ninth century and was well established by the twelfth, but it was very much a school for aspiring physicians, and there was scant regard for the practicalities of surgery. The practice of medicine, as conceived by the physicians of the day, was an intellectual activity in which reasoning was more important than empirical observation. They did see patients, of course, and might conduct a physical examination, but equally they might give a written opinion without actually seeing the patient. In the words of Sir George Clark, historian of the Royal College of Physicians, 'the physicians were prosperous, worldly-wise and respected, and in their dress and bearing they were much closer to the learned clerk than to the merchant or the man of action. In relations to the sick they may have stood somewhat aloof, as befitted the possessors of esoteric knowledge.'[14]

The physicians made an abortive attempt to form a College in 1423 which probably failed because they sought to gain some control over the activities of the surgeons, and the surgeons resisted. The physicians saw themselves as the premier group within what was to become the medical profession, but they were premature. The barber-surgeons did not have a high regard for these academic men who seldom dirtied their hands, and they were certainly not going to be subordinate to them. There were also very few physicians at that time compared with the barber-surgeons who were numerous, well-organized and possessed their own Company hall.

Towards the end of the fifteenth century there were signs that the physicians were gaining pre-eminence, and documents remain which indicate their rising authority over the surgeons and apothecaries. It was not the kind of power they were to enjoy later, but it was a beginning.[14]

Henry VIII and the doctors

In 1511, in the third year of the reign of Henry VIII, the Medical Act was passed by Parliament, for the first time regulating the practice of medicine by the state, as opposed to a royal charter or a local agreement.

The preamble to this Act (which, incidentally, was not repealed until 1948) indicates the interests of the petitioners to the king: interest in obtaining control over medical practice, raising standards of care, or both. The preamble also contains an early move to control the activities of women, hitherto accepted as providers of medical care – as indeed they are traditionally in all cultures unless deprived of that role by men.[15]

> Forasmuch as the Science and Cunning [i.e. art] of Physick and Surgery . . . is daily within this realm exercised by a great multitude of ignorant persons, of whom the greater part have no manner of Insight in the same, nor in any other kind of Learning; some also can no Letters on the Book, so far forth, that common Artificers, as Smiths, Weavers, and Women, boldly and accustomably take upon them great Cures, and things of great Difficulty, in the which they partly use Sorcery and Witchcraft, partly apply such Medicines unto the Disease as be very noious [i.e. vexatious], and [cause] . . . grievous Hurt, Damage, and Destruction of many of the King's liege People.[16]

Intending practitioners of physic or surgery had to be examined by a panel of physicians and surgeons, appointed by the bishop of the diocese. The bishop could then grant a licence to practise. This might seem like a return to ecclesiastical control over medical practice but it was a purely administrative arrangement, as the Church was the only body in England at the time capable of organizing anything at a national level. Physicians and surgeons evidently sat down together to examine candidates, but graduates of Oxford and Cambridge did not have to submit to these examinations.[16]

Although many practitioners were licensed, very few records remain to indicate how well the Act worked in practice, because a mere seven years later Henry VIII granted the charter which led to the creation of the College of Physicians and in effect superseded the 1511 Act. It may have been that the 1511 Act was unsatisfactory and needed drastic overhauling, or it may have been simply that the physicians judged that medical practice in England would be altogether better if it was controlled by themselves. With the benefit of 500 years of hindsight into medical politics, I would imagine that the physicians were more attracted to the latter view. The actual process by which it came about is interesting.

Most countries in Europe at the time, apart from England, had some professional organization for physicians. Henry VIII was prevailed upon to rectify this lack in England by six powerful physicians, three of whom happened to be his personal physicians. Thomas Linacre (1460–1524) was one of these three and was also personal physician to Cardinal Wolsey (1475–1530), then at the height of his power and a keen supporter of the physicians' proposal. As it happened, during 1518 the king was staying at Woodstock, seven miles north of Oxford, where there was an outbreak of plague. The air of crisis generated by this outbreak must have made the king extra sensitive to his subjects' petition, as the charter was granted promptly with a note to say that its ratification in Parliament was to take effect from the date of granting, even though Parliament did not happen to sit for another five years.[17]

The new College of Physicians acquired powers of licensing medical practitioners comparable with those hitherto enjoyed by the bishops; and in addition they were empowered to fine unlicensed practitioners, with half the fine going to the College and half to the king. The physicians were also exempted from jury service.

The six physicians had scored a major administrative triumph. They extracted a charter from the king, and then, so as not to be vulnerable to the fickleness of monarchs, they had their status ratified by Parliament in 1523. They had dealt a serious blow to the surgeons and the apothecaries, and had established their dominant position in medical power-politics which was to last for over five centuries. Considering how few physicians there were – a mere six to begin with, and only twelve by 1522 – their victory over the wealthy and long-established barber-surgeons was even more remarkable.

The barbers and surgeons, although in no way academic, should not be regarded as simpletons. The royal barber was held in high esteem at court and had even closer contact with the king than the physicians, as his terms of duty indicate:

ITEM it is ordained that the King's Barber shall be at the King's uprising, ready and attendant in the King's Privy Chamber, where being in readiness his Water, Basons, Knives, Combs, Scissors and such other stuff as to his room doth appertain for trimming and dressing of the King's head and beard. And that the said Barber take a special regard to the pure and clean keeping of his own person and apparel, using himself always honestly in his conversation without resorting to the company of vile persons or of misguided women in avoiding such danger as by that means he might do unto the King's most Royal Person . . .[18]

Henry VIII had cause to be grateful to his surgeon, Thomas Vicary, who had cured him of a 'soreleg', and whom he rewarded with the lease of a rectory and tithes from a dissolved abbey. Surgeons also had a special relationship with the king which the physicians did not, and that was in relation to war. The armies could not take to the field nor could warships set sail without surgeons present, however crude their methods might have been.

Doubtless the surgeons and barbers were furious at their defeat by the physicians, but it did prompt them to sink their internal rivalry, already mentioned, with the resulting union of the barber-surgeons and the Fellowship of Surgeons in 1540. The union was settled by Act of Parliament, and so another medical group had its privileges protected by law. A result of the union was a splitting of surgery from barbery. However, the barbers were allowed to go on pulling teeth although no surgeon was allowed to practise barbery. A strange, but, from the point of view of teaching anatomy, useful provision of the Act was that the surgeons might take the bodies of four executed criminals each year for the purpose of dissection.[19]

The physicians must have viewed the proposed union of the two groups of surgeons with dismay. It would have suited them better to have kept the opposition divided, so they came back with fresh legislation to defend their supremacy, which was enacted in 1540, just before the surgeons' union.

The physicians began by obtaining relief from watch and other civic duties which they claimed they had performed 'to their great fatigation and unquiet and to the great peril of their patients': a regular excuse of doctors down the ages. The physicians also managed to impose their will on the apothecaries, whom hitherto they had disregarded in their previous legislative ventures. In the 1540 Physicians Act they gained powers 'to enter the house of any apothecary in the City of London and to view his apothecary wares, drugs or stuffs', and to destroy anything they felt was defective or corrupted. If an apothecary refused the physician's entry, he was fined – half to the informer (the College) and half to the king.[20]

The third clause in the Physicians Act stated: 'the science of physick doth comprehend, include and contain the knowledge of surgery . . .', which would seem to mean in the minds of the physicians that they were licensed to practise surgery. And so the battle continued. Holbein's painting, commemorating the union of the two groups of surgeons in 1540, shows Henry VIII handing a document to Thomas Vicary who kneels in front of fourteen other barber-surgeons. The painting also depicts, on the king's right, two royal physicians and the king's apothecary.[21]

1540 was clearly a vintage year in medical politics, and it ended with the main protagonists evenly placed but with the apothecaries trailing. Henry VIII may have been as vulnerable as the next man to innuendoes from the medical profession about the dire consequences of not following their recommendations, but it is unlikely that he ever lost sight of the larger political game that was being played, a game which he could play more skilfully than any medicals. The medicals, for their part, worked politely together, served their king, and pursued their battles with gentlemanly discretion.

Physicians, surgeons, apothecaries

I had intended to give a brief outline of the machinations of the physicians, surgeons and apothecaries but soon found that I was being drawn into a labyrinth, and that it would require a whole book to chronicle the intrigues and rivalries of our professional ancestors. Sometimes the reading is hilarious, but mostly it is rather depressing to think of these able men devoting so much energy to enhancing their power and status. The histories of the (later) Royal College of Physicians,[22] the Barber-Surgeons,[23] the (later) Royal College of Surgeons[24] and the (later) Society of Apothecaries[25,26] contain detailed and sympathetic accounts of the endless struggles in which these gentlemen were embroiled. The historians were not writing histories of medicine, but there is so little mention of medical teaching and practice in these volumes that the uninformed reader might think the important medicals in any age were only really interested in their political manoeuvrings.

The political preoccupations continue, and become, if anything, more tortuous. Therefore, to simplify the story, I will merely describe the main turning points and legislative landmarks.

The apothecaries were granted a charter to form their own society in 1617, after repeated unsuccessful petitions. They met opposition from the physicians who wanted to perpetuate their ascendancy; from the Grocers' Company who would lose financially through no longer being able to sell drugs; and from certain apothecaries who felt they would be better off linked to the wealthy Grocers' Company. However, the seceding apothecaries, like the physicians a century before, had a powerful ally at

51

court, this time in the form of Francis Bacon (1561–1626), and he
happened to share their views about physicians.

The apothecaries were still to be subject to inspection by the College
of Physicians, but they were not forbidden to give advice or to supply
medicines. They were the ones who supplied medical care to the ordinary
people, and there is every reason to believe they did their work well. After
all, the apothecaries had each served seven years of apprenticeship and were
working all day with the sick, unlike the physicians who were scholarly
men, often unfamiliar with the common ailments of the populace.

In the view of the apothecaries' historians,[25,26] the Commonwealth
(1649–60) and subsequent events brought about a lasting shift in the
balance of power. The physicians were identified with the royalist faction
and so lost a good deal of their private wealth and influence, while the
apothecaries, being identified with the ordinary people, flourished. Then,
after the Restoration, the Great Plague in 1665 drove the king and his
attendant physicians out of London; and it is suggested that most of the
important physicians fled as well, leaving the apothecaries to cope with
the epidemic. The apothecaries' position was becoming consolidated,
and all the more so in 1704 when a judgment was given in the House of
Lords which gave them a legal right to practise. Thereafter their status
rose, and particularly towards the end of the eighteenth century with the
liberal ideas prevalent around that time. The culmination was the
Apothecaries Act of 1815 which enabled the Society of Apothecaries to
train what were in effect full medical practitioners, the prototype of the
modern general practitioner.

The physicians, barber-surgeons and apothecaries all had their official
premises burned down in the Great Fire of London in 1666: the apothecaries
and barber-surgeons both rebuilt quickly and grandly, along with other
City of London companies. Eventually the physicians rebuilt, and very
grandly indeed. The entrance arch, with carriage gates, led to a courtyard
about sixty feet (18 metres) square; and over the entrance arch was an
octagonal theatre (for demonstrations) with a gilded dome.[27] It moved
Sir Samuel Garth,[28] Fellow of the College and mediocre poet, to describe
it at the beginning of his satirical mock-epic, *The Dispensary*.

> There stands a Dome, Majestick to the Sight,
> And sumptuous Arches bear its oval Height;
> A golden Globe plac'd high with artful Skill,
> Seems, to the distant Sight, a gilded Pill.[29]

The Dispensary was largely about the conflict within the College of
Physicians, and the conflict between the College of Physicians and the
apothecaries over the provision of some kind of medical care for the poor

of London.[30] This battle with the apothecaries was evidence of the success of these now formidable rivals to the physicians.

The surgeons had been restive with the company of the barbers for some time, and in 1745 had legislation enacted which gave them their own Company. The split was inevitable because surgeons were becoming more effective and consequently their social standing increased. In the latter part of the eighteenth century there were considerable developments in surgery and there was the dominating figure of John Hunter (1728–93) who put surgery on to its present rational basis. It was only a matter of time until the surgeons had their own College: they had the prestige, they were rich, and in the memory of John Hunter they had a revered figure (comparable to William Harvey for the College of Physicians) who could add a numinous quality to their aspirations. Their royal charter was granted in 1800.

The end of this era, which had lasted in Britain since the fourteenth century, came in 1858. This was the year of the Medical Act, setting out plans for medical training on a national scale with the provision of a supervisory body in the form of the General Medical Council. The Society of Apothecaries had set the scene for this Act with the model of medical education they had been employing for a number of years. Unfortunately they were to lose out in the subsequent manoeuvrings of the Colleges of Physicians and Surgeons who, in the latter part of the nineteenth century, placed the energies formerly devoted to intrigue at court in the direction of medical education, or rather in medical examining and licensing.

The College of Physicians did little teaching, but the Society of Apothecaries, which certainly did teach, and still does, was relegated to a subordinate position. The College of Surgeons taught alongside the Society of Apothecaries for a long time, and from the end of the nineteenth century the surgeons have made a creditable contribution to teaching and research. The College of Physicians has had some forward-looking presidents in recent years and has campaigned on social issues, such as smoking and health. Nevertheless, there is a strong element that prefers the past, and when new premises were opened in 1964, these physicians once more had a building designed for ceremonial, and in which they could conduct themselves in the style of their illustrious forebears whose portraits line the walls.

The state joins in

In England, there has been some kind of social legislation since 1351, and the state has been involved with the care of the sick since the Elizabethan

Poor Laws of 1601.[31] Contributory insurance schemes date from the eighteenth century, and in the nineteenth they developed rapidly, being known then as friendly societies. They had about four million working-class members in the 1870s, who in return for a weekly contribution received a variety of benefits from simple burial grants to medical and unemployment payments. The friendly societies virtually employed their own doctors, and were rich and powerful organizations in their own right.

When David Lloyd George (1863–1945) tried to introduce his National Insurance Bill in 1911, he ran up against the friendly societies (and insurance companies which were in the same general line of business) as well as the doctors. He won over the friendly societies by telling them that they would operate any new scheme, but the doctors were more resistant. The British Medical Association organized a vigorous campaign against the Bill, claiming that there would be an increased employment of doctors on fixed salaries or by means of capitation fees, a lessening of freedom of choice of doctor, and the control of medical practice moving out of the hands of the doctors. The more affluent doctors feared that they would make less money if a greater proportion of the population became insured and no longer had to pay for each item of service, but doctors in working-class areas realized that they might look forward to more money and better conditions than they had endured in the service of the friendly societies.

Lloyd George dealt with the medical opposition by splitting it, then buying the parties off. He had the medical secretary of the British Medical Association appointed as deputy chairman of the Insurance Commissioners, so it would appear that there was a medical man in the new organization to see that the interests of the doctors were maintained. He then raised the capitation fee for each patient which was highly attractive to the ordinary practitioners up and down the country. There was passionate rhetoric, and a defence fund to compensate doctors who would suffer through the new scheme, but in the end the resistance collapsed and the Bill became law. No doubt the doctors could have obtained better terms if they had been less emotional and divided amongst themselves, but they were up against a political wizard, who, as it happened, had not previously revealed his skills.[32]

After the Second World War, the National Health Service was created, along with a great deal of other social legislation which comprised the modern British welfare state. The BMA, representing mainly the general practitioners, bitterly opposed it on grounds relating to money and conditions of work, namely, the sale of practices, the threat of a salaried service, dismissal procedures, and the possible direction of medical labour. To a great extent these were false anxieties, but there was no doubt about the frenzied opposition to the 'Health Scheme' as it was called. Aneurin Bevan was in charge this time. His strategy, like Lloyd George's before him in 1911, was to divide the doctors. Lloyd George had won over the ordinary GP with promises of more money: Bevan went for the elite doctors, and, as he said, 'stuffed their mouths with gold'.

Lord Moran was President of the Royal College of Physicians at the time. Bevan prevailed on him and the presidents of the Royal Colleges of Surgeons and of Obstetricians and Gynaecologists, with irresistible concessions such as part-time paid hospital appointments and the ability to continue with their private practices. Also, the teaching hospitals, where the most powerful doctors work, were allowed to keep their often considerable endowments, unlike the ordinary hospitals, which forfeited theirs to the state. The GPs at that time had an almost filial relationship towards the hospital specialists, especially the senior ones, so it was relatively easy for them to win over the GPs, and the National Health Service came into being.

Thirty-five years on, most doctors in Britain accept the National Health Service, and however much they find wrong with it, few would want to return to a fee-per-item-of-service arrangement.

For the present discussion the question is: how much has a national health service affected the doctor's authority? True there is a vast health-service bureaucracy, so that planning and decision-making become endlessly complicated and slow, but the doctors still have the last word. They are the ones who can bring about change or obstruct it as they wish, unless they are out-manoeuvred by an adroit politician. Also, the doctors are on average pretty well paid, they have almost complete security in employment and 'inflation-proof' pensions as well.

The medical establishment is flourishing under the National Health Service. The GPs are no longer, as in Lord Moran's view, simply the doctors who fell off the ladder to success; they are part of the system. They now have their own Royal College as do most of the other medically influential groups, such as the pathologists, psychiatrists, radiologists, etc. The doctors collectively wield enormous power, while the voices of the para-medical workers such as nurses and social workers, or of the ancillaries such as porters or ambulance drivers, are still scarcely audible where it matters. The medical political game goes on as ever. The royal patronage continues, and the older Royal Colleges can stage grand occasions with robes, mace and precious silver, in a way which would make an eighteenth-century monarch feel quite at home.

In 1982, the 150th anniversary of the British Medical Association was celebrated with a banquet for many of the important medical personages of the day. Prince Charles was President of the Association and their guest of honour, and he showed himself master of the occasion in the manner of some of his illustrious ancestors. Although having been grateful to doctors for the safe delivery of the heir to the throne earlier that year, he could tease the eminent doctors present; doctors whose political acumen had ensured them a position in the medical world which would guarantee an invitation to such a gathering. Prince Charles chose to lecture them about Paracelsus (1493–1541), of all people. He was the ultimate anti-establishment doctor, who spent most of his relatively short life challenging the very doctors whose ideological successors packed the BMA's Great Hall that night.[33,34] The Prince's points about what is needed in modern medicine may have been lost on many of those at the banquet, and some may not actually have heard of Paracelsus. However, the message was not lost on the wider public,[35] neither was the Prince's insight into the ways of the medical profession.

United States experience[36–38]

The English preoccupation with medical politics has a clear historical base. The various medical institutions have been in existence for a long time; their very similarities of objective have helped to keep them in conflict, and the habit is now so ingrained that it is hard to break. What then about the United States? Medical practice began there in the hands of people who wished to leave behind them many English institutions and habits. So how have they fared? Can the United States show us the way?

Medical practice became organized in colonial America quite early on, as there was legislation in Virginia in 1639 to regulate 'the immoderate and excessive rates and prices exacted by practitioners in physic and churyrgery'.[39] The guild philosophy still prevailed in the early seventeenth century, and legislation was enacted in Massachusetts in 1649 and in New York in 1664 to establish controls, but at that time there were few physicians (licentiates of the College of Physicians), so the control lay in the hands of the clergy. There was also a wariness about replicating English institutions. A century further on saw the development of medical societies in the colonies and the larger cities, and inevitably rules were set out to govern professional standards and scales of fees. Later the licensing was placed in the hands of government officials. However, none of this was very effective as there were no sanctions to suppress unlicensed practitioners, as there had been for some time in England. Part of the new ethic was to encourage individual enterprise and to avoid the restrictive practices of monopolies; thus all manner of irregular practitioners could flourish.

In 1765 an attempt was made to found in Philadelphia a licensing body modelled on the College of Physicians of London. John Fothergill, an eminent though liberal-minded London physician, wrote on this subject to Thomas Penn (son of William):

> There is a College of Physicians at Edinburgh, at Paris, in London, and other places. Experience does not clearly prove they have been of much utility. The pretence of founding these Societies was to countenance and support the regular Physician, to suppress Quackery; but the effect has generally ended in a sort of monopoly. A few have got into the management of these Societies, who have gradually found means in order to raise themselves, and lay others, not less knowing, able or honest, under great difficultys. All the advantages of a medical Society may be obtained without a Charter. There has been one in London several years, unconnected with the college, that has communicated more usefull knowledge to the world, than the colleges have done in their corporate capacity, since the time of their first foundation.[40,41]

This letter was written in 1768 and it sets out an anti-elitist view of a kind that was becoming more significant in England from the middle of the eighteenth century onwards. Fothergill's remarks were not disregarded in the new American colonies and no model of the College of Physicians was established. His own experience helps explain why. He had studied medicine in Edinburgh, since, being a Quaker, he had allegedly been debarred from obtaining a degree from Oxford or Cambridge; and although he had made important contributions to medical knowledge, he had independent views and he remained a licentiate of the College of Physicians and was never admitted as a fellow.[41]

After the American Revolution in 1776, the control of licensing by the College of Physicians ceased, although it had long been too remote to have been very effective. Free from external restraint, the new states were able to organize the medical profession as they chose. They almost all chose a system modelled on the old College of Physicians, and one after another of the old medical societies was incorporated and given monopolistic powers. By the middle of the nineteenth century county and state medical societies in New York, New Jersey, Rhode Island, New Hampshire, Massachusetts, Delaware, the District of Columbia, Ohio, Indiana, and Michigan were holding examinations and issuing licences. State boards fulfilled this function in Maryland, South Carolina, Georgia,

Alabama, Mississippi, Louisiana, and Tennessee; and joint licensing by medical society and state boards was employed in Connecticut and Maine.[42]

There was a proliferation of medical schools around this time and a great increase in the number of unorthodox practitioners. The influence of the medical societies declined and in due course licensing was taken over by the state boards. Control over the profession, particularly of the numbers allowed to practise, now became tighter than ever, and the means used were the raising of educational requirements for entry to medical school and the lengthening of courses. This was held necessary, and with some justification, in order to counter the 'hordes of quacks' who were thought to be roaming the country and from whom the American public needed protection; but the call to 'raise standards', when backed by legal sanctions, could be used equally well to stifle competition as to improve the quality of medical care.

The development of medical monopolies was proceeding at a time when there was a widespread resistance to monopolies in general.[43] Anti-trust legislation was designed to counter the efforts of large commercial organizations to gain control nationwide, whereas the doctors, who only function within a locality, were merely concerned with local arrangements. In this their interests coincided with those of local businessmen who wanted to avoid competition from the large organizations, and so tended to be sympathetic to the doctors' requests. The doctors argued that they were not engaged in trade so no such strictures should apply, and anyway they were not really monopolies at all since anyone with the required educational and other qualifications was free to enter the medical profession.

The American Medical Association was founded in 1847. It was to dominate medical practice in the United States henceforward and to become a paradigm of monopolistic enterprise.[36,44] The essential act which was to secure its power was the apparently innocuous separation of teaching from licensing. The medical schools would grant their diplomas but the holders of these would no longer be eligible to practise straight away; rather they would merely be eligible to submit themselves to the state which would grant them their licences. At first sight it seemed that this arrangement would break the monopoly of one organization both teaching and licensing, and so it was reassuring to the public, especially as it promised to raise medical standards at the same time. The state boards comprised teachers from the medical schools but mainly representatives from the medical societies who were practitioners. The composition of the medical profession, then, in size and in quality, was to rest in the hands of the ordinary practitioner. The supply of doctors was once again firmly in the hands of the medical profession, although this was no longer apparent.

The medical profession in the United States consolidated its position steadily. At best, for example at Johns Hopkins, the teaching and practice were excellent, but the standard was uneven and in many cases quite deplorable, as the Flexner report, published in 1910, was to show.[45] Abraham Flexner (1866–1959), who was not medically qualified but usually had with him an assistant who was, visited and graded 155 medical schools in the United States and Canada. His comments were at times severe, and as a result many medical schools eventually had to close down; especially the proprietary ones, and those, it is said, that admitted female, black and financially poor students. Thus the 104 medical schools in operation in 1904 fell to 66 in 1933; and where there had been one physician to 600 people in 1900, there was one to 768 in 1933 – a distinct benefit to the medical profession. Flexner's report praised the academic and technological aspects of medicine, and advocated the concentration of resources in large centres. This led to financial support from the large foundations, such as Carnegie and Rockefeller.[46]

Medical politics proceed quite independently of medical teaching, research and innovation, because in each of these areas there have been enormous advances in the nineteenth and twentieth centuries, and it would be wrong to give the impression that the whole of the medical profession was preoccupied with politics. On the other hand, the American Medical Association was a very powerful body, operating on a large scale, and there were people keen that it should maintain its position. The question of licensing was well under control in the early twentieth century, but a new threat was appearing in the form of health insurance schemes and group practice. These were seen as threats to the sanctity of the doctor-patient relationship and of the freedom of people to choose their doctor, but large numbers of American citizens nevertheless sought to protect themselves against the costs of illness through private insurance schemes.

The American Medical Association always seems to get a bad press, especially with regard to what it sees as its defence of freedom within the medical profession. In 1943 a judgment was given by the Supreme Court against the American Medical Association and the Medical Society of the District of Columbia because a number of doctors, who had been running a co-operative providing low-cost medical care for members, had been denied hospital privileges.[47] The AMA and the Medical Society of the District of Columbia were found guilty of conspiracy to engage in restraint of trade, and they were fined. The doctors concerned recovered their rights to use the hospital, but the AMA was left with the image of a rather reactionary body.

The 1960s and 1970s saw the AMA embroiled in an almost continuous battle over schemes for reducing the cost of medical care for ordinary people and the especially needy, such as the old, the very young and the disabled. From a European viewpoint, the AMA was taking up, or being forced into, an extreme right-wing position which was in danger of blinding its members to the realities of social change. The bogey of 'creeping socialism' could be seen behind quite elementary social measures to prevent illness causing destitution. To the outside observer changes were bound to come as a simple consequence of high-technology medicine which is just too expensive for ordinary people, let alone the especially needy.

The Medicare (for over 65s and the disabled) and Medicaid (for the 'medically needy') programmes generated powerful opposition, but they were forced through, and many doctors have found actual advantages in not being paid directly by the patient. They have also found that their authority has not been noticeably diminished, and that they can still make a great deal of money.

Doctors and power

Medical politicians in Britain and the United States have demonstrated how a small group within a profession can secure great advantages for themselves. On the whole I think the British doctors have been the more successful, and the reasons are partly historical and partly geographical.

In Britain, the monarch's court may no longer be the focus of power but the courtly style prevails where the main decisions are made by a small number of people in regular informal contact with one another. Medical power is vested in the hands of the Royal Colleges representing various specialties (including general practice), the medical schools and universities, the British Medical Association and the General Medical Council. In Britain, the power is all focused in London. All the important people are there, and decisions can be made which will be effective throughout the land. It also means that gifted politicians, such as Lloyd George and Aneurin Bevan, can manipulate this small group and know that the rest of the country will follow.

In a curious way British medicine benefited from these two able manipulators as they compelled the conservative medical profession to change and adapt itself to the twentieth century. In the United States, decisions made in the capital would never be carried out with the same speed throughout the nation for constitutional as well as geographical reasons, so any change is likely to be slow.

Because the medical profession in the United States was not forced to change in the same way, the upheavals associated with Medicare and Medicaid have been more protracted and emotional. Also such schemes conflict sharply with the American ethos of independence and self-sufficiency, and that has the effect of polarizing opinions and oversimplifying political issues in a way which astonishes Europeans. The result is that any alternative to singlehanded practitioners charging directly for each item of service is perceived as the thin end of the wedge of 'socialized medicine'; a barrier is erected and no serious attempt is made to differentiate passing fashions from fundamental social change. The realistic and pragmatic profession recognizes change which is inevitable and then bends with it, always just sufficiently to maintain its favoured position.

The British and American experience suggests that, given the chance, medicals will organize themselves into powerful and conservative groups with a deep feeling for the past. The American physicians copied the authoritarian style of their former masters as soon as independence had been secured, and they have not shown themselves to be in any hurry to innovate. The British medical profession has been compelled to change, yet even in a nationalized health service it is extraordinarily powerful, and the golden inner circle of doctors still enjoys great prestige and affluence.

Dominating professions

Is there something unique about the medical profession in its habit of creating restrictive organizations, or will all human groups try to do this if they have the power to impose their wishes on others?

There have been professionals of various kinds in many parts of the world for thousands of years, but the present-day professional, in this discussion, is a figure who came into being in medieval Europe.[48] In the eleventh and twelfth centuries associations were formed for crafts and trading, but anything 'academic' was under the control of the Church. The academic label, which may only have indicated a knowledge of Latin, distinguished the professional, who could be a lawyer, physician, civil servant or teacher, but he would be in holy orders first, with the profession simply as a specialized form of ecclesiastical activity.

The lawyers were the first to become secularized in England, and by the fourteenth century they had established themselves in what were to become the Inns of Court, from which bastions they were to flourish unimpeded. By the sixteenth century the other professions had left the mantle of the Church, and then, as knowledge and skills increased, new

61

professions appeared. That is to say, new activities which were somehow 'above' trade: architecture, for example. Even so, in the eighteenth century the principal professions were still divinity, law and physic; and they were to remain so for a long time to come.

The role of the professional had to conform to that of the 'gentleman', which meant in practice that he could not do anything with his hands, and this is one reason why surgeons were excluded for so long. The nineteenth century brought a complete change. The surgeons had their own Royal College by then and their skills were developing rapidly, so they were soon perceived as professional men. The dentists followed, and then the veterinary surgeons. Engineers were a new breed of expert vital to the expansion of the last century, so they became professional men as well, along with various other groups.

Nowadays anybody who lays any claim to special knowledge and skills wants to be described as 'professional', so the term is rather losing its meaning. Nursing is accepted as a profession (and has its own Royal College) and to a lesser extent so is pharmacy, but neither of these can function effectively in our society except in conjunction with the medical profession. So what then constitutes a profession?

Privilege and power are essential attributes, also a high degree of autonomy with a freedom to define one's working arrangements. All professionals have expertise of some kind, and their profession ensures a monopoly of that expertise, which, most importantly, is sanctioned by law. Entry into the profession is strictly controlled and new entrants are likely to endure years of privation and hard work before the full privileges can be experienced. A profession is something like a tribe, or a club, which is tolerant of its members, provided their conduct remains within certain unspoken boundaries, and provided they do nothing to weaken the prestige and authority of the profession. These guidelines are likely to be best understood by those who have grown up in a professional setting. A profession controls its own affairs and the conduct of its members, without any interference from outside.

The English bar, and in some countries the Roman Catholic Church, provide the best examples of professions, although the medical profession is not far behind. In the United States, the medical profession is probably ahead of the others; and in the minds of most people in the world, the medical profession is certainly perceived as the premier profession. One aspect of professionalism in medicine has already been discussed, and that concerns the excessive hours of work demanded of junior hospital doctors, which represents the final part of their initiation rite. Other aspects, such as autonomy, selection of entrants and socialization, will be taken up later.

Professions in general have been an object of interest to sociologists for some time,[48,49] although in the United States most of their attention has been directed towards the medical profession.[37,50–54] Max Weber, writing in Germany in the early years of this century, was interested in the broader question of how groups in society organize themselves for their private benefit.[55] Essentially, this is done by creating monopolies and then having the control legitimized by law. Weber's examples were drawn mainly from trade, and sadly he does not seem to have come across the Royal College of Physicians or the American Medical Association which would have supported his argument nobly, as the processes he describes apply so well to the medical profession. Actually, the professions have powerful advantages when forming associations that commercial concerns are denied, and which are vital if complete autonomy is to be maintained.

Another benefit professionals enjoy is that they do not advertise.[56] At first sight this might seem like an opportunity they forgo, being motivated by higher considerations than profit; but it also works to their advantage, besides giving them a feeling of moral superiority over the world of commerce. Advertising presupposes that the customer can make an intelligent choice, and this could lead to the patient determining the pattern of medical care, to the dismay of many doctors. Advertising would also generate competition among doctors which would divert their energies away from maintaining the unanimity of the professional group and encourage practitioners who would seek to give patients what they wanted, whether or not that was really in their best interest – a difficult question.

'The best interest' of the patient, or the client or the public, is a phrase of great importance in professional politics, and of absorbing interest to professional bodies. It can be an answer justifying whatever they choose to do, and until recently no one challenged them. Nowadays, consumer groups will ask by what means the professionals know so clearly what is in the public interest, especially when hardly any of the professional bodies have outsiders to help them define their objectives and determine policy.

The assumption that professionals know best is linked with their sense of high moral character, and the corollary that it is vital for the standing of their profession that high standards of moral conduct are maintained, and are seen to be maintained. It is almost as though the technical issues will take care of themselves provided the moral ones are upheld resolutely. Thus, we have elaborate machineries in the professions to discipline members who lapse in conduct.

The General Medical Council, for example, periodically pillories and 'strikes off' a lonely general practitioner who forms an emotional

63

attachment with a patient of the opposite sex, and the profession as a whole feels cleansed by the process. The person thus punished is usually of low professional standing, and I have never heard of a highly placed specialist being dealt with in such a manner. Other ancient professions have similar rituals for sacrificing those who challenge the tribal mores.

If a ship's captain runs his ship aground or an airline pilot crashes a large jet aircraft, the ensuing inquiry will be primarily interested in questions of competence and judgement. So-called moral lapses would not be of interest unless they could be shown to have a bearing on performance.

None of the ancient professions, by contrast, has comparable machinery for dealing with allegations of technical incompetence or negligence; nor, indeed, at least as far as the medical profession is concerned, is there much interest on the part of the profession in investigating these, although there are some encouraging signs.[57]

An interesting example of the ways of professions emerged in February 1986, and it received wide publicity as the 'Wendy Savage case'. Mrs Savage was a senior lecturer and consultant in the Department of Obstetrics and Gynaecology at the London Hospital. She had been perceived by those in power as a threat, because she had broken some of the rules of the medical tribe, and would therefore have to be extruded. This was partly on account of the person she was but mainly for what she had done. She was divorced, the mother of four, a vigorous campaigner, a feminist and a supporter of the Labour Party. More specifically unacceptable was her willingness to take maternity services out of hospital to the consumers. She therefore ran ante-natal clinics in general practitioners' surgeries.[58] She also allowed women a say in how they would like their babies delivered. This meant, for example, that women whose babies were in breech presentation would be allowed, if they so desired, to try a normal labour, instead of being told that the birth would *have* to be by a planned caesarean section.

In May 1984, a Bengali baby she had delivered died at nine days, possibly of a brain haemorrhage (autopsy was refused on religious grounds). The mother, who had already had one caesarean section, wanted to be allowed a trial of labour; it did not work, and the baby was delivered abdominally. The father complained to the Community Health Council, which exists to investigate such matters; and even though the substance of the complaint was not investigated, Mrs Savage, some time later, was suspended from clinical duties by the Health Authority. She was also suspended from university teaching duties.

To back up the administration's case, a search was made, without Mrs Savage's knowledge, of the records of 800 of her patients. This search was conducted by, or on behalf of, the professor in her department at the request of the Health Authority; and four more cases were found which were said to be examples of 'malpractice', although in none of these did the baby die.

All experienced doctors have seen, or have made, clinical errors. Many of these are understandable, though that does not make them excusable; yet how often is anything ever done to correct professional misdemeanours? It is the regular experience of the Patients' Association in Britain[59] that really substantial complaints received concerning professional competence are seldom investigated with any haste or vigour.

In the case of Wendy Savage we have a doctor of twenty-five years' experience being suspended from practice and then subjected to an inquiry into her professional competence, for clinical activities which fall comfortably within the range of accepted practice in contemporary Britain.[59] The case histories of the five patients (whose names were all made public) were used as evidence against her without the permission of the women concerned, and without them having made any complaint against her; one woman even came out publicly in her support.

The inquiry proceeded along rather farcical lines, and it was even shown that Mrs Savage's perinatal mortality rate was lower than that of the professor who was her main accuser.[60] The more evidence emerged at the inquiry, the more Mrs Savage appeared as someone genuinely trying to serve her patients; and the more her accusers at the hospital appeared as men under threat.

It is characteristic of this kind of behaviour that its proponents will react emotionally, ineptly and excessively, misconstruing events, while totally blind to the underlying issues.[61] They had used none of the accepted procedures (such as they were) for dealing with differences of opinion over management or doubts about a clinician's competence;[59] the cases which formed the basis of her suspension had not been discussed at a peer review of perinatal mortality, nor had there been any professional discussion of the clinical issues, so she had never had an opportunity to defend herself; the accusers had behaved almost subversively in their examination of the 800 case records, because they must have realized that no experienced clinician's competence could fairly be evaluated on the basis of a scrutiny of the five 'worst' cases; and they had suspended from teaching a university teacher who did not share their views. In view of the importance attached to academic freedom in universities, it says something about the power of the medical establishment that London University accepted this last action without demur.

It is a classic case of individual conduct being so threatening to the tribe that the person concerned must be eliminated by any means, yet the precise nature of the crime cannot be stated explicitly. Therefore some charge has to be found: virtually any charge will do. It is likely that Mrs Savage's colleagues had been waiting several years for such a moment.

It is reminiscent of Meursault in Albert Camus' novel, *The Outsider*. Meursault had been arrested because he had killed an Algerian – not, in those days, regarded as a very serious matter. His real crime, and the one which led the authorities to decide that he must be sentenced to death, was that he did not show the kind of grief they thought it proper for a man to show following the death of his mother. Mrs Savage had transgressed the unspoken mores of the tribe (the actual alleged offences being irrelevant) and she had to go.

Mrs Savage's opponents were good representatives of high-technology and interventionist medicine, private medical practice, and those who view doctors as an elite. And the chairman of the Health Authority, who actually wielded the axe, was equally firm in his views, even though he was not medically qualified. He is reported as saying: 'I was in the tea business: I was out in Bengal from 1946 to 1953. I don't want lectures from women on what Bengalis want.'[62]

And so it goes. An irony of the whole case is that the accusers made fools of themselves and turned their supposed victim into a national figure. These otherwise able and effective men had been so alarmed by the threat they perceived in Mrs Savage that their judgement was catastrophically distorted. Not only were they using quite irregular procedures in their attempt to suspend a doctor who was acting in strict accordance with government health policy and with the aspirations of many women and doctors, but they had chosen to attack someone who was a natural fighter and more than a match for them.

The outcome of the inquiry was that Mrs Savage was completely vindicated of the charges of incompetence, and it was recommended that she be reinstated to her former position.

I have described this case at some length because it captures so well the negative aspects of professions, the power they have and the way self-preservation comes before service, despite the noble ideals of caring for the sick. Ultimately, the whole issue is about power. The pursuit of power and the provision of good medical care may be incompatible. If there is a conflict of interests, the considerations of power usually win – in the 1980s just as they did in the Middle Ages.

5

Defensive Medical Attitudes

The medical profession is powerful. Individual doctors are also powerful, and face to face with patients they can behave in ways which enable them to enhance their power and avoid their various anxieties. Although doctors are largely unaware of the ways in which they maintain their ascendancy over those they are employed to help, the processes can be described; and this is the purpose of the present chapter.

The powerful position is established and perpetuated by what is called 'the medical persona', and by various strategies which will be dealt with under the heading of 'the medical virtuoso'. These refer to the maintenance of social distance between doctor and patient; the emphasis on the unique skills and knowledge of the doctor; the ability to generate an atmosphere of working against a background of imminent disaster, and the principle that proper medicine can be practised only in special places. The preoccupation with authority on the part of many male doctors is apparent from the way they treat women – either as colleagues or as patients; and all doctors can be unsettled when their power is repudiated, as it is by patients who develop illnesses which they cannot cure.

The medical persona

People need protection for their vulnerable inner selves against abrasive and intrusive interactions with other people. Also, people in responsible jobs need to present a consistent exterior, and to conduct themselves in ways which will facilitate their work; and they may also want to conform to the expectations of others.

Jung has called the result of this process the 'persona', and describes it as 'a complicated system of relations between individual consciousness and society, fittingly enough a kind of mask, designed on the one hand to make a definite impression upon others, and, on the other, to conceal the true nature of the individual'.[1,2]

Jung uses the term 'system' in the modern psychological sense, and the

67

components of this system are the inner person (actually Jung calls this the 'soul' but the term is confusing in ordinary usage), the outer world, and the persona itself, the persona being essentially the mediating factor. The word 'persona' is actually the Latin word for 'mask'. Doctors provide good examples of the workings of the persona because of their complicated natures and the demands made on them by society.

The newly qualified doctor feels insecure. He takes on the outward symbols of the profession – the white coat, stethoscope – which register him as a doctor and so evoke traditional responses from the public. His job would be harder if he wore casual clothes without the symbols. He may also copy the mannerisms, habits of speech and movements of influential teachers, much as a young person may copy the ways of a parent. The young doctor also seeks protection against the impact of the suffering he sees, and against the anger and guilt-laden emotion that distressed people are liable to unload onto those who are trying to help them.

As the doctor matures and gains confidence, the borrowed habits can be shed so that an individual style can emerge; the good qualities of the teachers may be retained, and the mannerisms dropped which betray a character still in thrall to another. Gradually an external image will evolve; if possible authentic, yet at the same time serving as a bulwark against the particular pressures of the medical life. The doctor, it is hoped, will learn to make good relationships with patients – developing an empathy with sick people, while at the same time maintaining the detachment required for logical clinical thought in a busy practice.

A reluctance to grapple with the emotional implications and practical demands of the doctor-patient relationship leads many doctors never to make any kind of relaxed empathic contact at all. Whether it is sought or not, a relationship of some kind exists between doctor and patient. The doctor who lacks awareness of the psychological processes operating in his personal and family relationships, and equally who does not try to become conscious of what is going on between himself and the patient, is likely to be harbouring unresolved prejudices and unconscious drives. These, then, are always in danger of erupting in some inappropriate way, and leading the doctor into painful conflicts with patients, or else into unsuitably close relationships with them.

Over-identification with the persona. Anyone who has worn a white coat in hospital will know the instant prestige it confers. It is a splendid boost for the doctor who is feeling low or unappreciated, and a spur to higher things when he is feeling good. The esteem is conferred on doctors by people who like to show respect, so the process is mutually satisfactory: heroes and admirers have reciprocal requirements. The danger point comes when the doctor begins to identify with his public image, so that

68

the public front displaces the real or private person. Such a doctor then carries his professional persona into every part of his life, authoritarian or avuncular as the case may be, and expects to control his personal and family relationships just as he does his professional ones.

The over-identification may lead to changes in outward appearances. We may see the large car, a dark suit, gold-rimmed spectacles on the tip of the nose, and a hand-made leather briefcase. An urgent manner with an air of preoccupation with important issues elsewhere reinforces the image, so that people feel they are in the presence of someone significant who is in great demand. The doctor responds in turn and the process spirals. There is nothing new in this, as George Crabbe (1754–1832) indicates, describing the style of a country doctor (apothecary) in 1783 in *The Village*:

> Anon, a figure enters, quaintly neat,
> All pride and business, bustle and conceit;
> With looks unaltered by these scenes of wo,
> With speed that, entering, speaks his haste to go . . .

Physicians, as the elite of the medical profession in the eighteenth century, often wore elaborate clothes as a mark of their special calling, and affected a grand demeanour which lives on to this day in the larger centres of medical influence. Thus the comments of John Gregory, professor in the Edinburgh medical school in the latter part of the eighteenth century, still apply two hundred years later:

> There is no natural propriety in a physician's wearing one dress in preference to another; it not being necessary that any particular respect or authority should be annexed to his office, independent of what his personal merit commands. Experience, indeed, has shewn, all our external formalities have been often used as snares to impose on the weakness and credulity of mankind; that in general they have been most scrupulously adhered to by the most ignorant and forward of the profession; that they frequently supplant real worth and genius; and that, so far from supporting the dignity of the profession, they often expose it to ridicule.[3]

One of the commonest arguments in favour of the doctor wearing smart clothes – that is, smart clothes by his middle-class standards – is that 'the patients expect it'. It is hard to know what other people expect, especially if they come from a totally different social group, and I take the statement to be more along the lines of: 'my idea of how the proper doctor ought to present himself is . . .' In other words, any statement about what the patient wants, I suspect, refers more to what the doctor wants: a common kind of rationalization where status-building is concerned. Similar arguments are advanced when a professional group is seeking to enhance its standing with the public: 'the public expects' a full-time course of study, a diploma, a uniform, letters after one's name, and so on.

The more highly developed the persona, and thus the more powerful and effective the outer self, the weaker, in all probability, will be the inner self. The outer development takes place at the expense of the inner. A strong persona can be cultivated to help overcome personal difficulties in relating to people. The brusque, academic doctor, with a reputation for irascibility, may have a real problem in making any kind of empathic relationship with another person, but he has intellectual gifts, so he can build a career upon these and ensure that he stays on ground where he is comfortably in control. At the same time he loses so much; and his relationships, both professional and personal, become arid because he never drops his mask sufficiently to reveal his humanity – weaknesses and all.

Young doctors of the 1980s are slightly less likely than their predecessors to introject traditional professional attitudes, and so inhibit their inner development and their capacity to make good relationships. That still leaves a great many who are using the professional persona as a way of avoiding confrontation with painful personal issues, and an even larger number of older doctors whose real selves have long since disappeared behind their dense personas. Nothing short of a major personal crisis is ever likely to bring about a fundamental change in such people. This kind of change is only likely to be precipitated by an exceptionally painful event, such as a divorce, serious illness or even a death in the family.

The medical virtuoso

One of the attractions of being a doctor is the regular opportunity which is offered to play a heroic role, without any personal danger or even unusual effort. Early in a doctor's career, such acts are good for boosting self-confidence and the development of a strong professional identity; later on, it can be reassuring and comforting to be able to play the hero and to dominate the scene with ease. These habits and strategies make up what has been called 'the virtuoso role',[4] and they show how the doctor, or anyone in a position of authority, can maintain a pre-eminent position. They are not desirable practices, but they are effective – in the short term, at any rate.

The virtuoso role does not apply, it must be said, to all doctors, most of whom are caring and conscientious. Rather, they are patterns of behaviour, like the medical persona, which certain types of doctor may adopt, or all types may adopt at times of difficulty. Therefore the succeeding pages provide a sketch of how things can be, rather than a description of the medical profession in general.

Social distance. At every point in the clinical cycle, doctors can distance themselves. The initial consultation may involve sitting comfortably in chairs face to face, or across a large desk cluttered with X-ray films, case records, diagnostic equipment – all of which proclaim the doctor's superiority. The atmosphere in the room may be calm, or there may be people hurrying back and forth, telephone calls and a general atmosphere of urgency which has an inhibiting effect so that the patient not only fails to ask pertinent questions but may forget the doctor's comments and instructions as well.

The doctor can create an impressive social distance from his patients on the traditional hospital ward round. He makes a stately or rapid progress past the ends of the beds of his patients, accompanied by as many junior doctors, visiting medicals, nursing staff, students and medical ancillaries as can be found. The occasion creates an insuperable barrier to communication, the patient is able to contribute little, and so the important decisions are made by the staff alone.

The surgeon needs his operating theatre and assistants in order to do his work. The operating theatre also provides him with a setting in which he can stand supreme and apart. The high point for surgical virtuosity was in the early years of this century when anaesthetic and antiseptic techniques permitted a great range of surgical interventions but high technology had not arrived. The surgeon then was often the only really skilled person present at the operation. If his helpers were all suddenly to disappear, he could still somehow complete the operation. The distance between surgeon and helpers therefore was enormous, his prestige soared and his helpers enjoyed the reflected glory.

Nowadays, there are many highly skilled people present in the operating theatre, on whom the surgeon depends totally; so he is now more the performing conductor of a small orchestra than a one-man band. Such a conductor must work in subtle relationship with his players if they are to give of their best. If from this position of leading yet participating he tries to place too much distance between himself and the rest of the orchestra and pretends he is back on the rostrum, the players will be dissatisfied and will not perform well. Unfortunately, the fantasy of the dramatic surgeon saving lives against all odds lingers on. There is more than a little longing for the status and privileges of a performing virtuoso, but acting like a prima donna does not make the surgeon into one.

Unique skills. The power of doctors rests ultimately on their ability to

71

intervene as no one else can in a medical crisis. All kinds of people can dispense remedies: nurses can treat common complaints; healers are associated with remarkable cures; but when a medical emergency is serious, it is the doctor who is sought. Only someone with full medical qualifications can deal with such a crisis, and so the only really reliable person to treat the sick is the doctor. Anything less is denying people their right to effective care, lowering standards and opening the door to all kinds of unscrupulous practitioners: at least this is the doctors' fantasy.

With nurses and other health professionals developing therapeutic skills so that they can act on their own initiative, and with para-medical workers in various parts of the world providing medical cover for whole communities, doctors can well feel that their unique status is under threat. In the Western world there are many instances when doctors will refuse to work with non-medically qualified people irrespective of their abilities, because even to acknowledge their existence calls into question the notion of the doctor as the possessor of unique skills. Therefore, if the doctor wants to maintain the illusion of being the only one with real competence, he will have to collect a retinue of passive people who allow their expertise to go unused.

Esoteric knowledge. It is the range of a doctor's knowledge which makes it distinctive, and at the time of passing the final medical examinations the emerging doctor really does know a very great deal indeed – and over a far broader range than any of the examiners. Much will be forgotten, and knowledge will be deepened in particular areas, yet the basic broad foundations will remain, enabling the doctor to comprehend medical concepts, principles and jargon in a way which is beyond the abilities of the vast majority of lay people. Doctors touch on many disciplines in the course of their training which they can never expect to master, and they develop the ability to extract what they want from them. Few have the knowledge to understand the chemistry of the drugs they use, yet almost all have the knack of knowing just what they need to know, and no more, about the use of a particular drug. It does make for a somewhat superficial and 'cookery-book' kind of knowledge, but it works.

This ability to deal with a wide range of information makes doctors appear to possess great wisdom, far beyond the grasp of ordinary people, and this impression can be used by doctors in managing their own affairs and maintaining control over their patients.

Medical services and institutions used to be run entirely by doctors for the simple reason, in their view, that no one else would be capable of comprehending the issues involved. Then, with the advent of technological medicine and medical care for all, health services became so complex that professional administrators had to be brought in. Initially there was a doctor at the helm, supposedly to guide his lay colleagues. Now, the non-medical administrators have established themselves powerfully in the system, and have demonstrated that they understand very well the intricacies of medical practice, and often with a clarity of vision denied their medical colleagues. All the same, doctors are still considerably more important than the experts or specialists in any large commercial organization, and they have enormous power to obstruct and initiate, provided they can agree amongst themselves.

Ignorant patients are easier to deal with than those who are well-informed, and the medical machine runs more smoothly if people do not ask questions, but place themselves, child-like and docile, in the hands of their doctors. The power of the doctor, then, may be related directly to how much or how little the patient knows about what is going on.

A physician's ability to preserve his power over the patient in the doctor-patient relationship depends largely on his ability to control the patient's uncertainty. The physician enhances his power to the extent that he can maintain the patient's uncertainty about the course of illness, efficacy of therapy, or specific future actions of the physician himself.[5]

This is a proposition based on the idea that 'the power of A over B depends on A's ability to predict B's behavior and on the uncertainty of B about A's behavior'.[5]

Doctors may not deliberately keep their patients in ignorance but they certainly want to maintain strict control over the clinical relationship. They are in an almost unassailable position since they possess all the information about the patients who, in turn, know practically nothing, yet are highly anxious; and that increases the doctors' power still further.

The issue of the control of information has come into prominence through the debate about who should hold patients' case records.[6-12] There are arguments in favour of patients holding their own medical records, and some of these are expressed in terms of human rights: that people have a right to know what is wrong with them and what, if anything, is going to be done. There are also practical arguments: that the records are more likely to be available when and where they are needed if they are in the patient's keeping, and health authorities will not have the bother and expense of handling them. Against the idea of patients holding or having access to their medical records, it is claimed that patients will be confused by information they cannot understand; that details and opinions (which the doctor is legally bound to record) about other people might cause difficulty if the record was seen by partners or by the other people mentioned therein; and that while it may be acceptable for patients

73

to hold their records on an obstetric unit, could the same be said with regard to an oncology unit? There is a fear that if records became, in effect, public, and thus open to criticism, it could vastly increase the amount of information which would be included; and behind this, of course, would lurk the fear of more malpractice litigation.

On the face of it, the question about who should hold the records is partly moral and partly practical. It is mentioned here because the possession of information in clinical medicine represents power, and since power is a sensitive matter in the medical profession, any discussion of access to case records will be loaded emotionally.

The disaster factor. Surgeons work against a background of disaster – one false move and the patient bleeds to death. To avoid this hypothetical catastrophe, everything must be to the surgeon's liking, since he alone holds life and death in the balance. He must therefore have the best available equipment, the best conditions for work, and the greatest consideration for his personal welfare. This is an agreeable aura for the surgeon to generate around himself, since it then becomes quite difficult for people to deny him whatever he wants in order to do his work; and his prestige out of hospital is also enhanced.

Surgeons can of course make the most effective use of this aspect of the virtuoso role – that *my* intervention, and *mine* alone, on *my* terms, will save the day. Other doctors are successful at it, generally according to the amount of high technology they employ. However, if this emotive stance is to succeed in an era of rising costs and increasingly shrewd and powerful hospital managers, it requires the back-up of public petitions and, if possible, media interest as well.

Medical temples. Technological medicine is so complicated and so expensive that it can only be practised in special places. Thus any threat to the doctor's traditional pre-eminence by the rise of skilled para-medical workers is more than offset by the appearance of superior medical establishments where the doctor naturally reigns supreme. A decline in the value placed on high-technology medicine would cause hospitals to lose their dominant position in the health services and would lead to a drop in status of hospital doctors. Actually, this process has already begun, not because technological medicine is no longer highly valued but because of the development of community services and the fact that the voice of the consumer is more powerful than it used to be. Also more and more of the best graduates from British medical schools are making a positive choice to work in the community, and not in hospitals.

The virtuoso role is attractive as the doctor enjoys it simply by belonging to a particular profession, and it is maintained merely by some members of the scientific community making headlines to supply the media's appetite for 'breakthroughs', 'wonder drugs' and 'miracle cures'.

Does the virtuoso role enhance the quality of medical care? Will people benefit more from being treated by doctors of manifestly high status? That depends on what is regarded as the proper kind of relationship between doctor and patient. If the doctor is all-powerful and the patient a passive recipient of medical care, then the more prestigious the doctor the more effective will be his attentions, as they will carry more powerful suggestion. If, on the other hand, the relationship between doctor and patient is seen more as a partnership, then equality is sought rather than social distance, and the virtuoso role will be an impediment.

Effects of power and prestige

High status and too much power mean that the doctor's personal peculiarities, prejudices and blind spots are unchallenged. Everybody has the tendency to become idiosyncratic if not exposed to some kind of criticism or control, such as occurs naturally in relaxed family settings or in working relationships. Doctors who have grown up in families and attended schools where relationships have been quite formal, with a ready acceptance of authority, are likely to model themselves on teachers and seniors who display authoritarian qualities. If young doctors from such backgrounds already lack confidence and have difficulty in relating to others, then the formal style of the medical persona is attractive and comforting.

The doctor who above all seeks high status and a position of power in the profession is liable to proceed, at a personal level, in a fairly predictable manner. He can come to believe that he possesses special wisdom, insight and competence.[13] He can come to see himself as the mainstay of his organization or department, and has long waiting lists to demonstrate that he is in great demand. It would be possible of course to refer patients to colleagues but he rarely does this, as he believes they are better off waiting for *his* opinion and skilled treatment; and he manages to work very long hours apparently to keep up with demands made on him. He may also come to believe that he can detect what is going on within people, plumb the depths of their psyches, and therefore know what is best for them. His conviction about the extent of his insight prompts him to offer opinions on all kinds of topics, and to correct his patients, even when they are talking on their own subjects. He has advice for everyone, and sees 'the meaning' behind world events and the activities of party politicians with the same clarity of thought that distinguishes him as a clinician. He feels particularly well placed to deal with medical events

75

which have ethical implications, such as abortion and sterilization, and he will offer categorical opinions where others appear to vacillate in uncertainty.

Over the years there is always some degree of matching of doctor and patient, so that when referring patients for further investigation, general practitioners find that certain kinds of patient get on better with a particular specialist. (And the primary-care doctor's list also may have a certain bias to it.) The ambitious doctor is most comfortable with those who respond positively to his high status, and he will attract the people to him who want to make sure they take their ailments to 'the best man'. The admiring patient meets the self-confident doctor and a mutually satisfying relationship ensues.

The medical consultation is always an intimate business, and a degree of closeness is established routinely in clinical medicine which would be exceptional in any other setting. Traditionally, it is a relationship in which one person reveals all and the other does not have to reveal anything. Furthermore, the one who reveals nothing can switch the relationship on and off at will, so that he has closeness when he feels like it and solitude when he does not.

This kind of doctor can easily find the clinical relationships more agreeable than the turmoil of his family life where his adolescent children have no respect for him and certainly do not do his bidding. The doctor can come, in effect, to live through his patients. They have their successes which he can enjoy, love affairs which he can look in upon, and he can feel genuine sympathy at their griefs and failures. The doctor thus can be closely involved at any one time in scores of personal dramas which he can find much more stimulating and less demanding than his own domestic life. He is always in charge and the patient knows it, playing up now and again, but always recognizing the doctor's dominant position. There is an emotional satisfaction here which makes virtually no demands, but it is a poor kind of living.

Such living at second hand carries with it certain complications. The power which the doctor has in these circumstances is in danger of being used to nourish him emotionally, even feeding his fantasies, sexual and otherwise, so that he has an interest in maintaining a close and dependent relationship with his patient. This type of practice can have a deadening effect on the doctor's personal and family life. Energy easily goes out of his domestic relationships for the simple reason that they are less convenient, as they cannot easily be controlled, and furthermore the problems connected with them will intensify if they are neglected. The busy doctor may come to see less and less of his wife. She complains that he is never at home and no longer talks to her about his work, and he responds by spending even longer in the company of people who do not complain about him. He may be grappling with difficult teenagers in his practice but he can walk off and leave them when he has had enough: he cannot do the same with his own children, and the more they protest the more he withdraws.

At the same time, provided the doctor does not hold on too firmly to his patients, they may get a very high quality of medical care from such a dedicated person. The doctor may be satisfied too. So, what then is wrong with this kind of total commitment to the patients' welfare? Is it not something of an ideal of service to others?

At a practical level, what is wrong is that the doctor is liable to become opinionated and paternalistic, his own personal relationships atrophy, and he ceases to develop as a person. He becomes a pathetic and even dangerous figure. Cut off from his family, friends and colleagues, he never meets anyone on a basis of equality, and avoids situations where people can speak their minds to him. It is as though any frank discussion is perceived as a threat. Thus we have the spectacle of 'the honoured scientist', which is Solzhenitsyn's term for the distinguished doctor who has lost contact with his humanity.

> If a man was called a Scientist during his lifetime and an Honoured one at that, it was the end of him as a doctor. The honour and glory of it would get in the way of his treatment of his patients, just as elaborate clothing hinders a man's movements. These Honoured Scientists went about with a suite of followers, like some new Christ with his apostles. They completely lost the right to make mistakes or not to know something, they lost the right to be allowed to think things over. The man might be self-satisfied, half-witted, behind the times, and trying to conceal the fact, and yet everyone would expect miracles from him.[14]

Solzhenitsyn was writing, in *Cancer Ward*, out of his own experience in hospital in Tashkent in Central Asia which is a very long way from the kinds of centre described here. Unintentionally, perhaps, he indicates the universal nature of these medical habits.

Attitudes to women

Women doctors. The attitudes in medical school most likely to be appreciated by the senior staff will be those that conform to the stereotype of the medical student: that is, a robust approach to life, little interest in ideas, never taking anything too seriously, playing hard, drinking hard, and having a good time with the girls. It is difficult to know whether the seniors really admire these attitudes or whether they have become so conditioned into their roles that they adopt them without thinking. It is even more difficult to know to what extent they are shared by today's medical students. However, there is certainly an awareness that these are safe attitudes, and any man wanting to impress his seniors that he is the 'right sort of chap for a job on the house' and 'not likely to rock the boat' has to pay some kind of homage to them.

This powerfully male ethos dominates an environment in which women doctors do exactly the same work as the men, yet the men often behave as though these women doctors simply are not there. Most hospitals, especially teaching hospitals, are dominated by men, and the women are expected to occupy a subordinate position. This ethos requires women to perceive themselves in the traditional way, as objects; and it is reinforced by the favourable position in which male doctors, and also medical students, find themselves in relation to nurses and other female staff in hospitals. Women who accept the role as passive objects are welcome, while those who seek to be treated as equals run up against deeply rooted opposition, as the history of women in medicine shows.

The high point for medical autonomy and prestige was in the 1940s and 1950s, culminating in the plans in the early 1960s for huge general hospitals in which would be concentrated the new technological resources. Sometimes these were built, sometimes they were partly built; often they remained as plans once their relevance was questioned in the harsher economic climate of the 1970s. Nevertheless there was a great expansion in the West of medical services of all kinds and a consequent demand for more doctors. Women were able to fill this gap (also doctors from poorer countries), and the cynic will argue that this has been an important reason for the rapid increase in the number of women admitted to medical schools in recent years.

The notion of women as second-class medical labour is worth examining. True, they are paid the same as men and work on a level with men early on in their careers. It is later that differences emerge, especially for women with domestic commitments, a term which usually refers to children, though not necessarily so.

A survey into the progress of medical women was conducted, based on a national sample of American physicians who graduated in 1960 and were followed up until 1976, when they were in their forties. Although the women did well in medical school and obtained prestigious intern posts, their level of professional attainment and satisfaction fell significantly behind that of their male colleagues.[15] The general message from this and other American surveys is that women are left with the lower-status jobs, usually in primary care (referring here to family practice, paediatrics, obstetrics and gynaecology) and less popular specialties such as psychiatry and anaesthetics.[16,17]

In Britain, the picture is much the same. The percentage of hospital consultants who are women rose from 8.7 in 1975 (the year of the Sex Discrimination Act) to 12 in 1983. Over the same period the percentage of all women doctors working in hospital rose from 16.4 to 22, although the percentage of women who are consultant surgeons has remained unchanged at 1.9.[18] It is often said that women in general practice are left with routine tasks that their male partners do not care for, such as family planning, cervical cytology and obstetrics; even though these activities provide a valuable source of extra income which the women doctors have to earn to make up for their smaller National Health Service lists.

A survey from a good sample of men and women doctors in Manchester showed that 'women and men have closely similar patterns of work and provide similar patterns of care',[19] and that the women spent on average only 1.8 hours per week less in the surgery than the male doctors. This survey was not set up to compare the ways of working of men and women doctors, and although the authors were aware that a number of the women held part-time contracts, they felt that the term 'part-time' might have 'more to do with status and financial reward than the actual number of hours worked in the consultations'. They also saw the married women doctors who had children as a relatively 'disadvantaged group'.[19]

The disadvantageous position of women doctors working in the community can be exacerbated by the presence of health professionals, such as nurse practitioners, health visitors, community psychiatric nurses, and physicians' assistants (in the USA).[20] The health professionals are often preferred by the traditional male doctors: they are cheaper to employ than doctors, most of them are women, and they do not challenge the male doctor's supremacy.

The position of women doctors in the United States, Great Britain and the Soviet Union has been compared, and their disadvantageous position is surprisingly similar, bearing in mind especially that three-quarters of Russian doctors are women. As in the other countries, they are mainly concentrated in the community, while the prestigious posts, and those where policy is made, remain in the hands of men.[21,22] The disadvantageous position of women extends throughout the industrialized world. A survey of the occupational attainments of women in general (agricultural and factory workers through to professional women) in twelve industrial countries (Austria, Denmark, Finland, West Germany, Great Britain, Israel, Japan, the Netherlands, Northern Ireland, Norway,

Sweden, and the United States) showed that all women, whether they were married with domestic commitments or single without domestic commitments, fared worse in terms of income and occupational attainment than men. However, the women who fell furthest behind were those with domestic responsibilities.[23]

In medicine, it is perhaps some consolation that a woman doctor without domestic commitments can plan her career as effectively as a man can, without the interruptions from having babies and moving house to follow her partner's employment. The domestically uncommitted woman, however, usually has to make her way in a male world because of the lack of women in positions of influence in medicine; so the chances are that she will have to depend on the sponsorship of men, and will be likely to adopt something of the male ethos.

Women doctors are faced with a choice: either to align themselves with the powerful medical establishment, adopt its ways and enjoy its privileges; or else to identify more with the consumers and health professionals, with the needs of the community in mind, rather than the needs of the profession – and perhaps with the women's movement in general and its freewheeling non-hierarchical style.

Women patients. It is, however, the women patients who are in the least favourable position with regard to these generally negative attitudes towards women, especially when they are combined with other immature and insensitive habits of doctors which deny the reality of a patient's experience and suffering. These two groups of adverse attitudes can cause great distress to women, who are the principal users of health services, and all the more so because many of their medical needs relate to their sexuality.

It is easy for a doctor in a busy hospital clinic to ignore the emotional significance of the uterus for a woman, when he is seeing the ninth patient in her late thirties who complains of heavy menstrual bleeding. It is understandable for him to take a purely pragmatic approach, offering her a quick and sure remedy (i.e. hysterectomy) for the presenting complaint; even though she may be left feeling resentful that she had not been listened to or understood.

Such denials of the woman's position, together with the judgemental tone that male doctors frequently adopt when dealing with matters relating to sexuality or childbearing, are rooted in the sense of paternalism which they bring to their work. Both women doctors and women patients suffer from these attitudes. If they are to be accepted as reasonable people they must deny their womanliness and behave as far as possible like men, always functioning at full stretch, regardless of the menstrual cycle, pregnancy or the demands of small children.

If the woman's physiology demands from time to time that she withdraw from full activity, there is a tendency to medicalize the matter. A woman working full-time who feels out of sorts in the days before a menstrual period may find that she has been caught up into the medical machine, and diagnosed as suffering from pre-menstrual tension – PMT for short – and then given a suitable drug to treat the abnormal condition. This medicalizing of the menstrual cycle amounts almost to a denial that women are different from men; and in a more general way, that they may have different aspirations and priorities from the majority of men.

Women doctors also suffer from these attitudes. The reluctance of medical employers to accede to the frequent requests from women doctors for more part-time employment and job sharing in the health services, particularly in the training grades, may be influenced by this denial of a woman's needs, even though the excuses are administrative and financial.

It is quite clear that in the not-too-distant future, most of the doctors in Britain, and possibly throughout the Western world, will be women, yet nothing is being done to create the kind of working arrangements that the majority of women seem to want. These working arrangements appeal to a fair number of male doctors, too, but these doctors are not of the kind who devote themselves to the campaigning and committee work which is necessary to bring about any medico-political change.

Denial of death

The whole question of power and control is extremely important in the transactions between doctors and patients, so that when the patient takes an initiative, it is often resented by the doctors. Patients who either refer themselves for help or engage in activities which will lead to medical referral are frequently unwelcome and may be treated as of secondary importance, compared with people who are referred with well-developed diseases for which, conventionally, they cannot be held responsible. Examples of conditions where the person plays a part in the referral are: self-injury of any kind; people who have harmed themselves by abuse of drugs and alcohol; people seeking cosmetic surgery, or who have had certain kinds of accident which in the opinion of the staff could have been avoided. They have all in a subtle way challenged the paternalistic authority of the medical profession.

The greatest challenge, however, comes not so much from people who arrive with conditions for which they might be held responsible, as from those who demonstrate that the doctor's power and expertise is limited. Someone suffering a terminal illness presents a great many doctors with a challenge to their authority and to their image of themselves as healers that they cannot handle. A dying person, enduring the despair and indignity of that state, can disconcert the most confident doctor.

Peter Maguire, by means of video-taped or audio-taped interviews, has studied the reactions of doctors (and nurses) to terminally ill people.[24]

SURGEON: Well, how are you today?

WOMAN (dying of breast cancer): I'm very worried about what is happening to me. I'm beginning to think I'm not going to get better this time. The pain in my hip is getting worse.

SURGEON: Tell me more about this pain in your hip.

DOCTOR: How are you today?

PATIENT (dying of lung cancer): I am not so good. I can't understand why I'm continuing to lose so much weight.

DOCTOR: Have you had any pain?

PATIENT: I'm not going to get out of here, am I?

DOCTOR: Have you had your bowels open since yesterday?

Doctors are always liable to disregard the possibility of death, and to reformulate the dying person's experience in terms of symptoms requiring treatment. Then follows the familiar sequence of antibiotics, blood transfusions, and even exploratory operations to see 'if anything can be done'. This latter strategy can break up the gentle departure from this life, and replace death in the setting of loving care at home by death in intensive care in hospital. It seems a heavy price for people to pay because of the doctors' difficulties in coping with the realities of death, but there it is.

Doctors can themselves suffer through the profession's collective anxiety about death. Those who have consulted colleagues about symptoms which may indicate serious illness, in particular cancer, have sometimes had less effective treatment than might be expected among those in the best position to obtain medical help. A number of studies have shown how the denial process can operate between colleagues.[25–27] In a way, it is not surprising. If doctors have profound anxieties about their own mortality, they will become uncomfortable when facing it in a patient. If the patient is one of them, mortality comes that much closer. Furthermore, while the doctors can usually shed patients who make them feel uneasy, that cannot always be done when the patient is a fellow doctor.

At the age of forty-five, David Rabin, then director of endocrinology at the Vanderbilt Medical Center in Nashville, Tennessee, developed amyotrophic lateral sclerosis. He had some neurological experience and he was able to suspect the diagnosis quite early on, but the time came

82

when he needed to confirm the diagnosis. This is how he describes the episode and his subsequent experiences.

> To confirm the diagnosis, I traveled to a prestigious medical center renowned for its experience with ALS. The diagnostic and technical skills of the people there were superb . . . The neurologist was rigorous in his examination and deft in reaching an unequivocal diagnosis. My disappointment stemmed from his impersonal manner. He exhibited no interest in me as a person, and did not make even a perfunctory inquiry about my work. . . The only time he seemed to come alive during our interview was when he drew the mortality curve among his collected [ALS] patients.

When Rabin developed a limp, he told his colleagues at the Medical Center that he had 'a disk'. They offered him advice and told him about their own back problems. Later, when he walked with a stick,

> the inquiries ceased and were replaced by a very obvious desire to avoid me. When I arrived at work in the morning I could see, from the corner of my eye, colleagues changing their pace or stopping in their tracks to spare themselves the embarrassment of bumping into me. This dramatic change in their behavior occurred when it became common knowledge that David Rabin had ALS. . .
> As the cane became inadequate and was replaced by a walker, so my isolation from my colleagues intensified . . . How often, as I struggled to open a door, would I see a colleague pretending to look the other way. On the other hand [it was] so natural for the non-physicians – the technicians, the secretaries, the cleaning women – to rush to open the door for me, even if it was the door to the men's toilet. . .
> One day, while crossing the courtyard outside the emergency room, I fell. A longtime colleague was walking by. He turned, and our eyes met as I lay sprawled on the ground. He quickly averted his eyes, pretended not to see me, and continued walking. He never even broke his stride. I suppose he ignored the obvious need for help out of embarrassment and discomfort, for I know him to be a compassionate and caring physician.[28]

Rabin described how he himself had avoided an older physican when he was mortally ill, although he attended the man's funeral. Rabin also pays tribute to some of his colleagues who were honest, supportive and practically very helpful to him.

I have three images in Bristol of the way doctors are treated by their tribe once they seem to be mortally ill. The first, in the 1960s, was of the then senior surgeon, a tall, powerfully built man, much respected personally and professionally. He had had a stroke; and the last I saw of him was as a patient in a wheelchair, in a row of other patients also in wheelchairs, waiting to get to the outpatient department at the Royal Infirmary – which only a few months before he dominated by his presence. Now, no one seemed to notice him at all.

The next image was in the 1970s of a more junior doctor who used to drop in at the local pub after his day's work. When it was discovered that his bladder tumour was malignant, his drinking companions would no longer look him in the eye or speak to him. Nothing had emerged formally about his diagnosis, but the others in the pub mostly worked in the hospital and news like that travels fast. Another colleague, around the same time, had a bladder tumour which turned out to be a benign papilloma, so he did not experience the same kind of rejection.

In 1985, a friend and colleague was having treatment for advanced ovarian cancer. Knowing my interest in the peculiarities of hospital life, she told me, with some irony, that she could confirm that in 1985 the traditional story that 'the only person in hospital who speaks to you as a person is the cleaner', is still precisely true.

Sick colleagues present the greatest emotional challenge to doctors. The professional persona and the various 'virtuoso' strategies are of no help at such a time, and are shown up for what they really are. True, they are of some help at the beginning of a medical career. The trouble is that very easily they become entrenched, so that doctors never have to grapple with whatever deep anxieties they may have about sickness and death. The result is that when people really need help, beyond the purely technological, the doctors fail them because they simply do not know what to do.

6

Doctors in the Making

How do doctors develop their bad habits? Are the doctors who appear to be so concerned with authority and the rational-intellectual aspects of medicine drawn to the medical profession because it provides a position in society and a life-style which permits those qualities to find expression; or are they essentially sensitive and socially aware men and women who have been moulded by the processes of medical education?

We can ask therefore: what kind of person chooses to study medicine in the first place; and then, what happens during the medical course to implant or to foster the notion of doctors as an elite in society, and medicine as a branch of mechanical science?

Choosing to study medicine

It is doubtful if we ever really know why we make the important choices in our lives, at least not at the time of making them. We can always produce a reason of sorts to satisfy people who casually ask 'why this . . . or that?', but the underlying motivation may take years to emerge, if it ever emerges at all. So there is no simple answer along the lines: 'I studied medicine because . . .'

Why did *I* study medicine? I ask myself. I have no doubt that it was a good decision, but how was the choice formed in the first place? There were immediate reasons largely determined by my middle-class professional background which ordained a career in one of the professions, although that was complicated for me by being at a school with a powerful military tradition where the army was regarded as the best possible career for just about everyone. My first step in selecting a career, therefore, was to avoid being dispatched into the army. That left the church, the law and medicine.

I had no leaning towards the church and was not thought strong enough at classics for the law, so medicine was the choice; and I studied physics, chemistry and biology as the necessary preliminaries. Looking back on those years in the late 1940s when the crucial decisions were being made, I find it hard to recollect how I imagined medicine. I had seen nothing of illness and had never looked after anyone, so that my immediate contact with medicine was with general practitioners treating various childhood medical conditions of mine.

The main influence was probably that of my father, who was a doctor. Because of the war, I saw him for only a few weeks out of five years of my teenage years, so the influence was mainly from my awareness of his life-style during my childhood, and from his personality. He was a psychiatrist, and as a ten-year-old I had little idea of what he actually did, having had no direct experience of mental disorder; and anyway he was not a doctor as a child might imagine one – going out to ill people and making them better. But then, how does a child imagine the doctor? We all have, or have had, our recollections and fantasies about doctors. He might be the kindly person who brought relief when one was ill. It might have been a doctor who sent one's mother away to hospital, from which she never returned. There may have been a doctor in the family; he may have been the one in the family who was prosperous or who drank, but whatever he was like, his influence would have been felt.

My experience was continuous in the early years, although indirect. My father was always busy on important matters. He went out early in the day and returned late; and at weekends the house had to be quiet because he was working. He was highly successful in his practice, which was largely private, as was the way in the 1930s and the 1940s after the war; he was in great demand, so had little time for his family – even if he had had the inclination to spend time with small children. He was seldom there but he dominated the household. So what does all this amount to? What message was being given to my brother and me about the profession of medicine? Whatever else it was, it was clear that medicine was an important activity: people respected doctors and deferred to them. The doctor's business came first, and it was apparent that the doctor always got his own way. The cynic might say it was a well-rewarded way of doing just as one pleased, but it was hard work and chancy, although in those days doctors, and most professional men for that matter, managed to live pretty well.

There was good sense in my studying medicine, as there is good sense in *anyone* studying medicine. It is one of the most 'sensible' careers anyone can pursue, and it was open to me if I passed the exams. I cannot even now evaluate the significance of paternal influence, either from the model I had of the professional life and the attractions I presume I then perceived therein, or from some desire to emulate my father. One thing I do know is that my brother and I, and a cousin who lived with us, all became doctors. That says something, but what?

A high proportion of medical students come from 'medical' families, and an even higher proportion are middle-class. From the point of view of most parents, medicine is an eminently wise choice of career, and it is understandable therefore if parents who are interested and able to promote their children's education encourage them in this direction.

Left-wing critics of the middle-class bias of medical schools argue that this is a device of the professional classes to maintain hegemony, as they put it, over society; not necessarily as a deliberate plot but rather as an implicit strategy of those who have nothing to gain from any change in the social order. These people, the argument goes, will ensure that the medical profession retains its power, but I am not aware to what extent the social origins of doctors determine their subsequent life-style and their attitudes to the medical monolith. Doctors from any background can become fascinated with the mystique of the medical profession, and others simply find they cannot avoid its ethos. In particular, doctors from working-class communities, whatever their early intentions, find inexorably that they become middle-class – although the feelings remain of not having been true to their origins.

In the middle teenage years a broad choice is made generally between 'science' and 'the humanities'. It is a choice with life-long implications which will close off a large range of possibilities and will steer the young person towards particular occupations about which there may be only limited, if any, information at school – as in the case of medicine. If the aspiring student does not come from a medical family, knowledge about medical careers will probably be negligible when the crucial decision is taken. Yet choices to study medicine or the sciences in general are often made around the age of fifteen, and made with an intuitive certainty unlikely to be seen amongst those selecting the humanities, whose guiding feeling may only be that they do not wish to study science.

Are there, then, any particular attributes which would make it possible to pick out the future medical students from a group of school boys and girls? Is there a profile of the future average medical student? Despite a good deal of interest and research in most of the developed countries of the East and West,[1,2] only broad trends emerge: that the applicant will be male (this is from the international surveys referred to, but the sex bias has now almost gone), from a professional family living in a town, and a high academic achiever with a leaning toward the sciences. But what kind of person is this who wants to study medicine, because alongside the advantages of a medical qualification there are a number of disadvantages to the medical life? After all, a medical training is long, with postponement of rewards, so that financial independence is unlikely before the age of twenty-five or even thirty; and women are unlikely to start their families before their late twenties. The medical course, and the now almost inevitable post-graduate training, involves a great deal of hard study and tolerance of assessments and examinations. The work, for the first few years after qualifying, involves, as already described, very long hours of work, day and night, enforced residence in hospitals and moves of house until the permanent job is obtained. There is also constant exposure to suffering, mutilation and death.

How many school boys and girls are aware of these realities, if indeed such realities are meaningful to teenagers? Or are they more influenced by an image of medicine and the medical life?

Medicine is a possible option for every school boy or girl who is academically bright and has a leaning towards the sciences, with the result that thousands apply overall but only hundreds are chosen. For instance, about 1,200 apply each year to the University of Bristol Medical School, 400 are interviewed and 120 are offered places. Throughout the country such large numbers of school leavers are involved that it would be unrealistic to expect to identify amongst these intending students a particular type of personality. Furthermore, medicine offers such a wide range of life-styles that there is no single type which could, or should, be sought.

It is inevitable, and good, that a wide range of personalities is to be found within the medical profession. The trouble comes from those who become preoccupied with power and prestige, and who devote their main energies to the kinds of political intrigue and personal status-seeking mentioned earlier.[3]

It would be interesting to know if there were among intending medical students some who revealed yearnings for high status and power early on, or whether these features appeared only as a result of the medical course.

It has been my regular experience that among the new medical students there is always a vocal group which takes a conspicuously hard line about the subject matter of the course. They prefer the apparent precision of anatomy, physiology and biochemistry, grounded as they are in the traditions of natural science, to what they regard as the 'woolliness' of discussions on human behaviour, which are based on psychological and social concepts.

The students who object to the study of human behaviour, or feel uncomfortable with it, often take up rather firm positions in relation to what they judge to be 'scientific' or 'unscientific'. In their view certain subjects are 'scientific', and therefore acceptable: examples are anatomy, physiology and biochemistry. 'Unscientific', and therefore to be treated with suspicion, is the study of human development and behaviour. These students, with their mistaken view of the nature of science, are ventilating attitudes and anxieties, and they can usually be led into the study of human behaviour by patient explanation of the principles underlying its study. However, their initial attitudes are quite striking; and even though while studying human behaviour they can become quite receptive (and the same processes occur in their clinical years when they study psychiatry), as soon as the particular course is finished, many of them revert to their traditional mechanistic position. In mechanistic medicine precise subject matter is preferred, and the closer it is to the physical sciences the better. The intolerance with the courses dealing with human behaviour suggests a mixture of impatience and anxiety at the ambiguities inherent in any study of people – even though clinical medicine is, by definition, all about people and the misfortunes that befall them.

Some of these same students adopt an unusually conservative style of dress and treat their teachers with deference, even addressing them as 'Sir'. They also give an impression of belonging already to a great profession, that they know exactly how to climb the ladder to success, and that they have a clear idea of what is necessary for their future careers and what is not.

Authoritarianism

A constellation of characteristics is apparent in certain medical students and junior doctors, particularly in those with ambitions for careers in the major specialties of surgery and internal medicine. These characteristics are even more noticeable among those seeking positions in the teaching hospitals, and thus likely to become generally influential in the medical profession, and in the training of future generations of medical students. This constellation of characteristics includes a predilection for subjects with a substantial body of precise information; a generally tough-minded attitude towards people, with a lack of sensitivity to their feelings; an identification with the powerful groups in society, with a consequent mistrust of minority groups (such as immigrants) and people who adopt unconventional life-styles (homosexuals); and very traditional attitudes towards the role of women.

When these qualities are set down together they are striking, because they correspond to the qualities which come under the heading of the 'Authoritarian Personality'.[4] This was a concept derived from an inquiry set up in the 1940s into the roots of prejudice and social discrimination, in an attempt to learn something about the origins of anti-Semitism.

The original concept of an 'authoritarian personality' has a commonsense validity; and during the thirty-five years since it was enunciated it has been subjected to intensive critical analysis,[5-10] and has emerged as a legitimate category. Adorno and his associates drew up a scale for measuring authoritarian tendencies, which was based on their survey of over two thousand American men and women of various social groups. Their interest was in political attitudes with special reference to anti-Semitism, and the result was their F scale.[11] 'F' actually stands for 'Fascism', although the concept of authoritarianism holds good (when applied to political attitudes) for extreme tendencies of the left as well as of the right.[5,6] The main features of the original F scale are reproduced here so that readers can decide for themselves to what extent they correspond with qualities they may have observed in members of the medical profession:

1 *Conventionalism*: a rigid adherence to conventional middle-class values.

2 *Authoritarian submission*: submissive, uncritical attitudes towards the idealized moral authorities of the in-group.

3 *Authoritarian aggression*: a tendency to be on the lookout for, and to condemn, reject, and punish people who violate conventional values.

4 *Anti-intraception*: that is, opposition to the subjective, the imaginative and the tender-minded.

5 *Superstition and stereotypy*: a belief in supernatural determinants of an individual's fate; and the disposition to think in rigid categories.

6 *Power and 'toughness'*: preoccupation with the dominance-submission, strong-weak, leader-follower dimension; identification with power figures; over-emphasis upon the conventionalized attributes of the ego; exaggerated assertion of strength and toughness.

7 *Destructiveness and cynicism*: Generalized hostility, and a vilification of the human.

8 *Projectivity*: that is, the disposition to believe that wild and dangerous things go on in the world; the projection outward of unconscious emotional impulses.

9 *Sex*: an exaggerated concern with sexual 'goings-on'.[11]

The interest of this scale is that a list of attributes which characterize holders of extreme political views can have anything at all in common with qualities to be found among leading members of a profession ostensibly devoted to caring for people in need. It seems like yet another of the paradoxes of the medical profession.

The F scale does in fact describe many of the qualities of doctors, especially of the kind noted in the last two chapters. For the present descriptive purposes I would like to paraphrase and develop the scale slightly. Therefore, a kind of medical version of the F scale – we might even call it an 'authoritarian syndrome' – would identify the following features:

– A rigid adherence to the conventional values of society (and to the mores of the medical profession – the in-group), and an acceptance of its authority on all matters. The authoritarian tends to identify with the existing social order, whatever it might be, and with the established institutions, such as the Church and the Law. The authoritarian will also change – even totally reverse – stoutly held beliefs when told to do so by a suitable figure in authority.

– A rejection of 'out-groups', for example, immigrants, people who harm themselves in various ways, and any groups that do not accept the profession's authority. A particular, and perhaps at first sight surprising, out-group is patients. Patients are, by definition, outside the medical profession; and in organizations, such as teaching hospitals, where issues of power are dominant, patients are perceived by the senior doctors, not so much as individuals as an outside group with preoccupations and needs that do not coincide with the doctors' – however dependent ultimately all doctors are upon the existence of patients.

– Corporal and capital punishment may be favoured, and a severe line will be taken towards sexual indulgence and drug abuse. Women seeking termination of pregnancy are not likely to be treated sympathetically if they are young, unmarried, or perceived as belonging to any peripheral group.

– The authoritarian also rejects attitudes of tenderness and displays of emotion; although at times this repressed aspect may break out in demonstrations of mawkish sentimentality, practical jokes and childish humour.

– The rigid personal style of the medical authoritarian is usually associated with a rigidity in thinking, so that his conceptual framework is implacably mechanistic, with little notion of alternative explanatory models of illness.[12]

This sketch of the medical authoritarian is intended to depict a certain pattern of behaviour which may be present throughout a person's life or may emerge only at times of uncertainty or extra pressure. It therefore simply describes what certain people do, and it is not an account of a set of basic attributes of personality, although the authoritarian tendency might happen to be such an attribute. The pattern of behaviour is familiar enough, and it is associated with a great deal of the dissatisfaction that people experience in their dealings with doctors. That seems to be a good reason for examining it, even if the behaviour cannot be explained.

It would be interesting to know when and how this pattern of behaviour becomes established. Is it present, for example, in school boys and girls and pre-clinical medical students, or only in qualified doctors? In other words, is it a variety of behaviour and a way of coping with difficulties which is established early on? If these tendencies were well established among pupils at school, it could lead certain budding authoritarians to choose a career in medicine because it would provide a milieu in which such tendencies could flourish – a poor motive for wanting to study medicine, but it may not be a rare one.

In an attempt to elucidate some of these questions, a colleague and I in the late 1960s constructed an *ad hoc* questionnaire which we gave to first-year students in psychology, philosophy, languages, history, mechanical engineering and, of course, medicine. The thirty-two questions explored attitudes towards punishment, social benefits, sex crimes, leadership and the like. It was no more than a pilot inquiry, and I would hesitate to offer it as evidence, but the authoritarian tendencies were much more pronounced among the first-year medicals than among the first-year students in the arts faculty, with the mechanical engineers in between but veering towards the attitudes of the medicals.

The underlying dispositions and attitudes of young people have been extensively studied by Liam Hudson with special reference to the concept of 'convergers' and 'divergers'.[13] Convergers, by definition, are those who do better at straightforward intelligence tests or tests of factual knowledge, as compared with open-ended tests where there is no single correct answer. They prefer exactness and precise entities, they are impatient with ambiguity, and tend to avoid expressions of emotion and opportunities to use their imaginative powers. They are ready to accept authority and the teaching of their elders, and they are likely to seek out courses of study where the body of factual information and the weight of accepted authority is greatest. The diverger, defined in terms of test scores, is the opposite in almost all these respects, and in the educational system is more likely to be found studying the humanities where empathy and the ability to evaluate ideas critically are qualities which would have more outlets than they would, say, in a medical course.

These convergent tendencies can appear as early as fifteen or sixteen years of age,[14] which is before the majority of eventual doctors have made their career decisions. (The convergent tendencies might appear earlier, but the tests were designed for use by teenagers.) The schoolboy (most of Hudson's work was done on boys) of a convergent disposition will find the science subjects more congenial than the humanities, and in many ways medicine has the largest body of uncritically accepted information of all. The medical course involves learning vast quantities of facts which are offered as the truth about the human body.

Undergraduate students of physics and chemistry probably also scored highly on the tests for convergent thinking, and they too have a good deal of factual material to cope with. However, physicists and chemists display more flexible thinking than doctors, so that when events demand it, they are prepared to seek fresh explanatory models. This does not happen in medicine, because the explanatory models are settled and not open to question, with the result that the apparent level of certainty is higher.

The only work I know of about attitudes among new medical students comes from Toronto, where entering medical students (total 877) were tested each year between 1967 and 1972.[15] Over some of this period they had comparative data from 94 students in the 'arts and sciences' in the University of Toronto, and from 2,031 'North American College norms', presumably representative of North American college men and women. The medical students scored significantly better than the arts and sciences students on cognitive testing (i.e. they were intellectually brighter). The medicals also scored significantly higher than the arts and sciences students and the 'North American norms' with regard to 'achievement' (defined by the adjectives 'striving, driving, competitive'), 'endurance' ('persistent, relentless, zealous'), 'order' ('systematic, consistent, methodical'), 'nurturance' ('sympathetic, consoling, assisting'), and 'understanding' ('analytical, rational, inquisitive'). The medicals scored significantly lower than the other groups with regard to 'play' ('fun-loving, gleeful, carefree'), and 'impulsivity' ('rash, impetuous, spontaneous').

The medicals also scored significantly lower than the other groups on their ability to tolerate change, uncertainty, and lack of structure. The authors thought this was a paradoxical finding because of 'the high degree of uncertainty associated with many diagnostic and therapeutic situations'. The authors also asked how this profile of traits in the Toronto medical students could result from a traditional selection system. The attributes of entering medical students may have changed in the years since this study was conducted, but the students in this study would now be reaching positions of real influence.

The Toronto study suggests that the medical students lean more in the direction of the convergers than the divergers, although the attributes they were measuring were rather different. The common factors would be a desire for certainty, structure and lack of change; and to a lesser extent, achievement and endurance.

There are parallels also between authoritarianism and convergence: for the authoritarian a central tenet is obedience to authority and the established order, and for the converger it is an attraction towards apparent order and precision. The two concepts seem to me to be very closely linked, indeed inseparable; and I would suggest that the convergent type, exposed to suitable influences, is more likely to become authoritarian in style than a divergent type. Again, it must be said that these labels, 'authoritarian', 'convergent', 'divergent', are merely descriptive of a way of thinking and behaving at a particular time: they are not necessarily enduring attributes of someone's personality.

Selection of medical students

In some countries all those wishing to train as doctors are allowed to start training, and the selection comes from the large numbers that drop out along the way. More common, in the developed countries, are selection procedures before entry, after which the great majority of those that start the medical course subsequently qualify. No one has yet devised a satisfactory way of deciding which seventeen-year-olds are going to make the best doctors, despite efforts to do so in many parts of the world[1,2] by means of interviews and special tests of various kinds, but it seems that 90–95 per cent of those selected subsequently qualify – and that is a pretty high success rate.

There is a commonsense academic base-line for students who are going to have to absorb a vast range of factual material; but academic excellence only seems to predict who will do well in the pre-clinical years, which is merely an extension of the kind of book work at which the students have already demonstrated their ability. The clinical years are less demanding intellectually, and other qualities are called for, and so a different group of students may lead the field then.

Liam Hudson found that 24 per cent of future winners of open scholarships and exhibitions to Oxford and Cambridge fell within the bottom 30 per cent for the measures of intelligence he used on his sample (admittedly a highly selected one); and that among fifteen-year-old schoolboys who go on to win open scholarships and take first-class degrees the relation between their test scores and their academic performance is 'very tenuous indeed'[16]. Hudson further found that high academic and professional achievement was by no means associated with outstanding performance at university. Among scientists, he compared those who became Fellows of the Royal Society and those who obtained the degree of Doctor of Science at Cambridge with those who did not obtain these distinctions, and found no significant difference in the quality of their undergraduate degrees. When he compared Cabinet Ministers with non-Cabinet Ministers and back-bench Members of Parliament, and then High Court Judges with County Court Judges, he found 'some slight relation between eminence and degree class, but . . . there were many striking exceptions'.[16,17]

Academic distinction is a relatively poor indicator of performance in final medical examinations, and personality factors such as might emerge from personality tests and skilled interviewing are even worse predictors,[18,19] so what are the selectors actually doing? They have numerous applicants with excellent academic records of whom they interview a selection. Some medical schools omitted a personal interview until recently, possibly for the good reason that it would accomplish nothing, but there is always pressure to have interviews because without them it can appear that the medical school does not really care.

It is possible that the reverse is true, and that the thankless task of trying to pick the best out of an excellent bunch might be misguided. There is a risk unwittingly of selecting students in one's own image, which may militate against women, the disabled, those from working-class homes, or those with odd quirks of personality. There is also a hint of hypocrisy about the interviewing: the selectors know that over two-thirds of their students will become general practitioners, yet they may resist any thought of involving a general practitioner in the selection. Universities guard their power jealously, so when it comes to having a general practitioner, or, worse still, a lay person – a representative of the consumers of medical care – influencing the selection of the community's doctors, it seems like taking democracy too far.

Socialization of medical students

'Socialization' is a process of social conditioning by which, in the case of medical students, the school-leaver changes into a conforming member of the medical profession who accepts the traditional ideals of that profession. The authoritarian types will respond well to the process, and for them it will be more a matter of enhancing what is already latent, rather than implanting anything fresh. For the rest, the experience will be variable.

The new student arrives at medical school with high ideals and plenty to be proud of, having won a place in the face of all the competition; and the students will form a group which will hold together for the next five years as they make their way through the system.

There is something peculiarly daunting about entering a medical school. There is the sheer bulk of the buildings, the mass of people with imposing titles, an atmosphere of confidence with the implicit message that if you do things our way you will be all right. The various departments are run by professors, affectionately known as 'medical barons', since they wield great power and are not generally keen on change, unless it is to increase the size of their departments or the amount of undergraduate teaching time they can have. They may be, or may have been, scholars but they are also locked in a perpetual struggle with their fellow professors. They are men of battle, and they bear the authority that comes from success on the battlefield. The students very quickly grasp that the medical school hierarchy has to be treated with respect.

The medical school's authority is augmented by an equally imposing teaching hospital, so there are in fact two powerful institutions to be negotiated. Bristol possesses typical examples of each. The Medical School was built as a result of the university expansion of the 1960s. It occupies a commanding position on a hill overlooking the whole of the centre of the city, and it is conspicuous by its size and dullness. Yet, planted there, dominating and without regard for its surroundings, it cannot pass unnoticed. The teaching hospital was founded in the eighteenth century. The original Infirmary was a large building by the standards of those days, but it related to its surroundings. Now the original building is dwarfed by the modern developments, and only remnants of the interior decorations remain. The new Infirmary buildings have spread up the hillside to match the bulk of the Medical School. They stand either side of St Michael's Hill, one of Bristol's most beautiful old streets, with a medieval church and a conglomeration of other buildings dating back to the seventeenth century, and which all now blend comfortably together. The modern medical constructions tower up behind the buildings of St Michael's Hill, and the huge horizontal concrete slabs of the new Maternity Hospital front directly onto it – in line with the old buildings but totally out of scale with them – as a final gesture of the ruthless authority of contemporary medicine.

The relationship of medicine to the society it elects to serve is eloquently stated to the students by the relationship between these groups of buildings. The message will be restated hundreds of times over the succeeding five years, but the students' views about the significance of these interrelated groups of buildings may mature and change fundamentally.

Meanwhile, the students have to survive the course they have chosen, to grapple with the work-load and all the extraneous influences to which they will be exposed. They will be expected to study more and learn more facts than is at all reasonable. There will be repeated assessments and examinations, and they will need to discover strategies to enable them to cope with this load. They will also encounter a number of disturbing experiences during their five years, starting on the first day of the course when they may have to face the formalinized cadaver in the anatomy room. In the clinical years, they will have to deal with the anxiety about developing all the diseases they see or hear of, and about contracting infections from patients. They will find themselves conducting intimate physical examinations on patients and discussing details of marital relationships; they will have to face chronic, disfiguring and disabling disease, sit with people who cannot be cured or who are actually dying, and then witness death itself. Afterwards there will be scenes in the post-mortem room where people reappear as pathological specimens, and where some clinicians will reveal unintentionally that they actually prefer diseased organs to whole people.

In the face of these anxieties, the students are bound to see their teachers and the members of staff in the departments where they are taught as people who are supremely successful at what they are doing; or at least as people who have learned how to deal with the problems inherent in medical work. This makes them attractive as models for uncertain medical students. If you are feeling unsure of yourself, it is tempting, almost inevitable, to copy people who seem to be managing well. Ally yourself with them and you will surmount the obstacles; better still, become like them and one day you will step into their shoes. Unfortunately, the spectacular models are often those of an authoritarian and elitist disposition who keep patients firmly in their place, and do not allow the comfortable rhythm of their clinical work to be disturbed by displays of emotion, or complicated by a consideration of the psychological and social factors in the illness.

The process of socialization is subtle and paradoxical for medical students who do not see themselves as future members of an authoritarian elite. Such students do not automatically fit into the desired pattern and have no desire to be broken down and reformed in the manner of recruits into the armed forces, yet they can gain confidence from copying the traditional styles of the medical profession, at least in the early years. These students come into medicine with high ideals about helping people, but what they see around them is the antithesis of caring. When they reach out to people they are criticized and mocked by their seniors for being soft-hearted and over-involved. By being caring and supportive they find they take upon themselves an accumulated weight of their patients' distress which they cannot handle, and nobody shows them how to manage this burden.

This is an unhappy dilemma for students who often see the difficulty in terms of their own shortcomings, on the grounds that there must be something wrong with them if they cannot share the viewpoint of these obviously successful doctors. Such students can become deeply troubled, to the extent that they seriously contemplate abandoning medicine as a career.

Socialization has been a topic of enormous interest to sociologists,[20-26] mainly in North America. They have demonstrated that the medical course has a profound effect on attitudes, and that the example of the teachers is very strong indeed. However, there is no question of the medical schools grinding out a uniform product. This was implied to some extent in the earlier studies done in the 1950s and 1960s, but twenty years on there is more questioning of established values, even in medical schools. The students are now much more aware socially, even though there is always a hard core among them who regard themselves as 'scientists' and display little interest in the human aspects of medicine. A greater number experience a gradual dissatisfaction with the medical course and disillusionment with the medical profession as they progress through their training, but in the 1980s the rising interest in holistic medicine and complementary or alternative systems of various kinds has indicated to disenchanted students that they are not alone in deploring the traditional habits. In fact, as students gain confidence towards the end of their course, there is a greater variation in attitudes than there is at the beginning of the pre-clinical and clinical courses when, presumably, anxiety is at its greatest.

The diversity of attitudes evident in the final years of the medical course is not long-lasting, because an even greater pressure awaits the students, and that is the intern year that follows the final medical examinations. Here there is a powerful need for any available aids to self-confidence, and also for protection from the tragedy around them. The student's dilemma begins all over again but now with more force, and so there is another shift towards conformity, to the traditional style, if only as a way of surviving the arduous duties of a junior hospital doctor; hence the need for a strong persona.[27]

Where and when does the process of socialization cease? The fully qualified doctor has the necessary knowledge and practical skills to practise medicine, and presumably has simultaneously acquired personal skills to help meet the strains of clinical work. What pressures then continue to prevail upon the doctor to conform to this or that mode of behaviour? In the British National Health Service there are two points after which, in theory, the doctor is secure and unassailable in employment, and so ought to be free of sanctions from outside. These positions are a partnership in general practice and a consultant post in a hospital specialty. These appointments are obtained about four to eight years after full qualification, but during the critical postgraduate years the trainees have had not only to obtain the required postgraduate diplomas and give evidence of clinical competence, but also to convince those in charge of the ultimate appointment that they are the kind of people that they want.

By the time the British doctor has reached this secure position, a dozen or so years after first entering medical school, it would be surprising if the subtle conditioning had not had some effect. After all the general practice partner, or the hospital consultant, has demonstrated the advantages of playing the game according to the unstated rules, and in some degree has been influenced by doing so, since it is hard to oppose a system which serves you well and lands you in a comfortable position. Still, there are some rebellious spirits, and to discourage them there is the system of Distinction Awards whereby doctors who distinguish themselves in various ways and make significant contributions to their National Health Service work (as opposed to private practice) may receive substantial extra remuneration. The system is not set up as a sanction to encourage doctors to stay in line, but doctors with heavy family and financial responsibilities will find it hard to forget that there is always someone looking over their shoulders. In entrepreneurial practice there are equally powerful pressures on doctors to conform to the public's image of the successful practitioner.

It is difficult to become a doctor, and once that position has been achieved, it is difficult to become anything else but a doctor. The rewards from a medical career are considerable, and so are the personal sacrifices.

7

Technology, Drugs and People

Many doctors fail to shake off the authoritarian style acquired or reinforced during training. The student who wants to become prominent in his chosen profession is likely to see himself as joining a group which can expect privileges, high status and handsome remuneration. If these expectations are fulfilled, the doctor can sustain the line of favoured practitioners and researchers: if, as often happens, they are not fulfilled, the doctor who has followed the precept and example of his eminent teachers can feel cheated of his proper rewards. In either event the doctor is in danger of going wrong.

Medical practice goes wrong when it ceases to fulfil its original objectives of service, and individual doctors err when they become preoccupied with matters other than, directly or indirectly, caring for people who are sick or in need. What constitutes proper medical care is, in the broadest sense, a political question. At one end of the spectrum, medicine is seen as a commodity, similar to food or a house, which is purchased according to an individual's ability to pay; and doctors have a right to respond to market pressures and opportunities like any other citizen. At the other end of the spectrum, medical care is regarded as a basic right of every man, woman or child in a caring society, and as a service which should be provided by the state.

The first two chapters in this part (Chapters 4 and 5) have dealt in a general way with the issue of doctors' authority at a collective and an individual level. The next three chapters will examine specific ways in which medical practice can go wrong. In this chapter academic and high-technology medicine will be discussed, along with medicine which is practised without reference to the real needs of the society the doctors are serving, and the subtle relationship that exists between the medical profession and the pharmaceutical industry. In the later chapters, there will be examples of the irrational element displacing commonsense in clinical judgement; and of how doctors, whether they realize it or not, can act on behalf of the state as agents of social control.

100

The academic-mechanistic-high-technology nexus

The great discoveries since the beginning of the sixteenth century find their logical fulfilment in the practice of academic medicine as it is seen in our centres of excellence. Here the Cartesian ideal of the truly objective observer, examining ever smaller parts with greater and greater precision, is manifested and admired; even if Descartes himself would not have approved of the Godless attitudes of such workers, and their belief that the great machine can run itself without His direction.

The highest status and greatest public kudos in medicine today goes to the doctor who engages in the most esoteric aspects of the subject. The doctor who studies some extremely rare disease or who is involved in dramatic developments, such as organ transplantation, or who works with a spectacular machine, such as a whole-body scanner, is going to receive more public and professional acclaim than a doctor who sets up a programme of community care for elderly people or the mentally handicapped.

The fascination of the higher flights of clinical medicine and surgery and of recondite medical studies is entirely understandable, since the human body is so endlessly fascinating; and it is valuable, too, as these studies can lead to discoveries which benefit the whole of humankind. But they do not provide examples of how the average doctor ought to behave. Certain themes run through these highly specialized activities which can distort good clinical practice and which are connected with many of the serious criticisms levelled at the medical profession in general. For example: there is the desire on the part of many of these doctors to be regarded in academic circles as scientists, there is a tendency to think in highly mechanistic terms, and an almost exclusive preoccupation with high technology and expensive medical machines.

The bogey of wanting to be regarded as scientific still haunts many academically-inclined doctors. Despite the immense successes in medical research, there is a feeling of being a poor relation alongside the 'real' scientists, that is, the physicists and the chemists. Of course, when judged by the standards of the physical sciences, clinical medical research can appear sloppy, and so medical investigators work hard to tighten up their methodology in an attempt to enhance their standing in the scientific community.

Experimental psychologists suffered from the same affliction – that is, the need to be seen as authentic scientists – and they had an additional problem, in their view, which was to shake off what they felt was contamination by Freud and his followers. Psychologists therefore retreated into areas where their methodology could be seen to be impeccable. They studied basic processes such as perception and memory, and accumulated valuable basic data; but gradually their insistence on a very strict methodology, often of a kind really only suited to the investigation of inanimate matter, stifled innovation, and in the long run reduced the relevance of certain schools of experimental psychology.[1]

There is no question of medical research drying up, because there will always be a plentiful supply of problems awaiting solution, but academic medicine, like experimental psychology, suffers from the methodological strait-jacket born of trying to imitate the physical scientists. Both academic doctors and experimental psychologists are involved in studying people, and both have frequently disregarded the person for the sake of the parts which happen to interest them. It is often to simplify problems in order to investigate them but there is a limit to over-simplification, and researchers of this kind can find themselves in absurd situations: for example, studying individual organs or bodily systems without reference to the whole person. This might be just what is needed to elucidate some patho-physiological detail, but equally it could be like a chemist studying the interaction of two substances without reference to the environment in which the reaction was occurring.

Academic doctors long to be taken seriously as scientists but they seem unable to avoid elementary traps. A particular trap lies in the notion of what science is. To the thinking world at large, science is a method: it is a particular way of handling information by making observations, creating hypotheses which are then tested and refined, and so on. Too often in medical circles, science is seen as a body of knowledge, so that certain subjects, or parts of subjects, are regarded as 'scientific', while other subjects are not.

People who run courses for doctors or who edit textbooks are aware of this idiosyncratic conception of science, and notices of postgraduate courses will often contain the word 'scientific' in the title to indicate that the subject matter will be substantial and reliable. Similarly there is a series of highly-regarded textbooks, the titles of which might amaze physicists and chemists. We have *The Scientific Basis of Surgery, Scientific Foundations of Obstetrics and Gynaecology, Scientific Foundations of Anaesthesia, Scientific Foundations of Orthopaedics and Traumatology,* even *Introduction to Scientific Psychiatry.* The emphasis in these books is on the basic disciplines underpinning clinical activities, such as the mechanics of lubrication and wear in synovial joints for the orthopaedic surgeons, and analysis of gases and vapours for the anaesthetists. The message is unequivocally reductionist, so much so that the editors of *Scientific Foundations of Oncology* found it necessary to explain what a chapter entitled 'The Challenge of Terminal Care' (by Cicely Saunders) was doing in a 'scientific' textbook.[2] Dame Cicely played the game admirably by including in her chapter graphs, a table, and photographs of patients before and after her interventions, but still her contribution was felt to be slightly anomalous since it concentrated on the whole person and not on the parts.

Doctors are sometimes upset when they feel that they are being criticized in the scientific community for doing merely what they have been taught to do by their teachers at medical school. It is as though they are being blamed for enjoying their jobs, working hard and possessing an abiding fascination with the workings of the human body. Ironically, it is this very fascination with the mechanisms of the body that can get in the way. 'If only', the academic doctors seem to say, 'diseases did not have to involve *people*. Then we could study all these processes without the unpredictable and confusing variable of the patient.' Clinical medicine without patients; that could indeed be an absorbing study.

When doctors talk about science, they are referring to what most people understand as technology. However, they imagine themselves as scientists, with the corollary that it is a good thing to be 'scientific'.

It is very easy for such a doctor to lose sight of the sick person altogether. He may never have been particularly interested in people, and a career in high-technology medicine is much more appealing. He thus enters the chronic conflict between the highly technological and the simple human. On one side are the high-spending departments, such as cardiology, cardiac surgery, those concerned with renal dialysis and transplantation; also all those that operate expensive equipment, such as scanners, fibre-optic instruments, and machines for automated blood counting and chemical analysis. On the other side are the lower-spending, community-orientated specialties such as psychiatry, geriatrics and general practice. The competition for resources is fierce and can lead to acrimonious disputes which further polarize opinions and over-simplify the very difficult issues arising in connection with expensive high-technology medicine.[3,4]

There is nothing wrong with the opportunities offered by high-technology medicine: there is often a great deal wrong with how these opportunities are used. Bryan Jennett sets out some of the misuses under five headings.[5]

Unnecessary, because the results could be achieved by simpler and less costly means; as would apply to the routine use of certain monitoring techniques in obstetrics, or the availability of head scanning by computerized tomography as a routine measure in hospital accident and emergency departments.

Unsuccessful, because the outcome cannot be influenced; as with fruitless attempts at the resuscitation of people who are moribund, and surgery and radiotherapy used more for the benefit of the family and the doctors than of the patient.

Unsafe, because the risks outweigh the likely benefits, as with arteriography of limbs, aorta or cerebral vessels; unless there is a reasonable probability of a lesion being present, which, if found, would be operated upon.

Unkind, because the quality of life is not good enough, or for long enough, to have justified the intervention; for example, after severe head injury.

Unwise, because it diverts resources from activities that would yield greater benefits – the eternal ethical dilemma about the allocation of money and expertise.

In the context of this book, the dangers lie in how the highly technological doctor, with, say, a whole-body scanner at his disposal or a kidney unit under his direction, views the people who come within his orbit. The technical flair which led him into this work in the first place may indicate a reluctance to engage with people. Also, whatever drive he may have towards power and status within the profession can easily be enhanced by having charge of hundreds of thousands of pounds' worth of sophisticated machinery: machines have become one of the newer symbols of worth in modern medicine, rather as a Rolls-Royce was a generation ago.

Losing touch with people's needs

People have fairly basic needs. True, the public has become familiar with medical discoveries and the achievements of high-technology medicine, and this publicity enhances the standing of those who work in these fields, but such developments are unlikely to improve the health of the population in any degree. As Thomas McKeown has shown,[6] the fatal effects of various diseases had begun to fall before the discovery of specific remedies. The decline in mortality from tuberculosis pre-dated the introduction of streptomycin and izoniazid, and the same is true of typhoid before chloramphenicol, and pneumonia before sulphonamides.

Improved housing, education, and above all clean water, have done, and still can do, more for the maintenance and improvement of the health of a population than any amount of medical care; and the more deprived the community the more this applies. If doctors (and drug companies, too, for that matter) really wanted to improve the health of the world they would sink wells, teach people to cultivate crops effectively and give them the resources to do this. When dealing with whole populations, as opposed to individuals, therapeutic medicine is a luxury, if these populations contain large numbers of people who do not have enough to eat, are inadequately housed or are uneducated. This is a simple fact that must be set beside our fascination with expensive high-technology medicine. That these basic priorities are not observed throughout the world is ultimately a political question, not a medical one; but there is no evidence that the medical profession as a whole (or the pharmaceutical industry) has made any effort to initiate fundamental change.

When the National Health Service was established in Britain in 1950, the end of inequalities in health care was in sight. Now, after thirty-five years of the welfare state, with essentially free medical care available to everyone in Britain, with a housing programme, compulsory education up to the age of sixteen with free meals at school where necessary, a system of social benefits designed to avoid the extremes of financial hardship, and no problem anywhere with clean water, how does the population stand?

What emerges from the large-scale review of the health of the population of Britain, known as the Black Report, published in 1980[7], is that while the overall mortality rates have fallen, decade by decade, over the past hundred years, serious inequalities in health still remain between the higher and the lower social classes.

> Most recent data show marked differences in mortality rates between the occupational classes, for both sexes and at all ages. At birth and in the first month of life, twice as many babies of 'unskilled manual' parents (class V) die as do babies of professional class parents (class I), and in the next eleven months four times as many girls and five times as many boys . . . A class gradient can be observed for most causes of death, being particularly steep in the case of diseases of the respiratory system . . . Self-reported rates of long-standing illness are twice as high among unskilled manual males and 2 times as high among their wives as among the professional classes.[8]

Despite an overall fall in infant mortality rates (deaths within the first year of life) in each class, the difference in rate between the highest and lowest group actually increased between 1959–63 and 1970–72. Working class people make more use of general-practitioner services for themselves (though not for their children) than do middle-class people, but they seem to receive inferior care. (They do of course go to their doctors to legitimize absence from work, and to gain access to social benefits, more than middle-class people, who tend to see their GP for more obviously medical matters.)[9] The least advantaged group in society makes the least use of preventive services such as ante-natal clinics, immunization of children, cervical screening and family planning; and a reason for this may be that the cost (bus fares) and effort involved (transporting small children and waiting in clinics) to obtain these services is not felt to be worthwhile.

Although the southern part of Britain (south of a line from the Wash to the Bristol Channel) is healthier than the northern part, the main differences in health are related to social class. These may depend in some degree on variations in life-style and diet, as the low-income groups eat more white bread, sugar and potatoes, and less fruit than the better off; and 'unskilled manual' men and women smoke twice as many cigarettes as the 'professional' classes. More important are the reasons for these variations. Poor education and low income can lead to inadequate nutrition; bad living and working conditions may lead people to smoke more; but despite all the social and economic factors, there is an inequitable distribution of medical resources in Britain today. Tudor Hart's 'inverse care law' applies as ever, that 'the availability of good medical care tends to vary inversely with the need of the population served'.[10]

The medical profession as a whole and doctors individually will tend to explain the inequalities of health in terms of medical resources, which is understandable enough since they are always on the trail of more equipment and better facilities. Doctors can read the Black Report and other studies on the variations of morbidity and mortality around the country,[11,12] yet still fight for a bigger slice of the cake for themselves and their service. They have little choice, in fact, because that is how the system works, and if they do not shout loudly they will get nothing. The individual doctors, practices, or clinical and research departments put in their bids, and the administration then allocates resources according to the overall needs of the district. At least that is how it is supposed to happen, provided the administration in a district or a region is sufficiently strong. In reality, there are angry battles which become ever more bitter on account of government restrictions on spending, and all too often the arguments polarize around technology: cardiac pacemakers will keep productive men in their forties and fifties alive, working, supporting their families and contributing to the general good; while geriatric services, so the argument goes, prolong the lives of unproductive people who are a burden on their families and the community.

These medical brawls reveal the naive attitude of so many specialists towards the broader objectives of medicine, particularly those concerning service to the community. They were brought up with the example of what one might call 'pure' medicine, that is, the study of disease, not only without reference to people, but also disregarding the social context of illness, and the fact that decisions about medical services are ultimately political. I am using the word 'political' here in the broadest sense. The health of a population depends mainly on the quality of housing, the water supply, transportation of food, education, and opportunities for work under reasonable conditions. The decisions which lead to the provision of these prerequisites for health are political, even in the simplest society. The decisions represent choices made by rulers or governments, therefore the political dimension cannot be excluded from any discussion of community health care.

This is an uncongenial idea for many of the leading figures in the medical profession, even though they may be astute politicians in their own field. Temperamentally, they are much more likely to be drawn to highly technological therapeutic medicine than to preventive medicine in the community. The vastly higher status of the super-specialist compared with that of the community physician indicates the material advantages that can come from disengaging oneself from the daily needs of people.

May I say again, there is nothing essentially wrong with high-technology medicine: great advances can be made in the centres of excellence which in time will benefit ordinary people. My objections are that they attract disproportionate prestige and resources, that people who work in them can easily come to see clinical medicine entirely in mechanistic terms, and that sick people can be treated with indifference.

These doctors may be unaware of the needs and aspirations of the society they are employed to serve, but the society is far from unaware of them. The extensive critical writing about the contemporary state of medical practice[6,13-16] poses specific challenges which are all but ignored by the majority of doctors.

Common interest with drug companies

The relationships of doctors with the pharmaceutical industry is ambiguous: they may have different immediate aims, but they share the same population of patients, they both strive to extend their influence, and the political climate which suits the medical profession also suits the drug industry. None of the activities of drug companies can be seen as totally separate from the medical profession, and doctors have to accept a large measure of responsibility for what these companies do. Doctors cannot stand back and condemn these companies, for there is no sense in which the medical profession is 'above' commerce; and there are scarcely any doctors who do not enjoy material benefits from the drug industry, in the form of meals, subsidized conferences, samples or outright gifts of various kinds. It is important, therefore, that doctors have a clear view of these companies which help them in so many ways and facilitate their work.

The drug companies are almost all aggressive organizations which have gained for themselves a formidable position in world commerce, and they can lay just claim to being the best (or the worst) examples of international capitalism in action. They have greater assets than many of the countries with which they do business, and they are so pervasive that almost any change in a country's or the world's fortunes is likely to benefit them in some way.

Drug companies do good by developing drugs of undoubted benefit.[17,18] They do harm by the way they promote certain of their products across the world, and appear to conceal the incidence of unwanted effects.[19-27] The sequence of scandals concerning the harmful effects of drugs began, in modern times, in 1937, with the deaths of over one hundred people who had taken a novel preparation of sulphanilamide which a Tennessee drug company had devised. It led to the setting up of the Federal Drugs Administration in the United States.

The list of drugs with harmful side-effects has continued, notable examples being chloramphenicol, steroids, clioquinol, and of course thalidomide. Thalidomide, more than any other drug tragedy, alerted the public to what can happen in the pharmaceutical world; but dangerous side-effects continue to occur from new drugs, as in the case of the non-steroidal anti-inflammatory drug benoxaprofen ('Opren').[28] These are powerful substances, and unwanted effects are inevitable. Too often the companies concerned have gone to great lengths to conceal the dangers, only making a full disclosure when forced to do so by a court of inquiry.

The practices of the multinational drug companies have been extensively documented,[21-27] and the charges have never been seriously challenged. For example, drug companies in Tanzania spend on drug promotion a sum greater than that spent by the Faculty of Medicine in that country to train its doctors in every branch of medical activity, including the use of drugs. In Tanzania, it is estimated that there is one drug-company representative for every four doctors; while in Nepal, Brazil, Guatemala and Mexico the ratio is closer to one representative for every three doctors.[26]

In Britain, where the ratio is about one representative to every eighteen doctors, and in the United States where it is about one to ten doctors, these people take up a disproportionate amount of many doctors' time. In the Third World, this intrusion is more serious, and it represents a significant loss in medical manpower because many of the representatives could themselves be doing useful work in the health field, since they often have medical skills. In fact, Dianna Melrose cites an example from North Yemen where an official in the government agency controlling drug marketing would supplement his income in the afternoons by acting as a representative for a number of leading drug manufacturers.[29]

The drug companies are such powerful multinational organizations that they could ruin the economies of many of the countries they are purporting to serve. On the other hand, they are in a position to give valuable aid, if they are allowed to market their goods as they choose. Sales promotion occurs on a level unknown in the West, and potent drugs are often sold directly to the public. This applies to drugs which may have been banned from sale in the Western world because of well-established harmful reactions: for example, clioquinol ('Entero-vioform' from Ciba-Geigy) against diarrhoea, anabolic steroids such as Orabolin (made by Organon) and Anapolon (ICI) sold for promoting growth in malnourished children, and amidopyrine (Ciba-Geigy) sold as a painkiller.

A survey was conducted on the promotion of twenty-eight prescription drugs (in the form of forty different products) which were marketed in the United States and Latin America by twenty-three multinational pharmaceutical companies. In the United States the indications listed for the drugs were generally few, and the warnings about contraindications and adverse reactions were detailed and extensive. In the Latin American countries, by contrast, numerous indications were given, and the risks minimized, if not totally ignored. For example, in the United States chloramphenicol was promoted for such serious infections as typhoid, Rocky Mountain spotted fever, *Hemophilus influenzae*, and a few other life-threatening conditions in which the causative organism could be shown to be susceptible to the drug. In Mexico, Ecuador and Colombia, the branded version – Chloromycetin – was promoted, not only for the life-threatening conditions, but also for tonsillitis, pharyngitis, bronchitis, urinary tract infections, ulcerative colitis, pneumonia, staphylococcus infections, streptococcus infections, eye infections, yaws and gonorrhoea.[26]

In many countries little is done by the medical profession to check obvious abuses; and even if the doctors did want to improve things, they would be hampered by the special agreements between the drug companies and the host governments. However, experience in the West has shown that these companies can be controlled without affecting the quality of treatment in any way; and some developing countries with socially committed governments are beginning to impose restrictions on the range and pricing of drugs,[30] the most successful being Sri Lanka and Mozambique. After independence in 1975, Mozambique reduced the number of branded drugs from 13,000 to 2,600, and the official formulary drugs from 1,100 to 380, with the proviso that only these (using generic not branded names) could be prescribed routinely.[31] The government of Mozambique is left-wing, and it is a sad fact that simple proposals to rationalize medical care so often conflict with the private interests of the medical profession.

A modest reduction in the range of prescribable drugs was proposed by the Department of Health in Britain in early 1985, and it provoked an entirely predictable response. The medical profession's objection was presented in terms of erosion of clinical freedom, on the assumption that each doctor is uniquely well-informed about which of the many thousands of drugs is most precisely suited to his patient's needs. Needless to say, the pharmaceutical industry objected also. The medical profession's objection has a good deal to do with its preoccupation with authority and control; and the right to prescribe any drug in the pharmacopoeia is one of the few absolute rights which doctors retain in what they see as a society increasingly dominated by state interference. Indeed, this clinical freedom to prescribe any drug at all may be a kind of compensation for the reduced economic circumstances of doctors in the British National Health Service.

A survey of general practitioners' prescribing habits published in 1976 showed that the main source of 'therapeutic knowledge', including side effects and contraindications, and of information sought during a consultation, was the publication called *MIMS* (Monthly Index of Medical Specialties), which is produced by the pharmaceutical industry. The next most popular source was the official British National Formulary. The majority of GPs learned of the *existence* of new drugs from the drug-company representatives, although they mostly looked to professional sources for information about a drug's *usefulness*.[32] Such information can be communicated by acknowledged experts at postgraduate study days, and these events are virtually always subsidized by the drug industry.

Postgraduate medical education in Britain is to a great extent financed by the drug industry,[33] and the representative's stall is accepted by most organizers of postgraduate events and conferences. The Royal Colleges receive handsome gifts from pharmaceutical companies and other companies that do business with the medical profession. In fact the Royal College of General Practitioners really only came into being through substantial cash payments from various drug companies. A company donated the presidential gold chain and pendant, and another presented some of its own shares to create an income for the College.[34,35] All the newer Royal Colleges have a heavy debt to the pharmaceutical industry, and the older ones, which are already wealthy, will allow the industry to help with renovation and expansion.

Many of the most important medical journals could not survive without the advertising of drugs, at least it is assumed that they could not. In the same way it is assumed in some countries, though not in others, that sport could not survive without sponsorship from the tobacco companies. The penetration of the drug companies into most aspects of medical professional life is much greater than that of the tobacco companies into the ordinary life of the country. Members of the public and politicians are unaware of the extent to which, in Professor Rawlins' words, 'we [doctors] accept (or even demand) rewards on a breathtaking scale'.[33]

8

Prejudices and Irrational Practice

Doctors are taught to take detailed histories from their patients, to make careful clinical observations, and then to supplement these by means of special investigations. The assembled data are scrutinized by the doctor, and by a process of induction the diagnosis is made. In practice, doctors are more likely to proceed by the hypothetico–deductive method in which a guess (or hypothesis) is made at an early stage about the likely diagnosis or diagnostic category. This guess is made from the pattern of presenting features combined with the observer's experience. The initial hypothesis is then tested by subsequent observations and investigations, and refined accordingly.

This is the intelligent and rational method by which doctors are supposed to reach their conclusions about patients, and most of the time that is how they work. There are other times when the doctor is fatigued from long hours of duty or is preoccupied about personal problems, and is not in a state to make any kind of subtle judgement.

There are yet other times when individual doctors, or even the medical profession as a whole, make decisions or hold opinions which, with hindsight at any rate, are clearly irrational. The decisions may have been quite logical; the danger lies in the initial speculative theories or false premises which led to them. For centuries innocent people, cast in the role of patient, have been tormented by treatments derived from false assumptions.

The masturbation story

Nothing better exemplifies the perverse power of the medical profession than the century and a half when the anxiety about masturbation prevailed in Europe.[1,2]

In about 1710, a man, thought to have been a clergyman turned quack, published anonymously a short book entitled, *Onania, or the Heinous Sin*

112

of Self-Pollution and All its Frightful Consequences in both sexes . . .[3] The
opening sentences give an idea of the author's viewpoint.

> Self-pollution is that unnatural Practice by which Persons, of either
> Sex, may defile their own Bodies without the Assistance of others,
> whilst yielding to filthy Imaginations they endeavour to imitate, and
> procure to themselves, that Sensation which God has ordered to attend
> the carnal Commerce of the two Sexes, for the Continuance of our
> Species.
>   It is almost impossible to treat of this Subject so as to be understood
> by the meanest Capacities, without trespassing, at the same Time,
> against the Rules of Decency, and making Use of Words and
> Expressions which Modesty forbids us to utter. But, as my great Aim
> is to promote Virtue and Christian Virtue, and to discourage Vice and
> Uncleanness, without giving Offence to any, I shall chuse rather to be
> less intelligible to some, and leave several Things to the Consideration
> of my Readers than by being too plain run Hazard of raising, in some
> corrupt Minds, what I would most endeavour to stifle and destroy.

The author appears to have had a lofty motive in drawing attention to
the supposed evils of this practice, although we may think again when we
discover that at the end of the book he advertises remedies for it. There
is 'The Prolifick Powder' and 'Strengthening Tincture', and these could
be purchased from Mr T. Crouch, who happened to be the publisher of
Onania.

The term 'onanism' was used by this author – who had a good ear for a
menacing name – as synonymous with masturbation; and it was based on
the probably erroneous assumption that this was the sin of Onan.[4]

These alarmist ideas had no widespread influence until they were taken
up by a Swiss professor of medicine, Samuel Auguste André David
Tissot (1728–97), with the publication in Lausanne in 1758 of a work he
wrote in Latin initially for reasons of modesty, but which, six years later,
he translated into French. In 1766 an English translation appeared under
the title of *Onanism: or, A Treatise upon the Disorders produced by Masturbation:
or, the Dangerous Effects of Secret and Excessive Venery*.[5] Much of the book is
devoted to descriptions of the terrible consequences of the habit.

> L. D—— was by profession a watchmaker; he had lived prudently, and
> had enjoyed a good state of health, till he was about seventeen years
> of age; at this period he gave himself up to masturbation, which he
> repeated every day, sometimes even to the third time . . . [Tissot then
> relates the history of the lad's affliction.]

113

I heard of his situation, and went to him; I found a being that less resembled a living creature, than a corpse, lying upon straw, meagre, pale, and filthy, casting forth an infectious stench; almost incapable of motion, a watry palish blood issued from his nose; slaver constantly flowed from his mouth: having a diarrhaea, he voided his excrement in the bed without knowing it: he had a continual flux of semen; his sore watry eyes were deadened to that degree, that he could not move them: his pulse was very small, quick, and frequent: it was with great difficulty he breathed, reduced almost to a skeleton, in every part except his feet, which became oedematous. The disorder of his mind was equal to that of his body; devoid of ideas and memory, incapable of connecting two sentences, without reflection, without any other sensation than pain . . .

He died at the end of a few weeks, in June 1757, his whole body having become dropsical.[6]

The victim here was clearly seriously ill, and the fact that he also masturbated seems to have blinded Tissot to the possibility of other explanations for his condition. The author of this extravagant clinical description was to become a most influential figure in European medicine and a Fellow of the Royal Society, and Tissot's book went through thirty editions before the end of the eighteenth century. Masturbation, hitherto a private sexual activity, had now become a matter of interest to doctors. Tissot had given the medical profession the gift of a totally non-existent disorder which, as soon as it was offered, was accepted uncritically; and the assumptions behind it would not be challenged effectively for the next hundred years. Doctors found themselves as agents for finding a target, not only for their own prejudices and unconscious anxieties, but for the sexual and other anxieties of society at large.

Tissot claimed that all sexual activity was dangerous, masturbation especially so as it could be practised in private so that excess was inevitable. Its dangerous effects were produced by a rush of blood to the brain which starved the nerves, rendering them more susceptible to damage and hence to general debility, melancholy, deterioration of eyesight, disorders of digestion, fits, impotence, dementia, paralysis and *tabes dorsalis*. Tissot formulated his ideas almost in the framework of Graeco-Roman medicine with semen regarded as a kind of vital spirit which flowed in a direct anatomical line between the brain, the spinal cord and the genitalia.[7] Semen for Tissot was 'the essential oil of the animal liquors . . . It is true that we are ignorant whether the animal[8] spirits and the genital liquor are the same thing; but observation teaches us . . . that these two fluids have a very strict analogy, and that the loss of one or the other produces the same ills.'[9]

Sexual intercourse, Tissot believed, involved a two-way flow of invisible substances, and so there was some replenishment not possible with masturbation. Thus the notion of loss of 'vital force' gave an almost archetypal power to Tissot's ideas, and this must be one reason why they held sway for so long. Spermatorrhoea, that is seminal loss other than during intercourse, was another supposed condition which engaged the energies of certain medical writers in the eighteenth century. It was 'clinically' and symbolically similar to masturbation, and was alleged to produce similar harmful effects.[10]

Masturbation caught the imagination of eminent physicians in Europe and America to a greater degree than any other irrational idea has ever done. They began to see around them the pitiful victims of the practice. A few independently minded men, such as John Hunter (1728–93), tried to introduce some reason into the frenzy but they were disregarded in the prevailing suspension of all critical evaluation. None of the protagonists stopped to ask whether the alleged ill-effects of masturbation – which comprised almost the entire range of medical symptomatology – might be the cause or the effect, or whether healthy people engaged in the practice, or why these harmful effects had only just come to light.

In 1812, Benjamin Rush (1745–1813), Professor of the Institutes of Medicine at Philadelphia, wrote in the first American textbook of psychiatry that onanism 'produces seminal weakness, impotence, dysury, *tabes dorsalis*, pulmonary consumption, dyspepsia, dimness of sight, vertigo, epilepsy, hypochondriasis, loss of memory, manalgia, fatuity and death'.[11] It was generally becoming accepted that masturbation caused epilepsy, 'fatuity' and dementia; and in 1863, a Scottish physician, David Skae, took the profession's preoccupation a great step further when he described, in a paper entitled 'A rational and practical classification of insanity', the condition of 'mania of masturbation'. Of his new clinical syndrome, he wrote:

> it cannot be denied that the vice produces a group of symptoms which are quite characteristic, and easily recognised, and give to the case a special natural history. The peculiar imbecility and shy habits of the very youthful victim, the suspicion, and fear, and dread, and suicidal impulses, and palpitations, and scared look, and feeble body of the older offenders, passing gradually into dementia or fatuity, with other characteristic features familiar to all.[12]

Women also, it was found, could fall victim to the habit of masturbation, and appliances were devised (for both sexes) to prevent the sufferers from handling their genitalia.[2] For more intractable cases, clitorectomy was carried out. A 'treatment' for men consisted of inserting a wire through the foreskin; and both sexes could be subjected to cauterization of the spine or genitalia. Later on, potassium bromide would be administered with its sedative effect on all function.

Two outstanding medical men of the nineteenth century fell under the spell of masturbation: they were Henry Maudsley (1835–1918), a distinguished early psychiatrist, after whom the Institute of Psychiatry in the University of London is named; and Sir Jonathan Hutchinson (1828–1913), a Fellow of the Royal Society and a President of the Royal College of Surgeons. They both made important contributions, respectively to psychiatry and surgery, for which they are still held in high regard.

In the course of an address to the Harverian Society of London, Henry Maudsley calmly discussed various types of insanity. When he came to disorders associated with self-abuse, which was the main topic of his address, his whole tone changed. He said 'the miserable sinner whose mind suffers by reason of self-abuse becomes offensively egotistic', and he continued over nine pages of the printed text, in emotive and extravagant language, with no attempt to separate clinical description from moral judgement.

We have degenerate beings produced . . . cunning, deceitful, liars, selfish, in fact, morally insane; while their physical and intellectual vigour is further damaged by the exhausting vice. [This leads on, Maudsley says, to] days of deep gloom, depression and wretchedness . . . in which he is a very pitiable object.

A later and still worse stage at which these degenerate beings arrive is one of moody and morose self-absorption, and extreme loss of mental power . . . It is needless to say that they have lost all healthy human feeling and every natural desire. The body is usually much emaciated, notwithstanding they eat well; and though they often last for a longer period than might be thought possible, they finally totter on to death through a complete prostration of the entire system, if they are not carried off by some intercurrent disease.

I have no faith in the employment of physical means to check what has become a serious mental disease; the sooner he sinks to his degraded rest the better for himself, and the better for the world which is well rid of him.[13]

In fairness to Maudsley, he did modify his moral censure in later writings, but for an appreciable time he was caught by the emotional implications of masturbation, and was quite unaware that in this area his judgement was impaired; while on other topics his commonsense and humane approach to mental disorder was quite admirable.

Sir Jonathan Hutchinson was an erudite and versatile surgeon in the very best traditions of the nineteenth century, and was a prolific recorder of what he saw and did. His memorandum 'On circumcision as preventive of masturbation' was prompted by a letter he had had from a fellow surgeon who for seven years past had been a patient in the 'refractory gallery' of a lunatic asylum. The surgeon concerned described himself as a 'confirmed masturbator' and sought Hutchinson's advice about circumcision as a possible remedy. Hutchinson did attempt to apply some reason to the matter, and cited the work of a late colleague who had sought to discover whether 'that habit' was less prevalent among Jews, but 'the distasteful nature of the inquiry' caused his colleague to abandon it. However, Hutchinson believed that circumcision might be beneficial, and

> I may indeed go further than this and avow my conviction that measures more radical than circumcision would, if public opinion permitted their adoption, be a true kindness to many patients of both sexes . . . I trust it will not be supposed from what I have written above that I believe that the removal of the testes or ovaries will either completely or in all cases subdue the sexual passion. All that I contend for is that such operations are often and in most persons conducive to that end.[14]

Medical students used frequently to be advised to read *Rest and Pain* by John Hilton, Fellow of the Royal Society and Fellow of the Royal College of Surgeons. Those who followed the advice would have encountered this passage:

> Surgeons are often consulted regarding onanism and its treatment, and it is a very important matter. It is a habit very difficult to contend with in practice. I know of no way to prevent onanism except by freely blistering the penis, in order to make it raw and so sore that it cannot be touched without pain. This plan of treatment is sure to cure onanism. I have adopted it during more than twenty years. Gentlemen have come to me and said, 'I have for many years suffered from this abominable, disgusting habit, and I have tried to cure myself of it, but I cannot; for my morbid inclination overcomes my disgust when awake, and when asleep I think I am sometimes pursuing it. Can you offer any suggestions?' I have said, 'Paint this strong solution of iodine over the whole of the skin of the penis every night; and if that does not make the

117

organ too sore to you to touch it, then apply in the same way a strong blistering fluid to the penis.' The result in practice of my experience has been that in almost every instance the continuance of the habit has thus been entirely prevented.[15]

This treatment might seem rather extreme, even for 1863, when Hilton's lectures were first published. What is more extraordinary is that this passage remains intact and without comment in the sixth edition of this classic work, published in 1950, and edited by a professor of anatomy and a president of the Royal College of Surgeons; even though these (and perhaps previous) editors had corrected Hilton on fine points of general topographical anatomy.[16].

Before Tissot, there was practically no medical writing about masturbation. After him there was a vast amount and practically all of it moralistic, with none of the intellectual rigour which would be found in the eighteenth and nineteenth centuries in other fields of inquiry.

Masturbation began to lose its grip on the medical imagination in the last fifteen years or so of the nineteenth century. More and more medical critics appeared who questioned the notion of masturbatory insanity; real evidence was never forthcoming about its dangerous effects, and the moral intensity of the protagonists began to decline. Around the same time, Charcot and Janet were proclaiming the importance of the neuroses; and then came Freud who at last provided a way of thinking psychologically, as opposed to morally, about the habit of masturbation. Even so it was many decades before the widespread guilt connected with the practice subsided. Over the same period, people began to marry younger and so perhaps there was less need for this outlet.

Doctors need to reflect that their colleagues of previous ages were not obviously cranks and misfits, quite the opposite in fact, as the ideas about the harmful effects of masturbation represented the generally accepted medical opinion for well over a century.

It may seem ludicrous today, but these prejudices and irrational attitudes were tragically real for those who had to suffer them and were made to feel guilty on their account. Have doctors learned any lessons from the misdeeds of their professional forebears? Is medical practice more rationally grounded in the twentieth century?

Further medical enthusiasms

As masturbation was gradually ceasing to generate such anxiety in doctors and educators, certain watchful authorities were turning their attention to the dangers of tea and coffee drinking.

The Regius Professor of Physic at Cambridge along with the most distinguished pharmacologist of the time described in a standard medical textbook the effects of excessive coffee consumption: 'the sufferer is tremulous and loses his self-command; he is subject to fits of agitation and depression. He has a haggard appearance.' Tea was no better: 'producing nightmares with . . . hallucinations which may be alarming in their intensity . . . Another peculiar quality of tea is to produce a strange and extreme degree of physical depression. An hour or two after breakfast at which tea has been taken . . . a grievous sinking . . . may seize upon the sufferer, so that to speak is an effort . . . The speech may become weak and vague . . . By miseries such as these, the best years of life may be spoiled.'[17]

This passage would have served quite well as a description of the evil consequences of masturbation. It was cited actually in a British government inquiry (the Wootton Report)[17] into the use of cannabis to make the point discreetly that public attitudes can change. Around the time this textbook was being written, cannabis was in the pharmacopoeia, and Weir Mitchell[18] and Havelock Ellis[19] were writing in the medical press about the benefits of mescaline. The Wootton Report appeared in 1968 when anxiety about the dangers of cannabis was at its height. No evidence was available at the time about harmful effects from its use but the judiciary would use emotive language when passing sentence on users of the drug. Many members of the medical profession also were convinced of the dangers of cannabis, and some ventured into print with more conviction than evidence to support them.[20]

To return now to more medical issues, there have been quite long-running examples in the twentieth century of emotion and fashion displacing reason in dispensing medical advice.

Circumcision. Virtually all societies circumcise their male children except the Indo-Germanic, Mongol, and Finno-Ugric-speaking peoples, but in the twentieth century it has been widely used by people with no traditional or ritualistic connection with the practice.[21-23]

In Britain, the United States and Australia, it was for a long time almost the norm. In the 1960s, Masters and Johnson found that only 35 out of 312 male volunteers for their studies of sexual behaviour had not been circumcised (and only 16 of the 231 aged between twenty-one and forty), the rest having been operated on 'routinely'. One of the reasons for this 'routine', say Masters and Johnson, was the 'phallic fantasy' that uncircumcised men have greater control over ejaculation, which presumably was regarded as a bad thing. However, Masters and Johnson tested this assumption and found it to be fallacious.[24] Some years earlier, in a sample of university students in England, 84 per cent of boys coming from independent schools and 50 per cent from state schools had been circumcised,[22] although this class difference was not apparent in the United States.[25]

Of course, medical reasons were given for the operation in terms of hygiene, difficulty in retracting the foreskin (it is now recognized that it frequently cannot be retracted before the third year) and the prevention of penile carcinoma (which is not now regarded as an indication, while the mortality from penile carcinoma is about the same as that from the operation of circumcision).[23] Critical evaluation of the procedure seems to have been lacking until Douglas Gairdner's paper in 1949.[22] It is almost as though there had been collusion on the part of the medical profession in a strange social practice, possibly initiated by mothers (some say as an act of retaliation against the male sex) and, for economic reasons, not resisted by surgeons. The practice increased in popularity until, in 1965, Dr Benjamin Spock could write in a book which has sold over sixteen million copies: 'I think circumcision is a good idea, especially if most boys in the neighborhood are circumcised – then a boy feels "regular".'[26]

Focal sepsis. The diagnosis of focal sepsis was used in the earlier years of the twentieth century as an explanation for pains in various sites, failure to thrive, arthritis, serious mental disorder and a variety of minor psychological disturbances. The idea was that the septic focus discharged toxins into the system and these caused the symptoms. The gall bladder, appendix, teeth, tonsils and adenoids could all become the seats of infection, throwing off the toxins, whether or not there were any symptoms directly referable to these organs. Any abdominal discomfort could throw suspicion on the gall bladder or appendix, any symptoms around the face, head or neck could incriminate the tonsils and adenoids. These structures could be removed in a more or less speculative way, hoping that the non-specific symptoms would be relieved. If the symptoms persisted, the next most likely organ could go, and so on. Thus, tonsils and teeth were sacrificed by those with psychological troubles or nebulous chronic physical symptoms. After any surgery, especially within the abdomen, later symptoms may be a complication of the initial operation, so a 'genuine' complaint could develop from what had, in the first instance, been a doubtful one.

The idea of focal sepsis is reasonable a priori; the real question, however, is whether or not it is true. With a mechanistic view of a human being it is easy to make the false assumption that if an abnormality is present, it must be the cause of any symptoms in the vicinity. If the patient has upper abdominal pain and there are gall stones on X-ray, then the stones are assumed to be the cause of the pain. This is perfectly reasonable until studies are done on the prevalence of gall stones, when the causal connection becomes more tenuous.[27] Here we have the logic of masturbatory insanity once more: the patient is undoubtedly sick, the patient is observed to masturbate (healthy people do it in private), masturbation is 'known' to produce disease, therefore masturbation is the cause of the patient's sickness. So much always depends on the untested assumptions of the doctor.

With tonsils, the apparent causal connection is more obvious, as the child is feverish and the tonsils can be seen to be inflamed and enlarged. Despite this, the decisions to operate seem to be more erratic than for any other surgical procedure;[28,29] and differential rates are reported for tonsillectomy in various parts of Britain,[30,31] even though the rate, overall, is dropping.

Sometimes the presence of one of these supposedly pathological conditions can lead to an increased likelihood of another of them being diagnosed. For example, in Newcastle upon Tyne, among boys under the age of four, 15 per cent of circumcised boys had had their tonsils removed, while only 2 per cent of the uncircumcised boys had, a difference of a factor of seven.[32] In a Canadian study, twice as many children who had had appendicectomy had had their tonsils removed (before or after appendicectomy) compared with those who had not had appendicectomy.[33]

Focal sepsis was an example of a mistaken theory being applied in an uncritical way – 'acted out' might be a better description. Recent medical history abounds with examples, and Alex Comfort has described many of these in his entertaining yet horrifying book *The Anxiety Makers*.[2]

One of the most spectacular examples of irrational clinical thinking is provided by Sir Arbuthnot Lane (1856–1943), who was unquestionably one of the great surgeons of his day. He was a pioneer of aseptic surgery, who developed the open fixation of fractures by plate and screws, and laid the foundations of operative orthopaedics as we know it today. However, he fell victim to the mistaken theory of alimentary stasis and toxaemia, and used it to explain all kinds of symptoms referable to the abdomen and, indeed, to the rest of the body. In Lane's words, from a paper delivered in 1913, 'The causation of stasis and consequent infection of the gastrointestinal contents are due to improper feeding in early life and to upright posture.'[34] Lane's biographer stated that Lane 'alleged that this resulted in peritoneal bands [developing] to counteract the tendency to downward displacement of the viscera'.

These bands were supposed to produce kinks at various points and thus stasis with inflammation, ulceration, or cancer. Lane claimed that stasis, largely by facilitating infection of the upper alimentary tract, was the cause of duodenal ulcer, cardio-spasm, pancreatitis, carcinoma of the pancreas, gall-stones, and cholangitis. In addition, as the result of the absorption of intestinal toxins, the following conditions arose: – degeneration of the heart, arteries, kidneys, and muscle; retroversion of the uterus, cystic degeneration of the breasts, *carcinoma mammae*, goitre – high or low blood pressure, and mental disturbances.[35]

This is a formidable list of complaints to ascribe to a single cause, and worthy of any quack dominated by an idea offering an explanation for so many human ills. Lane, however, saw himself as entirely rational: and of course he was, except for his initial false premise concerning the noxious effects of the imaginary condition – alimentary toxaemia. Excising the cause of serious illness was, and still is, reasonable treatment; and colectomy performed by a technical master such as Sir Arbuthnot Lane seems to have been tolerated quite well by his patients.

Another theory evolved to explain a variety of symptoms referable to the abdomen and back was based on the notion that organs can slip out of place and cause trouble. Hence we have retroversion of the uterus causing backache; and dropping down of the kidney(s) or stomach, known respectively as nephroptosis and gastroptosis. These alleged conditions were then dealt with by various operations to return the organs to their proper locations.[36]

As time goes on and stricter controls are imposed on researchers and those promoting novel treatments, and as patients become more critical and articulate, the likelihood of irrational treatments being perpetrated should decline. But has it really? Medical practice is more public, and the media are waiting to publicize any advance, however insubstantial, so it is less likely that an individual doctor or a group of doctors, within orthodox medicine, could persist long with any idiosyncratic and ineffective line of management. What we now have is public debate, and that can have the effect of leaving everybody – the profession and the public – rather bewildered.

Some dismay was experienced when H. G. Mather and his colleagues, as the result of a carefully planned survey in the south-west of England, found that, under certain circumstances, heart attacks were better treated at home than in hospital.[37-39] The claim was modest, the 'certain circumstances', such as normal cardiac rhythm, being all-important; yet it unleashed a storm because someone was suggesting that the coronary-care units, then coming into fashion, might not be automatically the best place for everyone suffering a heart attack. The ensuing row led to an over-simplifying polarization of opinion for and against technology,[37] and in particular it touched that forbidden topic among medical specialists – that hospital is not necessarily always best. A. L. Cochrane[40] relates an instance during this debate, when someone showed a coronary care unit enthusiast Mather's results, but with the figures reversed, so that it appeared that the mortality in the coronary care unit was lower than with home treatment. The enthusiast immediately declared that such a clinical trial was unethical and should be stopped at once. When he was shown the figures the correct way round he could not be persuaded that coronary care units under certain circumstances might be unjustified.

Cochrane gives a number of examples of treatments which were promoted with great enthusiasm. He cites the case of insulin, glucose and potassium in the treatment of ischaemic heart disease, and the statement by 'a member of the medical establishment that the evidence was so good that a randomized controlled trial would be unethical'.[41] A randomized controlled trial was carried out and the treatment has been dropped.

Controlled trials will eventually eliminate methods of treatment which have no rational basis, or at least do not have the rational basis claimed for them. For example, insulin comas were given as a routine treatment for schizophrenia for over twenty years before the basic assumption that a period of coma could somehow help the condition was ever put to the test. When a proper controlled trial was conducted,[42] the insulin coma was shown to have played no part in whatever improvement there was in the patient's condition, and this form of treatment gradually fell into disuse.

It might seem that with the widespread use of randomized controlled trials, as advocated by Cochrane,[43] the irrational element might disappear from clinical practice. This is a comforting thought but it would be dangerous to assume that human behaviour could ever become entirely rational.

Doctors' assumptions and beliefs

It is not possible simply to 'observe'. If a class of students was told to 'observe', and to write down what they had observed, they would have no idea where to begin, because before any observation is possible there must be certain assumptions about what is to be looked for; and also certain restrictions, because the amount of information in any scene is for practical purposes infinite.[44] Doctors, for example, make the assumption that the person they have been called to see may be ill; and, if they have been trained in orthodox medicine, they will further assume that illness may manifest itself by certain phenomena, called symptoms and signs, which indicate dysfunction in particular organs or systems within the body. Our theoretical framework determines the interpretation of what we see, and, in effect, what we see or do not see.

In addition to the effects of fatigue and anxiety on a doctor's perception and judgement,[45] there is a more subtle danger from the doctor's own prejudices. It can manifest itself in stereotyped thinking.

For example, if a girl goes to see her doctor, wearing a current garb of youthful protest – with dramatic make-up and hair-style, and a taciturn and slightly sullen manner – the prejudiced doctor is liable to make various assumptions about the girl, on sight and before listening to her. He may assume she uses drugs, is promiscuous, dishonest, lazy, and does not wash. He is generalizing from a few observations (about manner and appearance) and has made up his mind before he has got to know the person: a characteristic of stereotyped thinking. If the same girl turns out to be pregnant, the prejudiced doctor may lecture her on her moral turpitude and possibly try to 'teach her a lesson' by refusing her request for a termination of pregnancy.

This is an example, sadly not an uncommon one, to illustrate how a doctor's prejudices can distort proper medical judgement. Such stereotyped thinking (or reacting) is associated with the authoritarian style because it exemplifies the insider, who upholds the values of society, confronting the outsider, who challenges them. There is a clash of values, and the outsider is seen as a threat. Therefore, a well-meaning patient can be perceived by the doctor, on the basis of some misleading feature, as a threat to his authority and security. Such a patient can expect to be rejected.

Like the judiciary, doctors have an incorrigible habit of embellishing their observations with what are, in effect, moral judgements. Both uphold the conventional values of society, and both know that they will nearly always have the last word.

The examples in this chapter have been drawn from the main stream of orthodox medicine. In the case of masturbation, circumcision and tonsillectomy, I have related simply what was current medical practice over most of Europe or the English-speaking world at certain times. The individuals mentioned were men justly famous and influential in their day, yet whose rational judgement was at times clouded by emotion.

Doctors nowadays are trained to scrutinize data, to use statistical analysis, and to make a critical evaluation of all clinical information. This kind of intellectual superstructure can dazzle the public into believing that they are not vulnerable to prejudice, or into forgetting that their decisions may sometimes be imperfect. Doctors neglect the irrational element in themselves at their patients' peril.

9

Doctors as Agents of Social Control

There are times when doctors act on behalf of the state, either as formal agents or through their ability to influence social practices.

A great many medical decisions have political implications. A prescription for tranquillizing drugs can be seen as a means of suppressing a citizen's distress and dissatisfaction with an unjust social system; and a doctor who prescribes such drugs is, consciously or otherwise, promoting that system. Marxist critics of the medical profession regard doctors as inextricably bound up with the capitalist machine, keeping the public under control and clamouring for more and more expensive treatments which make fortunes for those who manufacture the drugs and medical equipment but do not meet the real needs of ordinary people.[1,2]

While most doctors will reject a Marxist view, they have to acknowledge the authoritarian streak in many of them which makes it easy for them to line up on the side of the state. The exact relationship varies, and its different aspects will be discussed in this chapter.

Doctors are in a position to influence all aspects of reproduction, and very occasionally to advise people to undergo brain operations which may permanently alter their mental state. Here the doctors are acting as independent professionals but their decisions have important social implications.

At other times doctors can act in a more formal capacity, such as when committing people against their will to psychiatric units, or in employment as a prison medical officer. Doctors in such work have to accept that they are carrying out the policies of a government, although it is possible for them to maintain their standards of professional ethics. Their position is more compromised if they work on defence contracts, and, most of all, if they become involved in the arrangements for torture of people under interrogation.

Women, sex and reproduction

Social control by doctors has been most conspicuous and effective with regard to women since they are the principal users of medical services. Most doctors are men, and the women are mainly seeking help in connection with sex and childbearing, so there is the added issue of male dominance of feminine activities. It is hard to say, therefore, which is the major force: male domination of women, or the medical profession's control of the business of reproduction. Whichever it is, any group that manages to control the process of reproduction in a society is in a very strong position indeed. With 98 per cent of births in 1977 in England and Wales taking place in hospital, the medical profession can claim almost total domination.[3]

The orthodox medical line in relation to women's needs is paternalistic in the extreme with the implication that the woman's primary function is to bear children and look after her man. This was demonstrated by two women who studied twenty-eight American textbooks of gynaecology to see if they had incorporated any of the findings of Kinsey and of Masters and Johnson concerning sexual behaviour. The textbooks virtually ignored these important contributions, and at the same time revealed fantasies about feminine sexuality which suggested that their authors had never allowed women to express their points of view, or to discuss their needs or aspirations.[4]

The medical control of reproduction was achieved by the same kinds of strategy that the profession has used down the years to deal with outside practitioners of any kind; and the case of the midwives provides an example of how the profession deals with its presumed rivals. Over the past century dentists, nurses, pharmacists and opticians have acquired the right to organize their own affairs, but the midwives – who are perceived as more direct competitors – have not. In Britain they are still precluded from holding a majority of seats on their controlling body, the Central Midwives Board; and the first midwife to be chairman of that board was only appointed in 1973.[5]

Currently, the battle for control of childbearing is focused on the issue of home versus hospital confinements. In Britain in 1980, the Peel Committee[6] advised 100 per cent hospital deliveries on grounds of safety for the mother and child, and so there was a running down of domiciliary midwifery services and the development of new maternity units.[3] Perinatal mortality rates were falling and the percentage of women having their babies in hospital was increasing, so the statistical association was assumed by the protagonists of hospital confinement to be causal, despite the fact that in the Netherlands, with a very low perinatal mortality rate, the majority of the babies were born out of hospital.

Practice is changing, however, as a result of pressure from women's groups; and innovators such as Frederick Leboyer and Michel Odent have made women aware that various methods of delivery are possible. The battle is likely to continue for some time, as fundamental issues of control are involved. If women are allowed to choose where they want to have their babies, to have the people around them they want, to select a posture which suits them, whether or not to have drugs, to have the labour induced surgically, or to try a normal labour even though there is a strong likelihood of eventual caesarean section; then the value of large maternity units may be called into question, and resources diverted towards the community.

All matters relating to sexuality and reproduction resonate with the doctor's own attitudes, so that in addition to medical paternalism, patients have to contend with the doctor's moral principles or prejudices. Consultations about contraception, abortion and sterilization, with their far-reaching social implications, are going to be affected by emotional considerations of which the doctors may not be aware.

Many women complain that advice about reproductive functions is often judgemental, and that they are liable to be categorized as 'deserving' or 'careless and irresponsible'. Certainly, doctors tend to add judgemental adjectives when describing women seeking advice about sexual matters, and the variations of practice with regard to abortion suggest that influences are operating beyond the purely medical and social. In England and Wales as a whole, in 1984, 36 per cent of women seeking abortion in their 'area of residence' had it performed under the National Health Service. In the north of England (Northern Regional Health Authority) the percentage was 98.8. In the five health districts which serve Birmingham, only 6.5 per cent had their abortions under the NHS, with 93.5 per cent going privately.[7] There are normally regional variations in clinical practice, but these are so great (and they have persisted for a number of years) that it is hard to understand them except in terms of medical attitudes.

Psychosurgery

In the 1940s and 1950s tens of thousands of people lost parts of the frontal lobes of their brains for a variety of psychological disorders.

For about a decade there was a bonanza of operating on the brains of people who had intractable psychological problems or who were chronic inmates of mental hospitals. There was euphoria that at last something could be done to help these people, and all the more so as the procedure was so simple. As a medical student in the 1940s, I witnessed a travelling neurosurgical team in action at a large mental hospital. (It was known as Wylie's circus after the surgeon involved.) Surgeon, assistant, theatre sister and anaesthetist arrived at the hospital and went straight to the operating theatre where the first patient was waiting for them. Under general anaesthetic, a hole was drilled with a brace and bit in one temporal region then a blunt needle was inserted 'freehand', angled up and down, then withdrawn. The patient was turned over and the procedure repeated. Three or four patients were dealt with thus, and then the team drove on to the next hospital. I did not like what I saw but could not avoid an admiration for the expertise involved.

Many were helped by operations of this kind but overall hundreds were rendered inert, disinhibited, aggressive, epileptic or incontinent as a result of what appear nowadays to have been unbelievably crude and dangerous interventions.

A simple medical technique had been introduced which promised to meet a genuine and widespread need. Whenever new hope is offered to the sick there is public clamour for it, and in this instance the medical profession was able to respond using ordinary skills and instruments. This instance, however, was unique, because minds and personalities were involved, rather than simply bodies. Furthermore, the requests came not so much from the sufferers as from their relatives, medical advisors, or those who had total charge of them in institutions. The doctors advising psychosurgery were doubtless being pragmatic as doctors always are, but just whose agents were they? Whose best interest were they serving? Were these decisions exclusively therapeutic, or were they, or could they have been seen as, actions on behalf of society by doctors who were acting in accordance with current values?

From the outset some church authorities condemned on moral grounds any interference with the brain for the purpose of altering the psychological state. Individual doctors also had misgivings at the time, but on the whole the medical profession responded to the public demand.

Nowadays psychosurgery has found a small and, as it now seems, legitimate place in the repertoire.[8-10] The indications and techniques are scrutinized closely, so that the operation is more of an ordinary therapeutic intervention and less of a medical assault which could precipitate a fundamental change in personality.

Psychiatry in democratic countries

All doctors, and psychiatrists in particular, can be called upon to sign forms which will cause citizens to be admitted to hospital against their will, if the doctors believe that, as a consequence of mental disorder, the people concerned are a danger to themselves or to others. In most instances there is little doubt in the minds of the doctors, family, neighbours and professional workers involved that committal to hospital is the correct course of action; and, in retrospect, patients whose liberty had been temporarily taken away will usually agree that the compulsory admission was reasonable in the circumstances.

There are other occasions when the doctor is asked to deprive people of their liberty for reasons which are more social than medical: someone may be causing a disturbance in the street, shouting in the night and keeping people awake; in the course of a family conflict a woman locks herself in the bathroom and refuses to come out or let anyone else in; an elderly man becomes convinced that his grown-up children are trying to get rid of him so as to take over his assets. General practitioners and psychiatrists are liable to be asked to intervene in these commotions in which intense passions are generated. They are urged to 'do something'; they fully agree that something should be done, but what, to whom and by whom, and on what authority?

At another time the people clamouring for action might well be campaigners for civil liberties; but in the heat of the moment will press for someone they regard as mentally ill to be admitted to a psychiatric unit. The doctors can organize this to everyone's satisfaction except, in the short term, the patient's, and the crisis is resolved.

There is more to this procedure than disposing expeditiously of awkward people. The doctors (one of whom must be a psychiatrist) are acting formally as agents of the state. They are depriving a person of liberty because a particular medical label has been applied. The label requires that the person be suffering from mental disorder where there is a substantial risk of causing harm to self or to others. In these conditions quite exceptional powers are vested in the medical profession, powers which transcend the normal processes of common law. In the ordinary way, if a citizen is thought to be unable to manage his financial or other affairs, then there is a judicial process leading to the appointment of others to act on his behalf. This is a basic requirement of the common law, but it does not apply once a psychiatrist has diagnosed mental disorder which is thought to carry a risk of self-harm or harm to others. In this instance, the citizen is judged 'incompetent' to make decisions. Even when the person is held to be competent, in that he is able to present his case rationally, if he expresses ideas of harming himself or others the judicial processes can be by-passed [11] These are sweeping powers which the state confers on doctors. The details vary from country to country but the broad principles prevail.

Needless to say, there are some articulate opponents of these practices; and none more so than Thomas Szasz, who, for twenty-five years, has argued passionately that mental illness simply does not exist.[12-14] He maintains either that people are suffering from a disease, like any physical disease, such as diabetes or hypertension (to give his examples), and so are in need of medical treatment; or else they are deviant, in which case they should be dealt with by the processes of law, where they will be assumed to be innocent until proven guilty. Szasz's extreme polemical approach is no help to those working in services that have some responsibility towards people who are defined by society as mentally disordered: his contribution serves mainly as an irritant to make psychiatrists and others keep their assumptions under constant review.

National security and defence

The term 'intimate body search' refers to the process of looking into orifices. Terrorists, drug traffickers and other criminals may be carrying illicit goods and articles inside their bodies: heroin, for example, secured in a contraceptive sheath, can be swallowed and retained for a while in the stomach. Objects can also be inserted into the rectum or vagina.

The doctor is called to make an examination. A medical case for examination may be made: the heroin in the condom in the stomach might leak and kill the carrier. More often the issue is clearly criminal. The doctor who becomes involved is likely to be a police doctor, that is a medical practitioner who undertakes to perform certain duties on behalf of the police – and hence on behalf of the state. It is a role accepted voluntarily; and the public benefit from the services of such doctors who, although identifying with the police, nonetheless normally act benignly in the interest of the person taken into custody.

Most doctors have worked in casualty departments of hospitals at some stage in their careers, and so will be familiar with the mutually supportive relationship that can exist with the police. They assist the police by taking certain people off their hands, and the police oblige the doctors by removing difficult people who cannot be helped in hospital departments, or who are creating a nuisance there.

Doctors and police have in part a common outlook which is a mixture of caring and controlling, and it generates a *bonhomie* between members of the two groups when they meet in a professional setting. It can lead doctors to expect special treatment and privileges from the police, which indeed they often receive. It also leads the police to expect special rights from doctors, such as access to patients' case notes or the right to interview patients informally in hospital. This cooperation can resonate with the authoritarian tendency in many doctors, who may feel quite uncomfortable when they realize they should say 'no' to certain police requests.

The intimate body search is a case in point. It is a disagreeable task, unethical perhaps, yet the doctor knows that if he does not do it, someone else will; and the people concerned are invariably suspected of serious crimes.

All doctors maintain that they put the interests of their patients first. But do they? Simply working for the police can place a doctor in a position where he is exposed to conflicting interests. Perhaps it is unlikely to become a major issue in a country like Britain (though see later), but it certainly has been an issue in South Africa; and the behaviour of doctors there is generally relevant because the position of the white doctors there is comparable with that of doctors in Britain and other Western countries. However, political affiliations and authoritarian attitudes are heightened by the policy of apartheid, so a police medical officer in South Africa can find himself beset with serious conflicts of interest; these emerged with great clarity in the case of Steve Biko. [15,16]

Steve Biko died, at the age of thirty-one, of wounds received while in police custody in Port Elizabeth. He was leader of the Black Consciousness movement in South Africa, and was perceived by the authorities as a dangerous person. The injuries which led to his death were probably sustained on the night of 6–7 September 1977, and he died on 12 September 1977. The medical management of his case demonstrates how doctors can place, or be compelled to place, the interests of the security forces above the interests of their patients. His death led to a public inquest in which various figures in the drama were exposed to hostile cross-examination. There were, however, no other judicial or professional disciplinary proceedings.

On the night of 6–7 September there was a violent scene in the cells in the course of which, according to the police, Biko fell and hit his head against a wall. The barrister appearing for his family argued that Biko was struck fatally on the head by police officers. On 7 September, Dr Ivor Lang, a district surgeon (equivalent of a police medical officer), was called to see Biko. He observed his lacerated lip, bruised sternum, and pigmented ring marks around his swollen wrists, ankles and feet. He thought his slurred speech was due to the lip laceration, and his difficulty in walking due to the leg irons he had been wearing. [17] Despite these findings Dr Lang, willingly or otherwise, wrote this report.

This is to testify that I have examined Steve Biko as a result of a request from Colonel Goosen of the Security Police who complains that the above-mentioned would not speak. I have found no evidence of any abnormality or pathology on the detainee. Signed: Dr. Lang. Time: 10.10 am, September 7 1977.[18]

These damning admissions emerged in the course of cross-examination, and Dr Lang admitted that it was the first time he had been overruled.[19] He also rather forlornly admitted:

I am a general practitioner. I have my limits and I know my limitations. Had I been permitted, I would have transferred him to the care of specialists with more knowledge than I have.[19]

As Biko's medical condition did not improve, Dr Benjamin Tucker, Chief District Surgeon in Port Elizabeth, also examined him and confirmed Dr Lang's findings. Specialists were called in or consulted, and Biko was removed to the prison hospital. On 11 September he was returned to the cells. Shortly afterwards he was found in a collapsed state.

By this point a number of clinical signs had been recorded by the various doctors who had seen him.

[Biko's] speech was incoherent and slurred, and he mumbled. He intermittently showed signs of weakness in the limbs, a possible ataxic gait, and extensor plantar reponse, symptoms of echolalia, weakness of his left arm and a slight limp. Red cells were found in his spinal fluid.[20]

Clearly proper hospital treatment, or at least hospital observation, was needed at this stage but the Security Police did not want Biko in a local civilian hospital. They therefore sent him by road, lying naked on mats in the back of a Land-Rover and without medical or nursing escort, 700 miles (1,100 km) to the prison at Pretoria, where there were said to be 'outstanding medical facilities'.[21] It was reported that during the twelve-hour journey, Biko did not speak or ask to relieve himself.

Biko died the next day, 12 September, in a cell in Pretoria prison. An autopsy was carried out on 13 September, and examination of the brain showed 'several areas of damage, mainly features of hemorrhage and necrosis, and that the lesions were "clearly indicative of severe traumatic brain contusions and contusional necrosis"'.[22]

Altogether there were five distinct lesions of mechanical origin in the brain. Injuries were also noted by the pathologists on the left side of the forehead and mouth. It was thought likely that the brain injuries would have been followed by a period of at least ten minutes' unconsciousness (possibly as long as one hour), and the injuries could have been sustained on the night of 6–7 September.[22]

Dr Tucker was also cross-examined, and this exchange illustrates the conflict of loyalties:

MR S. KENTRIDGE (counsel for the Biko family): Did you think the plantar reflex could be feigned?
DR B. TUCKER: No.
MR KENTRIDGE: Did you think a man could feign red blood cells in his cerebral spinal fluid?
DR TUCKER: No.
MR KENTRIDGE: In terms of the Hippocratic Oath are not the interests of your patients paramount?
DR TUCKER: Yes.
MR KENTRIDGE: But in this instance they were subordinated to the interests of Security?
DR TUCKER: Yes.
MR KENTRIDGE: The classic signs of brain damage are a deteriorating level of consciousness, an upgoing toe and blood in the cerebral spinal fluid.
DR TUCKER: Yes.
MR M. J. PRINS (Presiding Magistrate): In fairness I must point out that I have understood Dr Tucker to say that when he examined Mr Biko on the Sunday he had not been informed of the red cells in the fluid.
MR KENTRIDGE: Yes, but he was told before Mr Biko left for Pretoria.[23]

During their cross-examination, members of the Security Forces said that they were under the impression that Biko was shamming, a view which was confirmed by the early medical reports. What pressure was put upon the doctors to supply the kind of report that the Security Forces required is not known, but the overriding authority of these forces is clear from the following exchange at the inquest between counsel for the Biko family and the colonel in charge of Security Police in Port Elizabeth:

MR KENTRIDGE: Where do you get your authority from? Show me a piece of paper that gives you the right to keep a man in chains – or are you people above the law?
COLONEL P. J. GOOSEN: We have full authority. It is left to my sound discretion.
MR KENTRIDGE: Under what statutory authority?
COLONEL GOOSEN: We don't work under statutory authority.[24]

It is difficult for doctors to stand up against officers of a police force that can say such things in public. Of course one of the odd things about this case is that the inquest was held at all. Many people die in police custody in South Africa, as they do in most countries in the world today, and the basic questions never have to be answered. Doctors may be involved in these hidden cases, or they may not. At least in the Biko case most of the facts came out into the open.

At the end of thirteen days of evidence, the Presiding Magistrate found that:

> The available evidence does not prove that the death was brought about by any act or omission amounting to an offence on the part of any person. That completes this inquest. The Court will adjourn now.[25]

It was an extraordinary verdict, and all the more so because the Magistrate gave no reasons for his opinion.

As far as the medical profession was concerned, the matter did not rest there. The Magistrate evidently referred the records regarding Biko's medical treatment to the South African Medical and Dental Council.[26] The South African Medical and Dental Council has the Minister of Health as its political head; the government appoints two-thirds of its members and the medical profession one-third.[27] The Council reported that there was no evidence of improper or disgraceful conduct on the part of the doctors concerned in Biko's treatment. This finding led to an angry response from the Medical Faculty of the University of Witwatersrand,[28] but not, by 1980, from any other South African medical school.[29]

Some years passed, and Drs Lang and Tucker continued functioning as District Surgeons[30] (they had not, after all, been convicted of any offence, merely suspected of improper conduct). More recently (1985) the Supreme Court of South Africa ordered the South African Medical and Dental Council to hold a new inquiry. Dr Tucker was erased from the South African medical register, and Dr Lang was rebuked for improper conduct.[31]

It should be assumed that doctors who choose to work with police forces will take an interest in their work and share something of their ethos, otherwise the doctors would never undertake such work in the first place. The same applies to doctors who work in prisons, although there can be financial inducements here. There is no blame of course on doctors who take an interest in forensic medicine and the judicial processes: there are important medical as well as social implications in the care of offenders. (One must remember the stand taken by prison medical officers in Northern Ireland in 1977.)[32] The danger arises solely from the conflict of interests, as there should never be considerations which interfere with the doctor doing what seems to be in the patient's best interest. In too many countries this is a tragically unrealistic ideal.

A different kind of involvement with the interests of the state comes from the participation of doctors in defence contracts, in particular with some aspects of chemical and bacteriological warfare (CBW). Research in these areas has been active since the end of the First World War, and despite various treaties banning their development and use there is no reason to suppose that the great powers have abandoned their research programmes.

This kind of work requires people with medical training, and the accounts of the development of CBW do not show the medical participants in a good light.[33-36] Until fairly recently the medical practitioners concerned made little secret of the fact, the best known in the years around the Second World War being Sir Paul Fildes FRS, and Lord Stamp. More recently doctors involved have kept a lower profile; they have not published openly, and their involvement has been only indirectly apparent.

It is a matter of opinion whether *all* involvement with CBW programmes is beyond what is proper for a doctor. To develop methods of protection against these terrible chemical and bacteriological agents is a legitimate and necessary activity. Furthermore, the technologies relating to peace and to war are by no means separate. After all, the organo-phosphorous compounds comprising original 'nerve' gases (anticholinesterases) were derived from pesticides. During the 1957 Asian 'flu epidemic in Britain, the Microbiological Research Establishment at Porton Down, in Wiltshire, was able to produce 600,000 doses of vaccine against the Asian 'flu virus.[37]

There is always the possibility of a peaceful use for these destructive agents, and this led to a cooperative venture between doctors and scientists at Porton Down and St Thomas's Hospital, London.[38] It was an example of testing a hypothesis by clinical trial. The Langat and Kyasanur Forest disease viruses were known to reduce the level of white cells in the blood, and the researchers argued that these viruses might be beneficial if inoculated into people who were suffering from an excess of white blood cells, that is, patients with leukaemia. They therefore administered the viruses to ten patients with leukaemia, also to ten with bronchial carcinoma, and to eight with other malignant conditions. Eight out of the ten leukaemic patients showed a 'significant', though transient, fall in the white cell count; and four out of the whole group showed 'transient therapeutic benefit'. All the subjects subsequently died, some of their disease, and some as a result of the 'treatment'. However, the researchers felt that the results were 'sufficiently encouraging to justify continuation of the attempts'.

135

The Langat and Kyasanur Forest disease viruses are tick-borne, and were very likely being investigated at Porton Down for their suitability as agents in bacteriological warfare. The post-mortem findings from the patients in this series presumably have enlarged our knowledge about the effectiveness of these agents in warfare – against humans and animals – and also perhaps our knowledge about how to combat their dreadful effects.

In 1937, during their war with China, the Japanese established the notorious Pinfang Institute, near Haerbin in Manchuria.[39,40] It lasted until the Allied victory in 1945, and was the scene of horrific experiments on Chinese, Russian, American, Australian and British prisoners, who were forcibly inoculated with various pathogens and then left to die from their effects. Certain prisoners were 'sacrificed' before the disease had reached its natural end and examined by Japanese pathologists who were studying the pathological processes.

Bombs were devised to detonate and carry fragments infected with anthrax spores, which would injure and infect prisoners tied to stakes in the vicinity of the explosion.[41] The prisoners would subsequently develop and probably die of anthrax. Experiments were also conducted with the pathogens causing typhus, typhoid, cholera, plague, tetanus, botulism, gas gangrene, smallpox, tick encephalitis, tuberculosis, turalaemia and glanders.[42] When the Russians overran the Pinfang Institute in 1945, the buildings had been destroyed and the remaining prisoners murdered. Most of the senior personnel disappeared. In the West nothing more was heard of them, and they gradually filtered back into civilian life. None of these men was brought to trial in the West because a deal was struck with the Allies by the notorious General Ishii, who had created the Pinfang Institute. The deal was that the doctors and others working on bacteriological warfare would be given immunity from prosecution, provided they handed over their findings to the Allies. The Allies accepted the offer and the men were free to pursue prosperous careers. In 1985 a number of these men, now occupying positions of distinction in the medical profession in Japan, were interviewed for television, and several of them spoke with candour about their work.[40]

In the years after the Second World War, the research continued in the United States, Canada, Britain, most European countries, and the Soviet Union. The favoured agents were those causing anthrax, brucellosis, turalaemia and psittacosis: the last three of these are unlikely to be fatal to humans and so would be regarded by some as 'humane' weapons. In the meantime, however, the development of chemical weapons has been highly successful, and it seems that the populations of whole cities could be incapacitated by relatively small quantities of nerve gas, or even a hallucinogen in the drinking water. Bacteriological weapons appear cumbersome and slow by comparison, although they would continue to be useful against animals.

Participation in a programme of research connected with bacteriological warfare is a long way from conducting a medical examination in a police station. These activities represent the extreme points on a continuum covering a doctor's involvement with the interests of the state, at least when dealing with people who are judged to be of sound mind. At one end, the doctor is helping the police in the examination of a suspected criminal; at the other, he is helping to destroy the state's enemies.

Psychiatry in the Soviet Union

Prisoners of conscience are held in psychiatric hospitals in the Soviet Union for indefinite periods. Their offence has been to make some non-violent statement of protest against the regime on behalf of the human rights movement, or of religious or ethnic groups, or simply expressed a desire to emigrate. Having committed no obvious criminal act they cannot be tried in open court, at least not in parts of the country accessible to Western journalists; instead they are designated mentally ill, with the implication that they are not responsible for their actions. They can then be committed discreetly, and with no public proceedings, to psychiatric hospitals for treatment and when, in the minds of the authorities, they are better, they can be returned to society.

At least eighty-three such hospitals are known to house dissidents, seventeen of them in Moscow itself.[43] Some of these are called Special Psychiatric Hospitals which accommodate severely mentally disturbed offenders convicted of violent crimes, and to that extent they resemble Broadmoor, Rampton and Moss Side Hospitals in Britain. They also accommodate the more important dissidents; and several hundreds (possibly thousands) are being held against their will under penal conditions.

The activities of these institutions have been extensively documented,[44-49] and no systematic effort to refute the detailed accounts of the Special Psychiatric Hospitals has been made by the Soviet authorities; still less has there been any willingness to permit outside observers access to particular institutions, or give permission for them to examine named inmates. The dissidents live in close proximity with mentally disturbed inmates, even though none of the dissidents has been shown, in two surveys by Russian psychiatrists,[50,51] to be similarly disturbed and requiring compulsory hospitalization. They are in the immediate care of orderlies who are often recruited from the criminal population of civil prisons, so there is generally no vestige of hospital care as it is generally understood, but there is brutality and a need to pay bribes to maintain the barest level of comfort. There is frequent and haphazard medication with chlorpromazine, haloperidol and other sedative drugs which are administered by the orderlies, with the result that many of the prisoner-patients are over-sedated, disorientated and incoordinated for prolonged periods, and allowed to develop the side-effects associated with these drugs. There is, in addition, evidence of the use of injections of insulin, and of sulphazine (a preparation of one per cent elemental sulphur in oil, which causes a high fever and bodily pains). Both these drugs were once used in the management of mentally disturbed people but they have been dropped from ordinary psychiatric practice, sulphazine since the 1930s. Electroconvulsive therapy is not generally used in the Soviet Union but it is said to have been applied as a punishment.[51]

These practices could not occur without the active participation of doctors, who supervise the wards and prescribe drugs for people they know do not require medication and are even being harmed by it. Of course anyone can administer psychotropic drugs but some expertise is needed to judge how much a person can tolerate, as it is important that these people do not die in custody. What, then, is known about these doctors, in particular the medical staffs of the Special Psychiatric Hospitals? How do they view their role and how can they persist in procedures which defy the basic principles of medical practice?

The Special Psychiatric Hospitals are run by the Ministry of the Interior (MVD), not by the Ministry of Health (which runs the Ordinary Psychiatric Hospitals), and the senior psychiatrists hold rank in the MVD.[47,52] The MVD is interested in security and discipline rather than therapy, and these medical men and women can be relied upon to carry out the will of their political masters.

Soviet psychiatry is rigorously centralized and hierarchical; and the dominant figure for several decades has been Professor Andrei V. Snezhnevsky (born 1904), Director of the Institute of Psychiatry of the Academy of Medical Sciences. He is a full Academician and a man of some standing in the Soviet Union. He is one of the outstanding medical politicians of any age, and achieved his power, not only by the usual manipulation of medical organizations, but also by an adroit exploitation of ideologies and psychological theories. He was a zealous advocate of Pavlov's theories at a time when they were being taken up formally by Stalin in 1950, and when other points of view were being suppressed and their proponents retired or posted to inferior employment. Later on he broadened the concept of schizophrenia to an extreme degree until it could include even transient states of depression and anxiety. Dissidents, therefore, could be labelled 'schizophrenic' for the slenderest of reasons, and peculiar terms were used in reports; for example, 'sluggish' schizophrenia without 'clear symptoms', and even 'schizophrenia without schizophrenia'.[53-55] Snezhnevsky further maintained that schizophrenia could never be cured, with the result that once the label had been applied to someone, any out-of-the-ordinary behaviour could be interpreted in pathological terms and lead to immediate detention.[56,57]

Snezhnevsky was for some time Director of the Serbsky Institute for Forensic Psychiatry in Moscow – the principal centre for psychiatric abuse – and, more than anyone else, developed the techniques of using psychiatry for political ends. Around him at the Institute of Psychiatry, which advises the Ministry of Health and the Serbsky Institute and thus effectively controls the whole of psychiatric practice in the Soviet Union, is a small group of psychiatrists who have all been active in the political abuse of their profession.[45,46] These names and a very few others crop up repeatedly in the testimonies of dissidents.

It is impossible to know how many of this group believe wholeheartedly that what they are doing is in the best interests of the Party, but there certainly are material benefits from doing what they are told. They are all Party members and may be seeking high office within their profession and the Soviet system. In addition they can expect to earn three times the usual salary for a psychiatrist, have access to special shops, a cottage in the country and opportunities for foreign travel. This means that the same faces are seen at international conferences regardless of the special topic under discussion.

Until the mid-1970s, the average Russian psychiatrist probably had only a limited idea of what happened at the Special Psychiatric Hospitals, and did not want to know much more. Now it is harder to remain in ignorance of what is going on, but there is a strong tendency to conform in Russian society, nearly three generations after the Revolution. There is also a 'perfect understanding' about the kind of situation which it is wise to avoid, and the questions which one does not ask. If a patient appears in an Ordinary Psychiatric Hospital for reasons which do not seem to be medical, the event will be accepted tacitly, perhaps with the rationalization that if he is guilty of a crime against the state, he is better off in a hospital than in a labour camp.[58] To question the system is to put in lasting peril one's family, career, life-style and liberty. It is easy for Westerners to speak out against wrongs because they know that if their cause is just it will win support in the ensuing public debate. In the Soviet Union nothing is public, and the questioning doctor can be dismissed and prevented from seeking further congenial employment. Such a doctor will be harassed and threatened, ostracized by colleagues, and avoided by some friends as an awkward person to be seen talking to. The family can suffer similarly and the children be denied educational opportunities. There are likely to be arrests, interrogations, and then forcible detention or exile to a remote region. All this disappointment and suffering can follow the merest questioning of the system, and Westerners are naively disbelieving about the consequences that follow any dissent whatsoever.

A few brave Russian psychiatrists have spoken out publicly against the penal use of psychiatry. They have been and still are being persecuted for their actions. Notable among them are Dr Semyon Gluzman (born 1945),[59] who, shortly after completing his training as a psychiatrist in 1972, was sentenced to seven years in a strict-regime labour camp followed by three years' exile. This was for publishing an independent report about the mental health of Major-General Grigorenko, who was one of the most famous victims of recent psychiatric persecution, and for keeping secret the names of his co-authors. Gluzman also published with Vladimir Bukovsky, in 1974, *A Manual on Psychiatry for Dissenters.*[60] Dr Anatoly Koryagin (born 1938) published the results of his examinations of the mental state of dissidents who had been incarcerated in psychiatric hospitals (he could find no evidence or history of mental disorder in any of them),[50] and he was sentenced in 1981 to seven years' imprisonment followed by five years' exile in a remote area. By 1985 he was in a dangerous condition, having been weakened by repeated beatings to make him recant his findings, and weakened also by hunger strikes which were his only form of protest.[61,62]

Dr Alexander Voloshanovich was another psychiatrist who gave expert opinion about the mental health of dissidents whom the authorities claimed were suffering from mental disorder, but he was able to emigrate from the Soviet Union in 1980.[51] Both Koryagin and Voloshanovich assisted an extraordinarily brave small group who called themselves the Working Commission to Investigate the Use of Psychiatry for Political Purposes.[49,63] They collected information about the misuse of psychiatry and published a series of carefully documented *Information Bulletins* to publicize what was going on. Inevitably they were suppressed and the members imprisoned, but their activities have been partly responsible for the drop in the number of dissidents incarcerated in psychiatric hospitals for political reasons.

While individual doctors may be motivated by ideology, personal advancement or material gain, there is a background from which they cannot remain independent, and which may explain why the political abuses have become more institutionalized in the Soviet Union than in other totalitarian regimes. The explanation derives from a mixture of the Russian tradition, the Soviet political ideology, and the uncertainties about the boundaries of psychiatry.

As long ago as 1836 the reformist philosopher, Pyotr Chaadayev (1794–1856), was declared to be suffering from 'derangement and insanity' following the publication in Moscow of an article critical of Russia's backwardness compared with Western Europe. This angered Tsar Nicholas I who instigated the diagnosis of insanity and arranged for the treatment of 'this unfortunate person', and put him under house arrest as well.[64–66] It was an isolated, but well-known, incident which at a stroke removed and discredited a dangerous critic, all under the guise of benevolent paternalism.

Soon after the 1917 Revolution, while public opinion still mattered, the Bolsheviks managed to dispose of former comrades who were too well known to be shot by sending them to sanatoria where they would be silenced and discredited, and no longer a threat to the new regime.[67] These practices began in 1918, and proved to be so convenient that they soon became more widespread and formalized, and by the 1930s the first Special Hospitals were being created. As with the incarceration of dissidents in labour camps, the practice was established before the Revolution: the Soviets had merely to revive it.

There is also the peculiar logic of the Soviet system which insists that the Marxist-Leninist interpretation of history is the only correct one, and that anybody who disagrees with it must either be an agent of the West or suffering from mental illness. Dissent, therefore, cannot be accepted officially as a legitimate attitude in the Soviet Union. Added to this is the difficulty of deciding the point at which someone ceases to be merely eccentric and can be judged as suffering from mental illness (whatever mental illness might be); and also the point at which a person can no longer be held to be responsible for a particular opinion or action.

Doctors and torture

Vladimir Bukovsky has described a method of torture used in Soviet psychiatric hospitals in the 1960s.

> This involved the use of wet canvas – long pieces of it – in which the patient was rolled up from head to foot, and so tightly that it was difficult for him to breathe; as the canvas began to dry out it would get tighter and tighter and make the patient feel even worse. But that punishment was applied with some caution – there were medical men present while it was taking place who made sure that the patient did not

lose consciousness, and if his pulse began to weaken then the canvas would be eased.[68]

From several parts of the world, after terrible tortures have been inflicted on blindfold victims, there are accounts of a 'soft hand over the heart', which may be that of a doctor who is playing a part in the proceedings. Jacobo Timerman, in 1977, while editor of a Buenos Aires newspaper, was arrested without any charge being brought against him apart from that of being Jewish. He was brutally tortured and held in captivity for thirty months. He wrote of an episode in prison after two days without torture.

The doctor came to see me and removed the blindfold from my eyes. I asked him if he wasn't worried about my seeing his face. He acts surprised. 'I'm your friend. The one who takes care of you when they apply the machine. Have you something to eat?'

'I have trouble eating' [said Timerman]. 'I'm drinking water. They gave me an apple.'

'You're doing the right thing. Eat lightly. After all, Gandhi survived on much less. If you need something, call me.'

'My gums hurt. They applied the machine to my mouth.'

He examines my gums and advises me not to worry, I'm in perfect health. He tells me he's proud of the way I withstood it all. Some people die on their torturers, without a decision having been made to kill them; this is regarded as a professional failure.[69]

Solzhenitsyn has also written in *The Gulag Archipelago* about prison doctors, whom he regards as 'the interrogator's and executioner's right-hand man'.

The beaten prisoner would come to on the floor only to hear the doctor's voice: 'You can continue, the pulse is normal.' After a prisoner's five days and nights in a punishment cell the doctor inspects the frozen, naked body and says: 'You can continue.' If a prisoner is beaten to death, he signs the death certificate: 'Cirrhosis of the liver' or 'Coronary occlusion.' He gets an urgent call to a dying prisoner in a cell and he takes his time. And whoever behaves differently is not kept on in the prison.[70]

The first doctors publicly recognized as being involved in torture were those working in Nazi concentration camps. Dr Alexander Mitscherlich and Dr Fred Mielke have presented detailed testimony which was part of the evidence used in the Nuremberg Trials. They estimated that out of approximately 90,000 doctors working in Germany under National Socialism, 'some 350 committed medical crimes'.[71] They have described and documented these crimes under the following headings:

Low pressure and supercooling experiments; tests on the possibility of drinking sea-water; typhus vaccine experiments; epidemic hepatitis virus research; sulphonamide tests; experiments in bone transplantation; phlegmon experiments [i.e. effects of untreated infections]; mustard gas and phosgen[e] experiments; collection of the skeletons of Jews for Strasburg University; euthanasia of mentally afflicted; direct elimination of undesirable invalids and national elements; and experimental preparations for mass sterilization.

Only twenty doctors were actually charged at Nuremberg with medical crimes: four of these were sentenced to death, nine to varying terms of imprisonment, and seven were acquitted.[72]

In the forty years since the end of the Second World War, torture has become more widely practised in the world. Amnesty International have reported that 'between mid-1974 and 1979 Amnesty International interceded on behalf of 1,143 individuals in danger of torture (excluding mass arrests) in 32 countries; between January 1980 and mid-1983, Amnesty International made similar urgent appeals on behalf of 2,687 individuals in 45 countries'.[73]

There is every reason to believe that doctors have been closely concerned with these dreadful proceedings; and the whole question of the involvement of doctors and other health professionals has been described in detail by Eric Stover and Elena Nightingale in their book *The Breaking of Bodies and Minds*,[74] and by the British Medical Association in their *Torture Report*.[75] Outside the Soviet Union, where involvement of doctors in the maltreatment of detainees is on a much larger and more systematic scale than anywhere else, most of the examples come from Latin American countries, notably Chile, Uruguay and Brazil – Argentina having stopped these practices since the election of President Alfonsin in 1983. There are also examples from Portugal and Greece, during particularly repressive periods in their recent history.

According to the *Guardian* newspaper:

Doctors took part before, during, and after torture sessions, to examine prisoners and test their ability to resist further torture. Photographic records were kept for 'scientific purposes' so that the doctors could study the physical and psychological effects of the torture. . . Over 90 per cent of the torture victims suffered nervous breakdowns with hallucinations, acute states of anxiety and terror, and a complex disorientation of time and space. . .

The doctors helped the DGS [security police] at the Caxias detention centre in Oporto . . . Among the doctors are at least two psychiatrists who supervised the application of the most sophisticated method of sensory deprivation and the denial of sleep,[76]

In Greece, Pericles Korovessis, a victim of the military junta which held power between 1967 and 1974, described the tortures which he underwent in 'General Military Hospital No. 401'.

A nurse with an enormous starched cap, two soldiers and a male nurse loaded me on to a stretcher . . . We got to the doctor's consulting room. They placed me gently on a leather consulting couch; they tied me down with straps and buckles. A male nurse placed a rubber cushion full of water behind the nape of my neck, and a towel on top . . . next to my head there was a black machine with lots of dials . . . They gathered round me . . . all wearing white coats. Somebody examined my heart and said okay. Someone else adjusted the switches on the machine; he was holding something in his hand, like a needle with a screwdriver-type handle – it's called an electrode. He stuck it behind my ear.[77]

Korovessis, who had experienced other tortures before this electric torture, was bewildered by the proceedings, and thought perhaps they were performing experiments on him. He heard the senior man addressed as 'Mr Surgeon-Colonel', and he later discovered that this was the General Director of the Military Hospital.

Amnesty International have summarized the ways in which doctors become involved in the practice of torture. They may be expected –

– to perform medical examinations on suspects before they are subjected to forms of interrogation, which might include torture.

– to attend torture sessions in order to intervene . . . when the victim's life is in danger.

– to treat the direct physical effects of torture, and often to 'patch up' a seriously injured torture victim temporarily so that later on the interrogation can be continued.

– to develop, by means of their own techniques, methods which produce the results desired by their superiors, as when psychiatric methods are used.[78,79]

This chapter, and the whole of Part II of this book, has been devoted to descriptions of how doctors, singly or collectively, can behave under certain conditions. Where torture is concerned, a simple description would give an inaccurate picture, because the activities of these doctors cannot be separated from the repressive and ruthless regimes in which they live and work. The doctors, and other health professionals for that matter, are not free to make moral choices without the risk of serious harm to themselves or to their families. Unless we expect that all doctors will have the moral and physical courage, for example, of Anatoly Koryagin and Semyon Gluzman, compromises will be inevitable.

The issues surrounding torture are also much more complicated – even leaving aside the utilitarian argument that at times torture may be justified if it will lead to the saving of innocent lives,[80] and assuming that torture is in all circumstances morally wrong.

Four ways, indicated above, in which doctors could be involved in torture include services which might be in the interests of the victim. The doctor *might* be able to lessen the suffering, but that would only be through some subterfuge to make the torturers abandon their victim. There must be some kindly doctors caught up in these horrors who genuinely try to mitigate the torment of the prisoners, and the balance they try to strike between doing what they can for the prisoners and not antagonizing the guards must be respected.

Following the introduction of the Islamic *Shari'a* law in Mauritania in July 1980, four men found guilty of theft had their right hands amputated. These procedures were carried out without general anaesthetic by 'doctors or medical auxiliaries', despite protests from the Mauritanian medical association.[81] In Sudan, the official executioner and an assistant received, prior to a similar judicial amputation in 1983, 'four days of training in the surgical theater at Khartoum Hospital'.[81] It was not reported what the doctors concerned felt about their interventions. It is likely, however, that the victims fared better having had their mutilations performed surgically, rather than by a blow of an axe (or whatever traditional instrument may have been used).

The practicalities are terrible, and what, for example, is the right course of action for a doctor who finds himself caught up in events such as those reported in Mauritania in July 1980? True, the doctors involved probably would be Moslem (and might believe that physical mutilation was a proper form of punishment), but a dilemma exists which is independent of the prevailing religious ideology: namely, whether the victim's suffering can be alleviated by the skilled services of a doctor, whatever the doctor feels about the ethics of the punishment/torture; and therefore, to what extent should the doctor become involved? Or should the doctor

145

have nothing whatsoever to do with procedures he finds morally repugnant and which trangress any code of medical ethics?

A comparable dilemma exists in relation to clitorectomy (or female circumcision), and again doctors are called in as agents of authority, in this case, religious and social authority. In the radical procedure, called infibulation, the clitoris, *labia majora* and *minora* are excised and the raw surfaces of each side stitched together to leave a tiny orifice, just sufficient for urination and menstruation. Many women in those parts of Africa where this operation is performed feel that it amounts to torture, since it brings no benefit at all to the woman; merely the risk of haemorrhage, septicaemia, retention of urine and other urinary problems, the impossibility of sexual intercourse without first having cut through the scar tissue (and then no pleasure from the intercourse), and the likelihood of obstetric difficulties.[82,83]

If the doctor refuses to assist at female circumcision, the women will have it done by traditional means, with an increased risk of complications. On the other hand, if he does oblige, then the procedure acquires a false respectability. If the doctor refuses to participate in any way with the horrors of torture it will proceed without him, and he and his family may suffer persecution of various kinds. If he does allow himself to be involved, he again gives a false moral authority to what is being done; and the torturers can feel that they are engaged in a legitimate activity.

In democratic countries it is possible for doctors to speak out about abuses they witness or suspect, and there was an example of this in Northern Ireland when prison doctors noticed injuries among the prisoners which they believed were not self-inflicted. In 1977 the doctors concerned complained to the authorities and threatened to resign or seek transfer if nothing was done about what they regarded as improper treatment. Eventually, through national television attention and a visit from Amnesty International, changes were made.[84] These doctors knew that they would not be punished for taking their stand; even so their action took some courage, bearing in mind the strong feelings of the different groups, and it seems that they were considerably abused for the action they took.

Part III

Sources of Doctors' Problems

10

Thinking About Illness

Doctors do not often think about illness. They think about particular diseases but rarely about the nature and essence of illness or disease.[1] This is partly because the subject is extremely complex. At a metaphysical level, there is the whole question of the purpose of suffering; and there is the question of the meaning of the illness for the individual, its timing in relation to events in the person's life, and the consequences which might be expected to follow from having been ill. These issues are highly relevant for doctors wishing to look beyond the diseased organ, although they are not much favoured in orthodox medical circles, because psychological, social and even spiritual concepts are involved.

Another difficulty in asking fundamental questions about clinical medicine lies in its lack of a theoretical basis. There is no unifying theory of disease which can link human ailments in the way in which the elements are linked in the periodic table, or in which apparently different kinds of energy are linked within electro-magnetic theory. On top of this is the sheer urgency of clinical practice with sick people in need of attention. Thus there is little pressure on doctors to apply themselves to the more abstract issues when they can easily justify themselves at a practical level by offering symptomatic relief and quite often a cure.

Earlier chapters have indicated problems among doctors and in the medical profession. Some of these derive from the unsatisfactory ways in which doctors think about illness, its possible purpose, its essence, its meaning for patients and also for doctors. Hence there is a need to examine the models in use. This chapter is devoted to the dominant ideology in Western medicine – the mechanistic – and to its strengths and limitations. There are other approaches to understanding illness, notably those concerning its meaning, and some of these are taken up later in the book.

Before the modern era

In order to set contemporary thinking about illness in some context, I want to make three points about the past, under the headings: magico-religious medicine, empirico-rational medicine, and Galenism.

Magico-religious medicine. In ancient times little could be done for the sick; and people's relationship with the natural world was influenced by a cosmology which included capricious gods and all kinds of spirits, beneficial and malign. Primitive people thought about illness in terms of the interventions of these agents, and it was the task of medicine men – who were a mixture of priest, physician and sorcerer – to placate these supernatural forces and intercede with them.

The magico-religious approach persists in many parts of the world, in tribal societies, and the majority of the earth's population still adheres to such principles and practices, with or without the addition of Western medicine. There are remnants of this kind of thinking in the Western world itself. When some people speak of 'bugs going around', they are still using the language of spirit possession, with micro-organisms in the place of evil spirits[2] – even if the treatment prescribed belongs to the twentieth century.

Empirico-rational medicine. A great advance in medical thinking occurred when the focus of interest shifted from supernatural forces to the person who was sick. Illness could then be seen as a natural phenomenon accessible to study, and differentiated from divine or malevolent forces which it would be unwise to attempt to understand, let alone to conquer.

Empirico-rational medicine probably began in Egypt, at least that is where the oldest systematic literature has been found. There are fragments of medical texts written in the First Dynasty, about 3000 BC,[3] and the first direct evidence comes from the Kahun, the Edwin Smith and Ebers papyri dating respectively from 1900 BC, 1600 BC and 1550 BC.[4,5]

In the West, speculation about the mechanisms of illness began around the sixth century BC, along with the theories about the composition of the world of the Presocratic philosophers in Ionia (now western Turkey), Italy and Sicily.[6–9] By the time of Hippocrates (460–377 BC) an elaborate schema had been evolved which asserted that the human body, like everything else in the world, was made up of four elements (earth, water, fire and air), which were manifested in the body by four humours (respectively, black bile, phlegm, yellow bile and blood).[10] This is the humoral theory which originated in Asia[11] (where it still forms the basis of Ayurvedic, Unani and traditional Tibetan medicine) and dominated European medicine until the sixteenth century.

Galenism. Galen (AD 129–199) was the most influential doctor the world has ever known. He was born in Pergamon and his main work was in Rome. He was a meticulous observer, a clinical researcher of genius, and a prolific writer who had the good fortune to have most of his output survive.[12-21]

Unfortunately, Galen's teachings became petrifed into the dogma which became known as 'Galenism'.[22,23] It prevailed for fourteen centuries, flourishing through the era of scholasticism, when reasoning was generally regarded as a better way of discovering the truth than empirical observation; and, in its most rigid form, Galenism became a closed system. It provided the intellectual basis for the practice of most of the physicians who dominated European medicine, but it failed in the long run because it could not incorporate the advances in medical knowledge being made in Europe in the fifteenth and sixteenth centuries.

Evolution of the biomedical model

The anatomical studies of Vesalius[24] were published in 1543, and William Harvey's account of the circulation of the blood in 1628.[25] The ancient humoral theory could not accommodate discoveries such as these, and they were but part, albeit a very important part, of the widespread rise in empirical science in Europe at the time. There was a need for an explanatory model which could incorporate the new ideas about the structure and function of the body.

For centuries people had attended to the whole and to the harmonious interaction of the parts: now it was important to concentrate on the parts. In other words, there was need of a simple mechanical model, for example, a clock. Compare the body to the machine. Take it to pieces and see how each part works. Allow the mind to stand apart from the machine under observation.

René Descartes (1596–1650) perfectly expressed what was required, writing as a mathematician and philosopher; also, as was natural in that age, he held a firm belief in God. In his lucid and eminently sensible *Discourse on Method* (1637), Descartes insisted on the primacy of what he regarded as experience over logical argument, concentrating on what was actually there as opposed to what ought to be there. He enunciated four rules which laid the foundations for his new approach to knowledge, and which still dominate medical thinking three and a half centuries later.

> The first rule was to accept as true nothing that I did not know to be evidently so: that is to say, to avoid carefully precipitancy and prejudice, and to apply my judgements to nothing but that which showed itself so clearly and distinctly to my mind that I should never have occasion to doubt it.

151

The second was to divide each difficulty I should examine into as many parts as possible, and as would be required the better to solve it.

The third was to conduct my thoughts in an orderly fashion, starting with what was simplest and easiest to know, and rising little by little to the knowledge of the most complex, even supposing an order where there is no natural precedence among the objects of knowledge.

The last rule was to make so complete an enumeration of the links in an argument, and to pass them all so thoroughly under review, that I could be sure I had missed nothing.[26]

Dividing each subject into as many parts as possible, conducting one's thoughts in an orderly fashion, and enumerating the links in an argument, all became desirable features of the new scientific way of thinking. That is not to imply that in earlier ages people did not think in an orderly way. It is merely that the process of dividing the subject up into as many parts as possible, studying each, and then perhaps reassembling the whole, was something new; and it characterized thinking from the middle of the sixteenth century until the present day. It represents quite fairly the way contemporary doctors approach their patients.

Another preoccupation of Descartes' was the certainty that he felt he could achieve by means of mathematical proof.

My whole object was to achieve certainty, and to probe beneath the shifting soil and the sands to find the underlying rock or stone . . . [Of] the propositions I examined, not by feeble conjectures, but by clear and assured reasonings, I found none so dubious that I was unable to draw a sufficiently certain conclusion from it, even if this conclusion was simply that there was nothing certain about it.[27]

This quotation reveals that Descartes was rather more subtle than some people care to think, since he could allow uncertainty as an occasional object of his certainty. Descartes' quest for certainty, however, involved conceiving the human body as a machine, but it was a rather special kind of machine, because it had a soul and came 'from the hands of God'.[28] Descartes accepted the religion of his day, saying that 'He is the perfect being, and that whatever we possess comes from Him';[29] and philosophers and scientists in general in the sixteenth and seventeenth centuries had no difficulty in reconciling religious belief with empirical observations, even though these were gradually coming to replace speculation and reasoning as the primary way of discovering the truth and the secrets of nature.

This move towards empiricism was most clearly seen in astronomy, where the speculative cosmologies of ancient times gave way, after much prevarication on the part of the ecclesiastical authorities, to empirically based theories developed in the sixteenth and seventeenth centuries. In particular, Newton's theory of universal gravitation not only explained the nearly circular orbits of planets around the sun, but also the falling of objects to the ground, and the movement of ocean tides. He also unified the diverse theories about the nature and propagation of light.[30] Hitherto the writers on optics had been thinking in terms of a particular metaphysical system, often more interested in defending their position with regard to other schools than in the realities of nature. After Newton, in many areas of enquiry, there was but one theory, and disputes had to be expressed in relation to the actual phenomena rather than to the underlying systems of belief.

A good deal of blame is laid upon Descartes and Newton by well-meaning people who deplore contemporary mechanistic medicine. This is rather unfair on these two great men whose vision was much broader than that of the iatromechanists of today. If anyone could be 'blamed' for espousing a totally mechanistic view of humankind, albeit in the form of a personal belief, it would be Julien Offray de La Mettrie (1709–51).[31,32] In the course of his medical experience, including time as a military doctor, and also through his own illness, he became convinced of the primacy of physical experience over mental experience: an example of this for him is the way the effects of hunger or fever dominate an individual's mental state.

La Mettrie was also of a philosophical disposition, and in due course he developed his hypothesis that all mental events had a physical origin, in a polemic called *L'Homme Machine*, published in 1747.

> Since all the faculties of the soul depend to such a degree on the proper organization of the brain and of the whole body, that apparently they are but this organization itself, the soul is clearly an enlightened machine.[33]

> The human body is a clock, a large clock constructed with such skill and ingenuity, that if the wheel which marks the seconds happens to stop, the minute wheel turns and keeps on going its round, and in the same way the quarter-hour wheel, and all the others go on running when the first wheels have stopped because rusty or, for any reason, out of order. Is it not for a similar reason that the stoppage of a few blood vessels is not enough to destroy or suspend the strength of the movement which is in the heart as in the mainspring of the machine . . .?[34]

If La Mettrie had organized his ideas better and produced a coherent theory, he might have become the guiding spirit of mechanistic medicine,

153

and behavioural psychology as well. As it is, he remains an interesting medical *philosophe*.

Descartes had created a philosophy and a method which enabled the observer to stand back from the subject. Newton constructed mathematical theories which confirmed Descartes' view of the body and the world as a vast machine, so with these two men we have the mechanistic philosophy brought to fruition as the guiding model for medical thinking down to the present day.

The focus of medical interest had shifted from the careful history of the illness to a clinical description of the pathological appearances, from the biographical approach to the nosographical;[35] and from the time of the publication of Vesalius' *De Fabrica* in 1543, the tendency to describe illness in terms of bodily structure had been steadily gaining momentum.

The mechanistic approach is often equated with the biomedical model, or simply the medical model. It has been abundantly successful; and just as Newtonian mechanics explains very satisfactorily many of the phenomena encountered in the course of daily life, so mechanistic medicine enables doctors to deal adequately with most of the common medical complaints.

Most of the famous medical discoveries in the modern era validate the biomedical approach. At the end of the eighteenth century, Edward Jenner (1749–1823) observed that an attack of cowpox would render the patient immune to smallpox. He reasoned that matter from the cowpox lesion might be responsible for the immunity, so he inoculated a boy with some of this substance. When he subsequently inoculated the boy with smallpox matter, the boy did not develop smallpox.

In the 1860s, Pasteur demonstrated the role of bacteria in fermentation and disease, and how anthrax and rabies could be prevented by techniques similar to those used by Jenner. He established clearly the germ origin of disease, and finally disproved the idea that micro-organisms could generate spontaneously, setting an accepted biological process in place of something supernatural.

Another great figure from the nineteenth century was Robert Koch (1843–1910), and he typified the mechanistic view. He demonstrated the tubercle bacillus as the causative agent of tuberculosis. He also set out his four 'postulates', or conditions, which he judged necessary before an agent could be shown to be the *cause* of a particular disease, and which exemplify the rigorous mechanistic mood of the time with its insistence on a chain of cause-and-effect. Koch's conditions are: (1) The micro-organism is present and discoverable in every case of the disease; (2) it can be cultivated in a pure culture; (3) inoculation from this culture can reproduce the disease in a susceptible animal; and (4) the micro-organism must be obtained once more from the infected animal and again grown in a pure culture. These are stringent requirements indeed, and although they were enunciated with regard to infection by micro-organisms, they represent an ideal to which many academic doctors aspire; and any medical researcher meeting Koch's criteria for determining causation can be assured of a respectful hearing.

When the causative organism of syphilis, *Treponema pallidum*, was found in the brains of sufferers of what used to be called general paralysis of the insane,[36] it seemed as though a new era in a story of cause-and-effect had opened. Neurosyphilis, to use the contemporary name, had long been suspected of having a connection with syphilitic infection, but this clear demonstration showed for the first time how a physical process could cause a severe mental disturbance. In other words, here was a physical cause for a mental illness. Here was a mechanism to explain bizarre behaviour and gradual psychological deterioration.

To the nineteenth-century mechanist, it was easy to generalize this finding to all mental disorder, until the whole range of psychological disturbance could be regarded as having a physical basis: nothing necessarily as dramatic as syphilis, but something identifiably physical nonetheless, merely waiting for a sufficiently able researcher with sufficiently sensitive measuring instruments. This is the philosophy which, to this day, guides many psychiatrists, who prescribe psychotropic drugs for their patients as though they are treating what is primarily a disturbance of brain function.

A prime example of mechanistic medicine is found in the case of diabetes. In 1889 it had been discovered that a disorder in metabolism like diabetes could be produced by removing the pancreas; and then in 1921 it was shown that the administration of insulin could relieve the symptoms of diabetes. It was a clear demonstration of how disease could be due to a fault or a deficiency in the machine, something which could then be rectified by the administration of a specific substance. In the case of diabetes, it was insulin. Pernicious anaemia is another condition, previously fatal, which exemplified the same principles.

Workers in the biomedical field have concentrated on the smaller parts of the system because that is where the solutions to the unsolved problems are thought to lie. Problems at an organ level have been more or less worked out. Infections can be treated and tissues manipulated surgically; and even the challenges presented in organ transplantation have less to do with manual dexterity than with cellular physiology. The success of this approach has been demonstrated supremely well in modern times in the

155

elucidation of the structure of DNA (deoxyribonucleic acid). Yet, as the focus becomes narrower and more intense, relatively less is understood about the interconnections of the cells, the organs or the systems.

Limitations of the biomedical model

The greatest single weakness of the biomedical model stems from the fact that human beings are assumed to behave like machines when they are actually far more complex. Originally God was seen as directing these machines, but nowadays they are presumed to run entirely on their own.

People have attitudes, emotions and relationships which affect everything that happens to them, and although these can be disregarded some of the time, much of the time they are vital. These personal issues cannot be quantified in the way that biochemical data can, and in a mechanistic climate this can reduce their intellectual respectability. Neither can these personal reactions and experiences be replicated reliably, but they have a face validity which impresses thoughtful people outside the medical profession, and they can be studied rigorously using methodologies applicable to people rather than inanimate matter.

For example, a patient is experiencing severe anxiety on account of not being able to support his family while he is ill in hospital. He is worried about his employability later on, his future general health, and, as men frequently do when ill, about his future sexual capacity. He is worried about the man in the next bed who collapsed the night before and was taken away to 'Intensive Care'; and that his own father died in the same hospital from a condition which he feels is similar to his.

The biomedical model does not take account of subjective experience, which, from the patient's point of view, can be the most important aspect of being ill; nor does the model incorporate information which cannot be connected causally with the pathological findings, according to the precepts of orthodox medicine. Of course, anxiety may manifest itself in physiological changes, or the patient may have suffered a great personal trauma, such as the death of a close relative, but even such gross occurrences tend to be disregarded; not because mechanistic doctors think they are irrelevant but because they involve psychological concepts with which the doctors feel uncomfortable. They do not know how to evaluate them or how to combine them with formulations based on disturbed physical function.

The biomedical model encourages doctors to adopt an extreme Cartesian position about the separateness of the observer from the object under study. 'Objective detachment', as it is called, is regarded by some as a virtue, although of course it is a fiction. There is an intense interaction

156

between patient and doctor, whether or not it is admitted. Doctors who disregard it lose valuable clinical data, deprive their patients of empathic support, and in the long run deny themselves much of the personal satisfaction that is to be had in clinical work.

The division of a person into constituent parts makes it exceedingly difficult to imagine the whole. Indeed, Westerners scarcely have a language for describing the whole except in terms of the parts. So, however much doctors may want to view a patient as a whole and located in some kind of social context, they fall back on reductionist models because they are the only ones they have been taught.

The biomedical model predisposes doctors not only to see their patients' ailments in mechanistic terms, but to view just about everything that happens to them in medical terms as well. Childbearing becomes conceptualized in the language of pathology, even if most of the time it is 'normal', that is, without identifiable pathology. A patient in hospital who is frightened about an impending operation and reveals his worries to the staff may be diagnosed as suffering from an 'anxiety state' and prescribed a suitable tranquillizer. Grief has been discovered by doctors in the twentieth century and it has been duly medicalized, so that there are 'normal', 'abnormal' and even 'delayed' grief-reactions; and grief is now recognized as one of the 'causes' of depressive illness. Ultimately, death has come to be perceived by doctors, not as a natural process, but as a failure and a reflection on their clinical skill, or at any rate as a failure of resuscitation or life-support systems. Therefore, death must be fought to the last. This of course is the familiar medicalization of ordinary life and death which Ivan Illich has attacked so vigorously.[37]

Why change?

Although people are obviously more than machines, such a working assumption on the part of doctors does not prevent them from giving good medical care. The mechanistic model has its limitations but it does at least lead to rational medical practice, even if it lacks sensitivity. To deny this would be to deny the great progress of medicine. So why change anything?

There is nothing intrinsically wrong with the biomedical model, and people who see it at the centre of all that is wrong with clinical practice forget the great advantages it has over what went before. The problem is not that the biomedical model is intrinsically bad but that it is too restricted in its explanatory power, and that causes difficulties for doctors and patients alike.

Doctors, at least those who are sensitive to their patients' needs, are unhappy with the biomedical model because it does not explain many of the clinical problems they meet. They notice the psychological reactions of their patients and the social and economic problems that can surround illness, but there is no way of incorporating such information into the diagnostic formulation, still less of evaluating the importance of these non-physical factors.

Patients are unhappy with the biomedical model – and on the whole more frustrated by it than doctors – because it has the effect of denying them as responsible and feeling human beings. All that they know themselves to be, and all their personal experience, lies outside the range of the model.

At this point, the critics can say, 'Oh yes, it is nice to be sensitive to the patient's experience and psychosocial background. But does it really do any good? Does it make for better diagnosis and better treatment? And is it really justifiable to spend time on these refinements when resources are scarce?'

It does improve the accuracy of diagnosis and the quality of medical care to include something about the person who is ill. For example, people who have lost a close relative are more likely to die or to fall ill in the first twelve months of their bereavement than those who have not been bereaved.[38] This association has been demonstrated over and over again, and even the most sceptical clinician can be reassured that a recent bereavement is an item of information of potential clinical importance. Further, loss of any kind is likely to be significant – for example, after divorce or the material loss following disaster.

Put the other way round, illnesses are more likely to occur at times of personal distress. L. E. Hinkle and Harold Wolff found that the illnesses of a diverse population of New Yorkers, over a twenty-year period, clustered around times of personal difficulty, and that people had one-third of their illnesses during one-eighth of the twenty-year period. Furthermore, a quarter of the study population had half of the illnesses, while the quarter at the healthy end of the scale had only one-tenth of the illnesses. Hinkle and Wolff concluded:

> The great majority of clusters of illness episodes . . . occurred at times when [people] perceived their [lives] to be unsatisfying, threatening, overdemanding, and productive of conflict, and they could make no satisfactory adaptation to these situations. The situations were, in general, those which arose out of disturbed relations with family members and important associates, threats to security and status, and restrictions . . . which made it impossible to satisfy important needs and drives.[39]

This work was published in the 1950s, and methods have been refined since then, but the essential conclusion remains valid.

Another important early study was on 1,630 patients who had been admitted to a general hospital in Amsterdam, with a broad range of medical and surgical diagnoses. A forecast of outcome was made on the basis of conventional clinical information, and another forecast integrating this information with the results of a psychological and social assessment. The forecast based on the latter integrated assessment was more accurate than the forecast based on clinical data alone.[40]

There is now a well-known association between the restless, aggressive Type A personality and coronary artery disease. This also was first set out in the 1950s,[41] and it has stood the test of time and critical re-evaluations,[42,43]

The question in the 1980s is not *whether* incorporation of psychological and social factors can improve the quality of medical care, but *how* this important information can be handled and incorporated into routine practice.

Another reason for wanting doctors to change their approach to illness concerns the people who are ill. The biomedical model has a way of diminishing people, who feel devalued and so become dissatisfied. This is one of the prime reasons why so many people seek out complementary and alternative practitioners: they know they will be listened to, and what they have to say about their experiences can usually find a place in the theoretical systems employed by these practitioners.

Doctors at present lose much of the valuable information that comes their way because they do not know what to do with it. They need a wider framework into which to fit the diverse observations they make and the strange experiences they hear about in the course of their work. Patients also need doctors with a fuller understanding of what is being said to them. The biomedical model has served us well. It is now time to augment it.

11

The Doctor's Own Needs

It is hard to say which group has the greater need, the doctors or the patients. Patients, or rather potential patients, would not like to live in a society where there were no doctors, but they could, and they would survive. After all, far more people medicate themselves and advise their families and friends than ever go to see a doctor. Doctors, however, could not exist as such if there were no patients: they depend on patients for their identity.

What then are the needs of the doctor? And what in a doctor's past or present circumstances can render him vulnerable to the vicissitudes of professional and domestic life, and lead to some of the undesirable practices described earlier?

There are personality characteristics which may play a part in the decision to study medicine in the first place, and later may influence the choice of a particular specialty and a medical career that flourishes or flounders according to how satisfactorily the individual doctor's needs are met. Then there is the need to cope with the conflicting demands which all busy people encounter, and within that framework to find a life with meaning. There is the need for protection against the distressing realities of mutilation and death which are unavoidable in clinical medicine. There is also the perennial question of power, which intrudes so much into the professional life that it stands out as though it was a primary need.

Personalities

The question of what kind of people come into medicine was discussed in Chapter 6: teenage school boys who were attracted to subjects which contain a substantial body of precise and factual data, such as mathematics and the physical sciences (contrasted with the humanities), were labelled 'convergers'. I also extended this concept by linking it with the idea of the authoritarian personality which describes people who identify closely with the values of the group which is in control in any given society. This

160

added up to a profile of a person who favoured accurate information, who was more comfortable with facts than feelings, and who was concerned to establish and maintain a position of authority in society.

The convergent type, as described by Liam Hudson, and the profile of the authoritarian personality match very well the style of a great many doctors in our society, especially those in positions of greatest influence. It is not possible to prove causal connections here because of the difficulties of measurement and precise definition, but at a descriptive level these ideas are useful.

I would not have attempted to approach the elusive issue of the relationship between early childhood experiences and adult behaviour, had not the authors of a paper, described in Chapter 2, tried to answer this very question by empirical observation.[1] These authors, who followed up a cohort of doctors and controls for thirty years, found that the doctors had had more problems in their marriages and a higher incidence of alcohol and drug abuse than the controls. In trying to understand why this might be the case, they studied how data they had collected at the beginning of the survey about the childhoods of their respondents correlated with their subsequent progress in adult life.

They evaluated the childhood experiences of the respondents with regard to physical health, the quality of the relationships with parents, the extent to which the atmosphere in the home was warm and encouraging, and also with their performance at school, both academic and athletic. The researchers scored their findings and correlated them with the number of problems in adult life (in marriage, with alcohol and drugs), and also with the type of medical activity chosen (active, personal clinical involvement, as in internal medicine and paediatrics, compared with medical administration or surgery, where the authors judged that there was less direct personal involvement with patients).

The clinically involved doctors, they found, had many more problems in adult life than the others; and these clinically involved doctors had less happy childhoods than the other doctors. The controls scored lower than either group of doctors, but were fairly close to the less clinically involved doctors.

The authors, to their credit, addressed themselves directly to the thorny question: did the clinically involved doctors have more problems in their adult lives *because* they worked so hard, or did they work so hard and have problems in their lives as a consequence of their less happy childhoods? Put rather more crudely: were these doctors unhappy because they worked so hard, or did they work so hard because they were unhappy? It is a question one would like to be able to answer directly but there are formidable obstacles in the way of a simple answer.

First of all, the authors of this particular study were working within the Freudian framework which assumes that childhood experiences will determine adult patterns of living. Therefore, all that it is necessary to show is that the association between the childhood experiences and adult behaviour is statistically significant (which it was in this study) for a causal connection to be demonstrated.

It is not justifiable to generalize from one study, even such a good one as this, but the findings here and the principles about the relevance of childhood experiences are corroborated by a huge amount of empirical observation, in terms of a variety of psychological theories; and they conform with the experience of virtually all clinicians.

The whole question of proof or validation of findings in studies of human behaviour presents difficulties for many doctors. Sometimes they are suspicious of anyone making systematic studies of how people behave, and they may try to apply to those studies the criteria of the physical sciences, which is almost guaranteed to render the human studies meaningless. Proof can reasonably be sought in the physical sciences: the results of research into human behaviour usually have to be presented in terms of probability. It is possible to predict how a chemical reaction will proceed under various known conditions: it is not possible to predict the behaviour of a given person under various known conditions. The best that can be done is to take a good sample of people and match them with suitable controls, and hope that the individual variations will more or less cancel out.

Even with that proviso, studies of groups of people can only give a picture of the average, whereas one wants most of all to understand the unique person. Meaningful descriptions of people are possible, but they will be expressed in terms of quality rather than quantity. So the methodology must match the object of study. Chemical substances, groups of humans and individual humans require their own special approaches, and one method is not intrinsically superior to the others.

To return to studies about human behaviour, there is work to show how the quality of nurturing early in life can affect adult behaviour. It is based on a theory – all research must be based on a theory, whether the researcher realizes it or not – which, in this case, is a derivative of psychoanalytic theory. Adults with duodenal ulcers seem to reveal on tests that they have been more deprived emotionally as infants than adults who do not develop duodenal ulcers. This proposition has been tested extensively, to the extent that a 'deprivation scale' can be drawn up which can be used with reasonable success as a predictor of the likely outcome of surgery for duodenal ulcer.[2–4]

The detail of the theory upon which this work is based is that the adult is always striving to attain the unconditional maternal love and nurturing that was denied during infancy, with the result that this person is driven to strive throughout adult life towards better things – more money, higher status, greater success in general.[5]

A specific, although unproven, consequence of this early deprivation may be a powerful drive to care. It is as though there was a desire to give to others the caring that was never received as a child. As a scientific hypothesis, such an assertion would be virtually untestable. As a psychological idea, which might enable one to ask certain questions of those who go about their clinical practice in an almost compulsive manner, it is more useful. So it prompts me to consider the childhood experiences of those who make themselves compulsively busy; and my clinical impression is that it is a meaningful assertion.

Certain difficulties in looking for explanations of current behaviour in terms of remote events also arise from the assumption of the linear sequence of cause and effect – that the infantile deprivations were somehow causative of the duodenal ulcers; and that in the thirty-year follow-up study, the childhood deprivations were (possibly) causative in the adolescents' choice of medicine as a career, and were later causative in the choice of a highly involved clinical specialty. Such explanations also imply that the doctor's life is totally determined by what has gone before. Clues and insights can often be gained from looking at an individual's past, but not always. On the whole it can be more productive, when trying to understand people's behaviour, to examine their current circumstances and recent past events. In that way a coherent picture can be built up which makes sense of all the available information about the person, is meaningful to those accustomed to working with people, and, most important, gives insights about why the person had got into difficulties and what can be done to help.

Another approach to understanding why people act as they do is to examine, not so much the current and antecedent events in their lives, as the consequences of their actions. Male doctors can usually organize their lives to suit themselves, and it is reasonable to assume that any pattern they establish and in which they flourish is meeting their personal needs. (Women doctors who have domestic responsibilities have less autonomy within the existing social system, and therefore cannot be assumed to be creating a working environment which will accommodate their peculiarities.) By looking, then, at the gains doctors receive from their chosen pattern of life, it is possible to make inferences about their underlying motivation. There is an infinite range of possible kinds of behaviour open to the doctor, and I will confine the discussion here to two which pervade medical practice: the avoidance of anxiety, and the hankering after power.

Avoidance of anxiety

Fear about death is the extreme example. Related anxieties in the course of clinical work involve pain, mutilation and disability. Also there is anxiety about intimacy and sex, although it does not necessarily originate in the work or become intensified by it.

To point to specific anxieties is to make assumptions, but I feel this can be justified if some of the undesirable activities of doctors described in Part Two are thereby illuminated. The broad assumption is that death, pain, mutilation, disability, intimacy and sex have unusually powerful associations for certain doctors, which they find so disturbing that they cannot resolve them rationally in full consciousness. They therefore repress[6] the emotions surrounding the circumstances mentioned. They feel more comfortable once the disturbing emotion has been banished from consciousness, but it still continues to exist at an unconscious level and is liable to be activated by events which impinge on the doctor's consciousness.

For example, a doctor who has more than the usual anxieties about his own mortality, at the age of fifty, might be quite unable to discuss death or even use the word without qualifying it, making a joke about it, or using some euphemism to describe it. If he can avoid any discussion of death, he will. When he cannot avoid the subject, as when one of his patients has extensive malignant disease and is wasting away in one of his hospital beds, he resorts – quite unconsciously – to one of the familiar stratagems. He can simply pretend that the person is not dying, and repeat the tragically common charade which is acted out daily in every hospital in the Western world. The patient's condition is totally re-defined, so that the wasting is an indication for more nourishment and blood transfusion, the depression an indication for antidepressant drugs, and the abdominal pain an indication for further operation in case there is some intestinal obstruction.

Medical students and junior doctors who question the rationale of what is being done are in danger of being ridiculed and humiliated by their seniors at ward rounds or medical meetings, and may be criticized for being 'emotional' and failing to maintain 'true scientific objectivity'. This is a sorry and not uncommon occurrence, and it is embarrassing and confusing for juniors to witness an able person taken over by his unconscious anxieties.

Since many doctors act as though they have a real difficulty with the actuality of death, the question poses itself: do doctors have more anxiety than non-doctors about the reality and implications of death? I am inclined to believe that for many doctors this is true: a possible argument being that if the young person has deep anxieties about death, then one way of coping with them is to join those whose business it is to keep death at bay.

There are others also in the death business, so to speak. There are funeral directors, soldiers, priests, policemen, nurses, lawyers, life assurance workers, and various people who work against a background of death. Death is either the explicit basis of their work or else it is there by implication, but for all it has a particular significance, although this varies from group to group. Some will be accepting of death, others will be seeking it, causing it, or combating it. Perhaps these people have their own feelings about death which differentiate them from the rest of the population. However, the attitudes of doctors are of especial importance, because around half of the populations of the industrialized countries nowadays die in hospitals, and thus under the control of doctors.

This denial of death and medicalization of death has been the norm for so long in the West that many people regard it as inherent in institutional care, rather than as a defence mechanism of doctors, and, in many cases, also of nurses. It is not inherent in institutional care, and this is demonstrated by the kind of caring medical practice which can be observed in hospices and the better geriatric units.

Hospice care also highlights how far hospitals have gone to meet the emotional needs of the senior staff, rather than the needs of the patients. Once upon a time all hospitals performed the functions we now associate with hospices, but technological medicine has developed so far and many doctors have so redefined their roles that hospices and general hospitals now seem to be founded on almost opposite sets of principles.

In place of the impersonal, insensitive, detached and authoritarian style usual in general hospitals, hospices emphasize closeness between people and giving comfort through companionship. Patients are kept fully informed in hospices, whereas in general hospitals information is often withheld from them. Special attention is given in hospices to identifying the patient's needs, while in general hospitals individual needs are not normally considered at all. Hospice staff must have training in giving emotional support, but this is not part of the training of any staff in general hospitals.[7]

In his study of how various kinds of hospital workers cope with their anxieties, Keith Nichols,[7] a clinical psychologist, has argued that doctors deal with anxiety by becoming even more detached and physically orientated than usual. Nurses, by contrast, have their own, and different, anxieties to deal with,[8,9] and Nichols suggests that they are likely to respond in the opposite way to doctors, by becoming more personally involved with the patients, and by carrying out the doctors' orders even more automatically than usual.

Even though doctors may not have deep-seated anxieties about death, or abnormal fears about pain, mutilation and disability, they will have to work with patients for whom these are their immediate experience. They therefore have to develop adaptive mechanisms which will enable them to function consistently with people undergoing the great crises of their lives. Unfortunately doctors come virtually unprepared to cope with this aspect of medical practice. Specifically, junior doctors are ill-equipped to deal with people who are beyond cure, people who are emotionally distressed, and people in severe chronic pain – the techniques for proper pain relief are simple and are well understood in terminal care units, but they are not applied in general hospitals.[10]

Sexual anxieties in doctors have been, and still are, the source of widespread distress, especially to women. The masturbation story may seem absurd today, but it is a terrible example of how doctors, teachers, clergy and others can project their sexual guilts and unacceptable desires. Even today, in an incomparably freer sexual climate, many people feel that they cannot discuss sexual matters with their doctors. The patients may have some diffidence in opening up such topics; but it is the doctors really who inhibit the dialogue, as is apparent from the ready way people speak about their sexual concerns when given a chance. All operations around the pelvis, for example, and all afflictions of the heart, are likely to raise questions about subsequent sexual activity, yet far too few patients, and their partners, are allowed to discuss them.

Where sexual anxieties or anxieties about mortality actually 'come from', I hesitate to say. It is likely that attitudes implanted early on will be important, and also family habits and the socializing process in medical school, but that is very general. The only practical way to discover the origin of these anxieties is in relation to particular individuals – by observation of the quality of their reaction to specific patients (reactions of outrage, a salacious interest in the details of the person's experience, a visible display of heightened emotion), or by a willing and open-ended discussion of the doctor's attitudes and experiences regarding sexual matters and mortality.

Compulsive busyness can be seen as another avoidance mechanism. It implies a constant searching after something, even though, paradoxically, it often seems that the doctor is urgently trying to get away from whatever he happens to be doing. In a more general sense, excessive busyness suggests dissatisfaction with the present moment and a preoccupation with the future, and with what has not yet been accomplished. The style exemplifies the competitive and aggressive 'Type A' personality.

Being busy in medical practice means being in constant demand. I am not referring here to the situation of general practitioners in an influenza epidemic or to the routines of junior hospital doctors, as they are responding to circumstances outside their control; but rather to doctors who consciously or otherwise create a style of living in which every moment is assiduously filled. Engagements are scheduled close to one another so that there is inevitably a rush between them, and yet there always seems to be time for one more consultation before the end of the evening, when there will be papers waiting that have to be read before the start of the following day.

A doctor like this does not allow space in the day to ask himself what he is doing, and will see little need to do so because the response of those around him confirms his value. His energy generates keenness in others. His supporting staff feel that they are part of an exciting enterprise, packed with action and variety, and patients will be impressed by the sheer momentum of the busy doctor. Relationships, superficially at any rate, with supporting staff and patients can be very good. The doctor is emanating enthusiasm which stimulates staff and patients alike, and enables them in turn to nourish the doctor.

Along with perpetual busyness can go the grand manner and other appurtenances of authority and success, and they enable a doctor to avoid just about any situation he chooses. Apart from the specific anxieties mentioned, about death, pain, mutilation, disability and sexuality, he can avoid virtually all real contact with people. This is commonly seen in doctors who never see any patient without assistants of various kinds being present, who always interview their patients across a large desk, who never willingly halt their forward movement during the ward round, and who certainly never approach closer than the foot of the bed.

These are avoidance strategies. They keep the doctor sufficiently well insulated from the patients to protect him from the disturbing effects their distress would have upon him. He is not real to his patients because they perceive no evidence of a genuine person. He gives them nothing but his expertise – which may be very well worth having on its own – and he remains untouched.

Attraction of power

Issues of power, authority and control permeate into all aspects of the medical profession and personal medical care. Of course, it is what left-wing critics have said all along, with regard to powerful groups in capitalist society, but I had not expected to see these issues so dominant in medicine, nor so persistent throughout the history of the profession.

The question is why the preoccupation with power should have such a firm hold on so many members of the medical profession. There is a social or political answer: that it is an innate tendency of all groups to form themselves into powerful organizations if they get a chance. Certainly history seems to bear this out, but I would add the proviso that probably it applies more to organizations run by men than to those run by women.

At an individual level, there is no need to explain why people set themselves up comfortably if they are in a position to do so; and it is understandable if doctors organize their lives to their advantage. I am more concerned about the doctor who comes into medicine with the object of achieving a powerful niche in society, and I suspect that this kind of person is either materially ambitious or has introjected values of authoritarian parents and medical teachers. This suggestion makes the behaviour of authoritarian doctors intelligible to me, although it is not encouraging from the point of view of bringing about change.

Another, larger, group comprises those whose authoritarian style (using this term in a general way, not necessarily corresponding with Adorno's classification) represents a defence against the consequences of open relationships with patients. In an open relationship the doctor has to reveal his humanity and vulnerability, and also whatever anxieties he may have are liable to be exposed for honest discussion.

For yet another group, preoccupation with power and prestige within the medical profession becomes a substitute for enthusiasm. After a decade. of so of clinical practice, without the intellectual stimulus that comes from teaching and research, and in the case of academic doctors when the pure subject has lost its excitement for them, many doctors become disillusioned. Their work has lost the meaning it once held for them, and they re-direct their energies into medical politics and administration. They may do well in this new field, and make a useful contribution; on the other hand it may just become an outlet for frustrated energy, and never bring any lasting satisfaction.

Mid-life and meaning

A change of direction, which is likely to happen about ten or fifteen years after qualification, coincides with a phase – at any rate in the lives of men – popularly known as the mid-life period. This is the time, in the late thirties and early forties (or even into the fifties), when men characteristically take stock of the point they have reached in their lives. By then, doctors are usually well placed materially and have families.

At the mid-point of his life, the doctor wakes one morning with the realization that his life is in the Now, in what he is currently doing, not in what one day he hopes to do. For some it is a comforting thought; for others it can be devastating, especially those who have cherished fantasies about abundant success and distinction, but whose daily reality is one of professional and domestic routine.

This moment induces a crisis of meaning. The doctor is compelled to take stock of his life and judge its worth. For those with modest aims there is no problem. Others will begin to realize that their early expectations are now unlikely to be fulfilled. Many will find that they are living in a measure of conflict, with a constant need to balance opposing demands: notably those of personal life with professional life, and the inner and spiritual longings with the external practicalities.

Sometimes these contrary demands can be resolved. Sometimes the doctor has to learn that true resolution is not possible, and the best that can be hoped for is to be able to hold the opposing demands in a gentle tension.[11]

Often reactions to this inner challenge take the form of external activity. There may be a fundamental change in direction, taking up a new type of work altogether, which will be successful according to how well the new realities match the expectations and fantasies. There may be diversions, temporary or otherwise, such as love affairs, fast cars and yachts. There may also be some of the less desirable developments described in earlier chapters. Many of these will be associated with becoming an important person in society, with a re-channelling of effort away from people and towards organizations, with the inevitable fascination with power.

There is of course nothing wrong in a change of direction, quite the reverse. The trouble comes when changes are misplaced, and initiated by a crisis of meaning leading to a sudden jump away from a previously satisfactory way of life into another unknown way of life. It may work or it may not; it depends on the conjunction of the fantasies and the practicalities.

The search for meaning is perhaps the main preoccupation of people in the second half of life. Indeed Jung has said that *all* the people who came to see him in the second half of their lives (over thirty-five) had essentially a spiritual problem.[12] That is, they were experiencing a crisis of meaning in their lives. To many people outside medicine, this seems odd, since medicine, par excellence, should provide a life with abundant meaning. But it does not seem to do so for many doctors, which is sad, and also unnecessary.

This section touching on mid-life crises is related to men, because the concept applies in its usual form to men. Women have the menopause, but by that time they are usually settled into the second half of life, and it is hard to identify a comparable crisis point for women. Their lives tend to be more directly affected by domestic and family events than men's do. A man may carry on with his professional activities regardless of how many children he has; and illness, moving house, taking care of elderly relatives, and so on, may not affect his work at all; nor will most people expect these events to divert him. If women have domestic commitments they are often so occupied by them that they may not contemplate their own destiny until the children are about to leave home. If they do not have domestic commitments, then there are emotional hurdles at thirty, and again at forty when the likelihood of having children has more or less passed.

Whatever may be the reasons, the crisis of meaning is fundamental, and a successful transition into the second half of life will make for more contented doctors and much more satisfied patients.

Some word is needed about the position of doctors in countries where there are repressive regimes. Quite different criteria apply here. The pursuit of power in, say, the Soviet Union has a very different significance from the pursuit of professional power in Britain or the United States. Equally, doctors in totalitarian countries cannot be expected to speak out on moral questions. If they are brave enough to do so, the rest of us can listen with respect.

At the same time we can reflect that in the West there may be professional freedom for doctors to say what they like, but, to frightened patients, the medical profession can sometimes seem uncaring – almost like a totalitarian regime.

Part IV

Images of Medicine

12

Early Medical Alternatives

The biomedical approach has been dominant for more than three hundred years. Its advantages and shortcomings are well understood. It needs to be improved, but how?

One way is to look beyond the main stream of Western, or cosmopolitan,[1] medicine, to what has been going on concurrently in the same society at different periods in history. Another is to examine the origins of medical thinking in our culture, and the ideas which were displaced in Europe in the sixteenth century; and also medical thinking in other cultures.

This chapter is devoted to describing a series of unusual doctors who practised in the main stream of medicine, yet who maintained individual positions at odds with strict biomedicine. In the next chapter there is a brief account of some of the background to the principles underlying ancient medicine in Europe, and a note about their origins in the Indian sub-continent. Traditional Chinese ideas are the subject of Chapter 14: it deserves special consideration because of the potential of Chinese thought to enhance our understanding of health and illness.

The transition from medieval to modern encompasses a broad shift of interest from the whole to the parts. In the humoral theories of the Hippocratics and Galen, health was defined as a state of balance in the human system, and illness as imbalance. Thus to consider the person as a whole was fundamental to the theory. Once these ancient ideas were rejected, and once it became possible to imagine individual diseases and diseased organs, it became relatively easy to forget the person and direct all one's attention to the specific disorder.

One solution to this fragmentation came in part from a mixture of orthodox Christianity and the Renaissance hermetic tradition.[2] The Christian culture could reject the system of the heathen Greeks and Romans, and replace it with one based on God's revelation, which was to be found in the Bible, and also in God's creation, which was nature. From the hermetic tradition came alchemy, astrology and various occult ideas and practices. Alchemy was ostensibly concerned with the transmutability of elements, but in the twentieth century we can make more sense of it by regarding it as primarily concerned with individual spiritual or psychological transformation.[3,4] Astrology was (and serious astrology still is) mainly concerned with the relationship between humankind and the cosmos, and it relates to the macrocosmic-microcosmic analogy in which every part of the external world and the universe (macrocosm) was held to have its counterpart within the human being (microcosm). It is an idea that is important in early Chinese thought, and in our civilization was first recorded by Democritus.[5]

The dominating figure of the early period of change was Paracelsus (1493–1541).[6–12] He propounded an enormously complicated medical system derived from Germanic folk medicine, his own clinical observations, astrology, alchemy, the Renaissance hermetic tradition, and his particular Christian vision. He was thus a holistic practitioner, although he was volatile, suspicious, and temperamentally incapable of working with any other person. He was a passionate opponent of the old ways, of Galenism and humoral theory, and the idea that contraries cure. Paracelsus fought almost all the eminent doctors of his day in order to establish his own ideas, notably that disease was a real and independent entity (as opposed to mere imbalance of humours) and needed to be treated with specific, often chemical, remedies.

Paracelsus was a decidedly eccentric character. For a while he held an academic post in Basle which entitled him to give lectures on medicine. These turned out not to be on Hippocratic or Galenic medicine, as the authorities would have expected, but on his own experiences and ideas about unravelling the secrets of nature and disease. He dispensed with the customary robes of his office and appeared in public in a leather jerkin. To make matters worse, he lectured in German instead of Latin, which was a drastic break with tradition, since it meant that non-academic barber-surgeons could now attend his lectures as they would be able to understand what was being said. It was as though, in our own day, a lecturer in medicine appointed to one of our ancient seats of learning violently rejected orthodox medicine, and taught instead from an idiosyncratic school of alternative medicine, wore the clothes of a farm labourer and spoke in a thick regional accent, addressing himself to anyone who cared to come along.

All medical historians are agreed that Paracelsus is a figure of major importance, and today he is sometimes held up as an example of the complete physician.[13] But what precisely is the basis of this importance? And why, more than 450 years after his death, is he the object of so much interest?

Paracelsus' practical contributions included the conservative treatment of wounds and chronic ulcers, based on his belief in natural healing powers; the introduction of laudanum (tincture of opium) into medical practice; the use of carefully prepared compounds of mercury in the treatment of syphilis and dropsy; the recognition of cretinism and goitre as due to mineral deficiency; and the first treatise on occupational medicine, recognizing conditions, now known as silicosis and tuberculosis, as occupational hazards for miners.

This is an impressive list of achievements but it does not account for the fascination Paracelsus holds for so many people. More important is the way he could combine practical medicine based on empirical research with his religious view of life and his sense of the relatedness of all things. In particular, he saw the essential union between the sick person, the physician, the rest of humanity, the material world and the realm of the spirit.

In his medieval mentality Paracelsus felt the identity between subject and object. It was a projection of the idea of interconnectedness. He could not treat the human body (the microcosm) without reference to the macrocosm. 'Medicine can do nothing without heaven, it must be guided by heaven.'[14] This, and his spiritual approach to his practice, characterize the man, and they come out in these quotations from his works: 'Where there is no love, there is no art.' 'Thus the physician must be endowed with no less compassion and love than God intends towards man.' 'The practice of this art lies in the heart: if your heart is false, the physician within you will be false.'[15]

The influence of Paracelsus grew after his death, and many of his later medical admirers occupied positions in the main stream of medicine, practised in an outwardly conventional way and kept up with the new developments.

Early in this line of unusual practitioners, about one hundred years after Paracelsus, was Robert Fludd (1574–1627)[16–18] and he provides a bridge between the Renaissance figure of Paracelsus, steeped in the hermetic tradition, and the new chemical philosophies of the sixteenth and seventeenth centuries. He was a highly successful London physician, an advocate of the new chemical remedies, and wealthy enough to employ his own secretary and an apothecary to ensure the proper preparation of the medicaments. His outspoken opposition to Galenism caused him some difficulty with the College of Physicians, and he was only admitted as a Fellow on his fifth attempt.[19] Nevertheless, he went on to become a censor of the College, which must later have confirmed his respectability. He was a friend and colleague of William Harvey (1578–1657) and was the first to accept in print Harvey's views about the circulation of the blood.[20]

Harvey and Fludd shared something of an animistic view of nature, and Fludd's almost magical views about the circulation of vital spirits may have given Harvey ideas which led to his discovery of the circulation of the blood.[21] The two men were judged together on equal terms in their day on the continent of Europe, even though one was concerned with mystical–alchemical symbolism and the other with direct observation and experiment.

Fludd was also an astrologer given to producing complicated and beautiful drawings of the relationship of man to the cosmos,[18] an occultist and a practitioner of esoteric religion, notably Rosicrucianism.[22] This open mixture of interests might seem unusual to some people today, but in the sixteenth century, when knowledge was seen as a whole and no distinction had yet arisen between the arts and what is now called science, it was quite ordinary for someone to approach the study of nature using not only his rational faculties but his feeling and intuitive functions as well.

Jean-Baptiste van Helmont (1579–1644)[23,24] was born in Belgium, a contemporary of Fludd and sharing many of his ideas, yet more straightforward and analytical in his thinking, and easier for us to comprehend. He was one of the outstanding scientists and physicians of the seventeenth century. His ideas are said to have influenced Newton in the formulation of his third law of motion (that action and reaction are equal and opposite),[25] and that Goethe used him as the model for Faust's father.[26] Van Helmont's distinctive position is summed up well by Walter Pagel:

> The separation of components of complex bodies, the building-up of composites from simples, measuring and weighing – in short, chemical analysis and manipulation – were his deliberate choice, combined with meditation at the site of the still (the *athanar*), in a quest for intellectual union with the objects of his research and the divine power which had created them.[27]

Van Helmont believed that chemistry, which he called 'the art of fire', would provide the key to the secrets of nature. It led him to recognize the existence of discrete gases (in particular, carbon dioxide), and it is for this that he is best remembered in the history of science. However, van Helmont's conception of a gas is rather different from that of most contemporary scientists. He saw the gas as the 'wild spirit' which is released when a substance is forced by heat or chemical change to give up its fixed state. The gas is a spiritual form of matter which contains the essential nature of the substance, the *archeus* in his terminology.[28,29]

The most important of van Helmont's contributions to medicine concerns his concept of diseases as entities which had their own existence and were classifiable. This radical departure from humoralism had been initiated by Paracelsus, but with the greater knowledge, based on empirical studies, available in the seventeenth century, attention could be directed to specific pathological changes which were now accessible to anatomical and chemical analysis.

Although van Helmont was a brilliant observer and experimenter, he retained a vision of the union of all things, material and spiritual. He formulated it in external terms – the union of everything in the world with God. He was a cultivated and retiring person, the very antithesis of the bombastic Paracelsus who was always in the midst of practical medicine and controversy; and also of Robert Fludd who was constantly engaged in disputes, although of a more metaphysical nature.[30] Both Fludd and van Helmont had been deeply influenced by Paracelsus, Fludd pursuing the hermetic aspects and van Helmont the chemical. Van Helmont is closer to contemporary thinking than Fludd, although Fludd's vision may in time become more meaningful as people become more adept at taking in the whole.

The term 'Chemical Philosophy' refers to the activities of people in the sixteenth and seventeenth centuries who saw a way to understanding nature through chemical analysis. From the medical point of view, this involved an opposition to Galenism with its emphasis on herbal remedies and its intellectual rigidity. They were a diverse group, and gradually they separated into two main streams. One followed in the main Paracelsian tradition with an essentially mystical and holistic view of the world. The other stream was more practical and mechanistic, investigating the size, shape and motion of things rather than their essence.

All scientific activity in the latter part of the seventeenth century was dominated by Isaac Newton (1642–1727), and he is commonly portrayed as the arch-mechanist who gave mathematical form to Descartes' propositions. That is an over-simplification, as is indicated by the 1.3 million words Newton wrote on biblical and theological topics, and 650,000 words on alchemy.[31] These writings caused something of a shock when they first came under public scrutiny in the middle of the nineteenth century, as is indicated by the reaction of an early biographer, Sir David Brewster.

We cannot understand how a mind of such power, and nobly occupied with the abstractions of geometry, and the study of the material world, could stoop to be even the copyist of the most contemptible alchemical poetry, and the annotator of a work, the obvious product of a fool and a knave.[32]

177

Scholars have debated the value or otherwise of Newton's hermetic writings.[31,33-36] The most convincing view to me is that his religious and hermetic ideas enabled him to transcend the limitations of the mechanistic philosophy of his time. To advance his theory of universal gravitation and of specific attractions, he required some concept of force acting at a distance, and simple mechanics could not help him. His hermetic ideas about the interrelatedness of all things, and his belief that every material body is immediately present to God who actually moves the bodies about as though they were spontaneously attracted to each other, enabled him to formulate his theories, even though he did not publish these particular ideas in his scientific works.[37]

Newton had a deep belief in the wisdom of the ancients – *prisca sapientia*, truths about nature which had been revealed long ago but which were preserved in an enigmatic form to conceal them from the vulgar; but Newton was aware, as indeed was Descartes writing fifty or sixty years before him, of the explanatory power of the hermetic ideas which embraced the whole. It is a pity that these men are remembered mainly for trying to split up our universe so that we can better study the parts.

J. M. Keynes made these remarks after reading Newton's hermetic writings:

> In the eighteenth century and since, Newton came to be thought of as the first and greatest of the modern age of scientists, a rationalist, one who taught us to think on the lines of cold and untinctured reason. I do not see him in this light . . . Newton was not the first of the age of reason. He was the last of the magicians, the last of the Babylonians and Sumerians, the last great mind which looked out on the visible and intellectual world with the same eyes as those who began to build our intellectual inheritance rather less than 10,000 years ago.[38]

It was, however, the work of the public Newton that was to prevail over science during the eighteenth and nineteenth centuries, and the mechanistic philosophy in general was to predominate over all others. In the seventeenth century it was quite usual for men such as Fludd and van Helmont to blend their hermetic studies with their more orthodox medical and scientific studies and practice. By the eighteenth century this blending of the spiritual and the material was uncommon. That is not to say that people in the eighteenth century were not religious, rather that the hermetic style had become unfashionable.

The hermetic tradition continued, as Allen Debus, historian of science and medicine in the sixteenth and seventeenth centuries, has indicated.[39,40] There was a sequence of medical men, through the eighteenth century, who kept this tradition alive while practising orthodox medicine. Then, with the coming of the Romantic movement at the end of the eighteenth century, there was an upsurge of interest in occult matters, secret societies and the like, and a doctor attracted to the values of the hermetic tradition would again feel more comfortable.

In our own time this esoteric medical tradition is well represented by the followers of Rudolf Steiner (1861–1925).[41,42] Steiner was not medically qualified but he was a dedicated student of the works of Goethe, and was greatly interested in medical matters. He imagined several levels of being, so that in addition to the physical body and the ego (the conscious self), he described an *etheric body* (formative and developmental forces) and an *astral body* (instincts and emotions). This model enables those working in anthroposophical medicine, as Steiner's medical system is called, to take account of a greater range of phenomena than can be incorporated into the strict mechanistic models. The system has a certain amount in common with the teachings of Paracelsus, with which Steiner was acquainted,[43] and, as with Paracelsus, the spiritual component is fundamental – being, in Steiner's case, basically Christian with certain ideas grafted on from Hinduism.

Nowadays we are seeing a blossoming of complementary and alternative medicine. Some of these merely involve practical methods to remove symptoms by gentle or what are regarded as 'natural' means. Some are based on larger philosophical systems or cosmologies which can attend to the whole person by setting the person's sufferings, in body or mind, in some kind of metaphysical framework. This seems to be the essential advantage the complementary and alternative systems have over orthodox medicine, and it is at the root of the huge appeal of these approaches. Many people have a deep yearning to understand their afflictions – the meaning of their illness and the purpose of their suffering. Orthodox medicine fails people here. The complementary and alternative therapies succeed in part because they acknowledge the psychological and spiritual dimensions as well as the physical.

During his presidency of the British Medical Association (1982–83), Prince Charles tried to heal the split between orthodox medicine and the complementary and alternative medical systems, and this led to an inquiry into the practice of complementary and alternative medicine.[44] Unfortunately the BMA selected a working party of specialist doctors which did not include any complementary or alternative practitioners, or even any doctor working in primary care. These doctors judged various of the complementary and alternative therapies according to the strict criteria of reductionist medicine, and not according to the principles on which these therapies are based, so the resulting report, predictably, is

179

meaningless. However, the British Holistic Medical Association has produced a detailed critique of the BMA report which should help set the record straight.[45]

The esoteric tradition in medicine which has run quietly in parallel with the great technological advances is now emerging into the open, so that a dialogue between the orthodox-mechanistic and the complementary-alternative-holistic may become possible, just as it was in the seventeenth century, when there was an easy communication between representatives of each camp, such as Harvey and Fludd.

Although it is customary in the twentieth century to talk about the 'whole person', there is little room in orthodox medicine for such a concept. An awareness of the whole person, and in particular the spiritual dimension, is the distinctive feature of the esoteric tradition, and also of many of the complementary and alternative systems. It is this dimension, along with the psychological, which is connected with so much of the discontent with orthodox medicine, and which represents a major part of the contribution that can be made by inheritors of the esoteric tradition and the complementary and alternative practitioners.

13

Harmony and Balance in the Human System

Some concept of the whole has to precede any study of the parts; and even today when medical scientists are preoccupied with the parts, they have to retain a vague awareness that the parts are components of something larger.

Long ago, when it was not possible to study the parts very effectively, there was a relatively greater interest in the whole. Health was conceived in terms of the harmonious functioning of the organism, and hence the idea of balance. Illness, by contrast, was seen as a state of imbalance. In the past there have been valid objections to thinking about health and illness exclusively in terms of balance and imbalance of forces – as opposed to the biomedical or ontological view of illness as a distinct entity – but the actual idea of harmony and balance deserves further consideration.

It seems basically desirable to be in harmony with oneself and one's environment. Bodily systems, notably the endocrine system, function to maintain a balance of hormones; and disorders in that system are almost always due to imbalance – that is, deficiency or excess of one or more of the constituents. So what about these ideas of balance? Where did they come from and how did they develop? What lessons may there still be for us in this aspect of the Hippocratic and Galenic systems? And then, how did the Hippocratic and Galenic systems evolve?

Early Greek philosophy

To answer these questions properly would be to write the history of early Greek philosophy.[1-14] That would be out of place here, and I am not equipped to write such an account. Instead I will refer to five outstanding figures in the early Greek period: Heraclitus, Pythagoras, Alcmeon, Empedocles, and Hippocrates.

Heraclitus[5-7] (540–480 BC) came from Ephesus in Ionia (western Turkey). He was one of the early Presocratic philosophers who were constructing speculative theories about the composition and structure of the Earth and universe. For Heraclitus, fire was the primary element from which everything we know is derived, and he identified it with the deity. (Previous writers had claimed that everything was derived from water, or from air.) Fire, of course, is constantly changing, hence the notion that everything in the world is in a permanent state of flux.

> This world-order, the same for all [men],
> no one of gods or men has made,
> but it always was and is and shall be:
> an ever-living fire, kindling in measures and
>   going out in measures. [fragment 30][8]

Heraclitus conceived everything in the world in relation to its opposite. This story about his end exemplifies his philosophy, and also his eccentric habits.

Finally [Heraclitus] became a misanthrope, withdrew from the world, and lived in the mountains feeding on grasses and plants. However, having fallen in this way into a dropsy he came down to town and asked the doctors in a riddle if they could make a drought out of rainy weather. When they did not understand he buried himself in a farmyard (lit. cow-stall), expecting that the dropsy would be evaporated off by the heat of the manure; but even so he failed to effect anything, and ended his life at the age of sixty.[9]

Heraclitus had a predilection for riddles, paradox and ambiguity; and his writings read more like oracles or poetry than philosophy. The opposites could exist in a dynamic equilibrium, as is seen with the forces operating when a bow or a lyre is fully strung.

> Men do not know how what is at variance agrees
>   with itself.
> It is an attunement of opposite tensions, like
>   that of the bow or the lyre. [fragment 51][10]

The opposites could also succeed one another as do night and day, and they were not seen as separate or different entities but rather as two aspects of one thing.

God is
day and night, winter and summer;
war and peace, satiety and hunger;
and he takes various shapes (or undergoes
    alteration) just as fire does,
which, when it is mingled with spices,
is named according to the scent of each of them.
    [fragment 67]

Heraclitus' conception of opposites was different from that of Pythagoras (580–500), an older contemporary and native of Ionia who migrated on account of persecution to Croton (now Crotone) in southern Italy. Pythagoras saw the opposites as blending together by a law of proportion so that their oppositions were neutralized and they produced, for example, harmony in music and health in the body, and *cosmos* – that is, order and beauty – in the universe as a whole.[11] Heraclitus rejected this on the grounds that the opposites must be continually pulling apart and resisting each other. Heat and cold, wet and dry cannot exist together. Harmony, to Heraclitus, did not mean a blending of opposing forces, but merely indicated that these forces were temporarily in balance; and any disturbance would lead immediately to imbalance. Heraclitus' philosophy is dialectical to an extreme degree, and it envisaged an existence of permanent strife. He is quoted as saying: 'Rest and quiet? Leave them to the dead, where they belong.'[11]

In our age we experience the idea of the opposites overtly in debates about defence: whether we can ever achieve true harmony between East and West, or whether the best we can hope for is a balance of terror, with the proviso that the strife will break out once the opposing forces slip out of balance. In the Christian tradition, some groups see the conflict between God and the Devil in the same light – a struggle demanding life-long vigilance, with no possibility of resolution. Jung gained a great deal from Heraclitus, and felt a personal affinity with him, too.[12]

Old Heraclitus, who was indeed a very great sage, discovered the most marvellous of all psychological laws: the regulative function of opposites. He called it *enantiodromia*, a running contrariwise, by which he meant that sooner or later everything runs into its opposite. Thus the rational attitude of culture necessarily runs into its opposite, namely the irrational devastation of culture.[13]

What does the idea of opposites and continuous change have to contribute to our thinking about health and illness? Can the human

183

organism never reach a state of harmony, as Heraclitus suggests, or is some continuing balance possible?

The first writer in our culture explicitly to introduce ideas of balance into thinking about health and disease was Alcmeon (c. 500 BC). He was another younger contemporary of Pythagoras, and he also lived in Croton, where there existed what might be the prototype of holistic medical practice as we know it today. Pythagoras and his followers aspired to the good life, through meditation, good diet and moderation in all things;[14] and yet they were close enough to the well-established medical school at Croton to be able, if they chose, to take advantage of orthodox medical techniques when these would be more expedient.

Alcmeon's views can be summarized in a quotation from Aetius, commenting in the first or second century AD:

> Alcmeon maintains that the bond of health is the 'equal balance' of the powers, moist and dry, cold and hot, bitter and sweet, and the rest, while the 'monarchy' of one of them is the cause of disease; for the monarchy of either is destructive. Illness comes about directly through excess of heat or cold, indirectly through surfeit or deficiency of nourishment; and its centre is either the blood or the marrow or the brain. It sometimes arises in these centres from external causes, moisture of some sort or environment or exhaustion or hardship or similar causes. Health on the other hand is the proportionate admixture of the qualities.[15]

The 'proportionate admixture' (*crasis*), in other words, balance, is all-important in Alcmeon's system. Balance implies the interaction of two or more forces or factors in the genesis of disease. Alcmeon liked to make an analogy between medicine and politics, between the animal body and the body politic: each requiring a delicate set of controls to maintain it within its proper limits.

Perhaps Alcmeon reconciles the more decisive views of Pythagoras and Heraclitus. He does not see humankind moving towards an enduring state of harmony, nor does he envisage the permanent strife of Heraclitus. Alcmeon also takes account, not merely of two opposing forces, but of a number of forces, usually in pairs, so that we have the beginning of the idea of a system in which many forces are acting simultaneously upon the individual.

Empedocles (490–430 BC), a native of Acragas in Sicily, is generally credited with having formulated the theory that the world was made up of four elements, and not of a single element as some of his predecessors had maintained. The four elements – fire, earth, water, air – existed together and on equal terms.[16] This theory formed the basis in Europe of the elemental theory that was to dominate medical thinking for the next two millennia. The theory was considerably elaborated by later generations, and reached its full development by the time of Hippocrates, after which it continued more or less unchanged until the sixteenth century AD. The elements were manifested in the body by particular humours (*umor* is the Latin word for moisture), and associated with seasons of the year: fire was manifested by yellow bile and the season of summer; earth by black bile[17] and autumn; water by phlegm and winter; and air by blood and spring. There were also qualities connected with the elements: fire was hot and dry; earth dry and cold; water moist and cold; and air moist and hot.

Health, in this system, was said to exist when the humours were in balance, indeed this amounted to a definition of health. Disease, conversely, was the expression of imbalance. Physicians varied in the strictness with which they interpreted the humoral theory, and some were quite ready to admit the possibility of outside agents, such as poisons, as the cause of illness. Others interpreted the theory rigorously, the only exceptions being injuries.

Henry Sigerist has described humoral theory, and in terms that might have been used by any physician practising in Europe between the third century BC and the sixteenth century AD:

These humors are not fictitious, not mere principles, but are very real. Wound the body anywhere and you will see blood. Give a drug that acts on phlegm and the individual will vomit phlegm, or bile if you give him a cholagogic remedy. Similarly he will evacuate black bile in response to certain drugs. This happens in every season, no matter how old the individual is. The physician must always consider the seasons, since they have a definite influence upon the humors. Phlegm, the coldest of all humors, increases in winter. At that time therefore phlegm diseases are prevalent, and you see people sneezing and blowing their noses. In the spring phlegm still is powerful but the blood increases, for it is moist and hot like spring. Dysenteries, bleeding from the nose, and other hemorrhages are not infrequent at that time. The hot and dry summer sets the bile in motion, and bile dominates until autumn. People vomit bile, their stools are bilious, fevers have a bilious character, and the skin is frequently yellow. Autumn is a dry season, beginning to be cold. At that time the black bile dominates in the body. Thus the four humors are always present in man just as the qualities hot, cold, dry, and moist are always present in nature, but the blend is not always the same, and this explains the different disposition of man toward diseases according to the seasons of the year.[18]

The basic principle of medical treatment which follows from humoral theory is that of 'contraries', that is, treatment by an agent 'opposite' to that which caused the disease in the first place. If the disease was due to an excess of blood, then the treatment involved removing blood. If the disease was caused by heat, then cold was applied.

Humoral theory is depicted schematically in the diagram. There are detailed weaknesses in such a theory but these do not matter in the present discussion, and humoral theory and the ideas which led to it are only under consideration with regard to the ideas about harmony and balance within the individual.

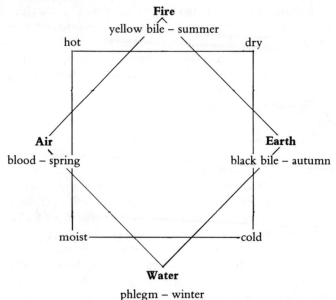

The fully-developed Hippocratic schema incorporating the four elements, their humours and related seasons. Between each of these are the qualities that relate to each pair.

Traditional Indian medicine

It is tempting to suppose that the Greeks, who created so much, also created, on their own, the whole of their theories about the origin and composition of the world. The sixth and fifth centuries BC certainly were a period of great intellectual growth, but Indian medicine during the same

186

era employed a comparable humoral theory, and so also did Tibetan and, to some extent, Chinese medicine. In India it was the time of the Buddha; and in China of Lao Zi[19] whose liking for paradox and acceptance of the inevitability of change (albeit gentler change) is reminiscent of Heraclitus.

Early Indian medicine, which developed into the Ayurvedic system, had a recognizable humoral structure a good five hundred to a thousand years before Greek medicine;[20,21] and there is good evidence of its spread westwards to ancient Greece.[22]

The Ayurveda is a great and elaborate system of medicine,[23-29] with two principal texts, the *Caraka Samhita*[30] and the *Susruta Samhita*.[31] In its original conception it was primarily concerned with the maintenance of health and spiritual development, and only secondarily with the elimination of disease. In fact the word 'Ayurveda' in Sanskrit means literally the science of life or longevity (*ayu* meaning life, longevity; *veda* meaning knowledge, science).[26,27]

The related system, the Unani-Tibb[26,32-34] (meaning Graeco-Arab), is widely represented in the Indian sub-continent and the Arab world; and it relates to the Moslem religion in the same way as Ayurveda relates to Hinduism. It is directly descended from Galenic medicine, which spread to the Near East in the second century AD, and which survived the collapse of the Roman Empire. It was then developed by Arab physicians, notably Avicenna (980–1036), and his *Canon* is still the traditional text in the Unani (or Yunani) system.

Ayurvedic medicine is based on an elemental theory involving five elements: in addition to air, fire, water and earth of the Greeks, there is space (or ether). These elements are manifested by three humours, called *dosas*: space and air are manifested by *vata* (or *vayu*) (motion); fire by *pitta* (energy); and water and earth by *kapha* (inertia). They are conventionally spoken of, respectively, as wind, bile and phlegm; and while this may not describe the concepts accurately, it does relate them to the more familiar Greek system. The three *dosas* are not quite comparable to the humours of ancient Greek and medieval European medicine,[35] which anyway had a fourth humour in the form of blood, but the differences do not matter here. What matters is how the Ayurvedic humoral theory operates as a whole, and in that respect the Indian system matches the Greek. Disease occurs when the humours are out of balance, and treatment is directed to restoring the balance: undesirable ingredients are eliminated (removed by surgery if necessary) and replaced by desirable ones. Infections are recognized as real but not as the essential cause of diseases, rather they are seen as external agents which upset the balance of humours. Unani

187

medicine is also based on humoral theory, and, although there are differences in detail,[36] for the present purpose they can be taken together.

In the clinical examination of the patient the Ayurvedic practitioner (*vaid*) is looking for evidence of imbalance of the three humours.[37] Very detailed accounts exist about the particular signs associated with excess or deficiency of this or that humour. Careful note is taken of the physical constitution, and there is a classification of body builds resembling the somatic typologies of Kretschmer and Sheldon.[38] This leads to a formulation about the specific imbalance of a bodily system and also about the personality of the patient – about the pathological state and about the person who is affected. The Unani system leads to similar formulations, this time expressed in terms of what are called the four temperaments (similar to those used in medieval Europe), so that their patients are described as sanguine, phlegmatic, choleric or melancholic, according to the respective preponderance of the humours.[39]

At first sight this can seem to Westerners like a step backwards to the humoral theories of sixteenth-century Europe, even though most of the population of the Indian sub-continent are currently treated by Ayurvedic and Unani practitioners.[40] These systems have proved flexible enough to incorporate, where necessary, knowledge and methods from cosmopolitan medicine; and many Indian practitioners are qualified in cosmopolitan *and* Ayurvedic medicine, and the two systems can coexist, even in the approach to a single case.[27]

Because of this flexibility we can concentrate on those parts of the system which have most to teach us. One of the strengths of Ayurvedic and Unani medicine lies in how, as a natural part of the clinical approach, the practitioners can take account of the whole person. To learn from these systems we do not have to accept humoral theory as an empirical truth. Rather we can accept it at a metaphorical level, and, through its idea of the harmony of the whole, think more realistically about the whole person than is possible in the Western system based purely on organ and system pathology. Furthermore, we can incorporate into our own thinking the implied categories of body, mind and spirit. In Ayurvedic and Unani medicine the uniqueness of the individual is valued; this contrasts with the Western approach where the main interest lies in what each patient has in common with others, as the diagnosis of diseases depends upon finding common patterns. The main aim of clinical research is also to find patterns so as to be able to make predictions, and these naturally will be expressed in terms of probability. There is benefit for the majority from this approach, but at the same time we diminish the significance of the individual we are supposed to be treating.

Regarding the person as unique can make evaluations of treatments

188

difficult. The question is not, does this particular treatment 'work' – that is, for the majority of patients; but will it work for this particular patient, with *these* personal problems, at *this* time in his life, in *this* environment, at *this* season of the year, in *this* part of the country, and so on, and in the hands of *this particular* practitioner? This is the true whole-person approach, and is familiar in the West in some of the complementary and alternative systems. It can make systematic study difficult, because of the large numbers of variables involved, but not impossible.

It can be argued that these a priori systems once fulfilled a useful function, but after the rise of empirical science they became superfluous and can now safely be discarded. The detailed practice of ancient Greek medicine, and in modern times of Ayurvedic and Unani medicine, can seem questionable, as a Western-trained doctor is likely to be sceptical about any system not based on anatomy, physiology and pathology. But such a judgement would miss the point. What these systems have to offer us lies in their conception of the whole person. We do not, in the West, need any help in understanding the parts. We do need help in comprehending the whole and comprehending how the parts interact. We do need help with the spiritual aspect of illness, or, to simplify that concept, with the aspect of illness that has to do with meaning.

14

The Dao and Chinese Medicine

Cosmopolitan, or Western, medicine is linked to no explicit philosophical system, and its advocates like to imagine themselves as purely empirical. Ayurvedic medicine, because of its great antiquity, has developed its own philosophical basis although it rests firmly in Hinduism. Traditional Chinese medicine is so intimately bound up with its philosophical roots that it cannot be comprehended without reference to Daoism (Taoism)[1] and, to a lesser extent, to Confucianism.

In Chinese medicine we are dealing with a highly developed theoretical system, so the practice – as traditionally described – is closely integrated with the theory. The theory, in turn, derives from the special Chinese type of thinking and cognition. I believe the Chinese mode of thinking has a great deal to offer us in the West in our attempts to comprehend people and their ailments, and I will concentrate therefore more on these psychological processes than on the medical theory, and more on the medical theory than on the daily practice. Thus there will be little mention of acupuncture, for which Chinese medicine is best known in the West.

The categories of ideas which characterize Chinese thinking, and hence medical practice, are those concerned with the interrelationship of all things; the inevitability of change; and the pre-eminent interest in function as opposed to structure – 'what is happening?' rather than 'what is it made of?'

The Dao

The term 'Dao' (Tao) is fundamental in all Chinese thought, including the Confucian. The Chinese character for 'Dao' is the picture of a head (symbolizing a person) *heading* somewhere on a road, hence 'way', and hence 'the right way'.[2] 'Dao' is usually translated as 'the way', and may

190

also be understood as 'reason', '*logos*', 'meaning', 'providence', and even 'God'.[3] The Dao refers to codes of behaviour, to individual conduct, to a spiritual discipline, to that which unites nature and man, and to the universal force in the cosmos.

Daoism is the religio-philosophical tradition surrounding the notion of the Dao. Tradition says that it was founded by the sage Lao Zi (Lao Tzu) in the sixth century BC, and three of the works in which its teaching is set out are well known in the West. These are the *Dao de Jing*[4] (*Tao te Ching*), also known as the *Lao Zi* after its supposed author; the *Zhuang Zi*[5] (*Chuang Tzu*), which again is the name of its supposed author; and the best known of all, the oracle, the *Yi Jing*[6] (*I Ching*).

The nature of Daoism is such as to elude attempts at precise description, so I will merely refer to a few of the principal ideas and give some quotations which I hope will catch its spirit.

A fundamental idea in Daoism is change. Change and transformation is inevitable and systematized, as in the transformations of the five elements (or Evolutive Phases) – *wu-xing* (*wu hsing*) – fire, earth, metal, water, and wood. The *yin-yang* polarity also implies continual movement between the poles, and change in weighting one way or the other. The *Yi Jing* is known also as the *Book of Changes*. It evaluates the petitioner's question *in the moment* of asking. A moment later, because of the inevitability of change, the circumstances would be different, and the same question might receive a different answer. The moment is unique just as it is unique in the world of sub-atomic particles. Thus when trying to function within the conceptual framework of Daoism we have to abandon our Cartesian-Newtonian view of life, with its neat sequence of cause and effect.[7] That is not to say that there is no notion of causality in Daoism, or in Chinese medicine. There is, of course, but it is more subtle. It involves networks of influence, a range of relevant factors rather than a single, unvarying cause.

In the processes of change all being comes from the Dao and everything returns to it. 'Returning is the motion of the Dao',[8] and this applies especially to anything which develops extreme qualities, for it will reach a point where it can only move by turning into its opposite. This is similar to the *enantiodromia* in the writings of Heraclitus. The Daoist version of change was more gentle than that of Heraclitus, since it was possible to attain a state of balance in which happiness, health and good order could be achieved,[9] whereas Heraclitus saw permanent strife as the norm.

The idea of negative action pervades the *Dao de Jing*. It sounds like the very antithesis of how Westerners are taught to conduct themselves in life, although it is anything but a prescription for idleness.

In the pursuit of learning, every day something is acquired.
In the pursuit of Dao, every day something is dropped.
Less and less is done
Until non-action is achieved.
When nothing is done, nothing is left undone.
The world is ruled by letting things take their course.
It cannot be ruled by interfering.[10]

Those who know do not talk.
Those who talk do not know.[11]

The Dao of heaven does not strive, yet it overcomes.
It does not speak, and yet is answered.
It does not ask, yet is supplied with all its needs.
It seems at ease, and yet it follows a plan.[12]

Confucianism existed comfortably alongside Daoism from the earliest times until the beginning of the Han dynasty in 221 BC, when it became the state orthodoxy, and the differences between the two approaches became more pronounced. Where Daoism pursues the inner way, Confucianism looks outward to society, and is concerned with social control, the smooth running of human affairs, education and administration. It was to dominate Chinese life for two millennia, and led to a complacency similar to that engendered in the West by the advances in technology in the nineteenth century.[13] The Confucianists felt that they could solve all the problems of mankind by using their proven methods. This led them to apply their humanistic and sociological approach to the solution of biological and medical problems, which led, in the long run, 'to a perversion of theoretical speculation and an erosion of clinical and empirical research'.[13]

Chinese medicine had been declining because of the 'deleterious influence of Confucian values'[13] from the thirteenth century, and reached its nadir in the nineteenth. Confucianism, with its extreme paternalism, had an equally stifling effect on Chinese society in general, but this discussion of Chinese medicine deals with the ideas current before the decline. The account is based to a great extent on the work of Manfred Porkert in his book *The Theoretical Foundations of Chinese Medicine*;[14] and also, of course, on the prodigious contribution of Joseph Needham,[15] in his still-growing series of volumes entitled *Science and Civilisation in China*. For a more clinical and less theoretical view, I have referred to Ted Kaptchuk's book *Chinese Medicine*.[16]

As one who cannot make use of primary Chinese sources, I am struck by how different these and other accounts are from one another. It is not always clear that they are all, in fact, describing the same system. Perhaps it is like the Dao: there is no one true version, and all approaches have their own distinctive value.

The Chinese approach

Acausal thinking. Traditional Chinese thinking and cognition is fundamentally different from Western thinking and cognition. In the West we think about something – say, a disease – in causal terms. That is, we look for a logical sequence of cause and effect. Chinese thinking does not operate that way, and various words have been used to describe it. Jung writes of the 'synchronistic principle',[17] and has coined the term 'synchronicity', which he calls the 'acausal connecting principle'.[18] Joseph Needham uses the terms 'correlative',[19] 'coordinative' or 'associative thinking'.[20]

In coordinative thinking, conceptions are not subsumed under one another, but placed side by side in a *pattern*, and things influence one another not by acts of mechanical causation, but by a kind of 'inductance'. . . The symbolic correlations or correspondences all formed part of one colossal pattern. Things behaved in particular ways not necessarily because of prior actions or impulsions of other things, but because their position in the ever-moving cyclical universe was such that they were endowed with intrinsic natures which made that behaviour inevitable for them. If they did not behave in those particular ways they would lose their relational positions in the whole (which made them what they were), and turn them into something other than themselves. They were thus parts in existential dependence upon the whole world-organism. And they reacted upon one another not so much by mechanical impulsion or causation as by a kind of mysterious resonance.[21]

The idea of correspondence has great significance and replaces the idea of causality, for things are *connected* rather than caused.[22]

Needham also uses the metaphor of the dance to make his point.

[The universe] was an ordered harmony of wills without an ordainer; it was like the spontaneous yet ordered, in the sense of patterned, movements of dancers in a country dance of figures, none of whom are bound by law to do what they do, nor yet pushed by others coming behind, but cooperate in a voluntary harmony of wills.[23]

In the *Zhuang Zi* the connectedness is expressed in terms of the interactions of the different parts of the body.

The hundred parts of the human body, with its nine orifices and six viscera, are all complete in their places. Which should one prefer? Do you like them all equally? Or do you like some more than others? Are they all servants? Are these servants unable to control each other, but need another as ruler? Or do they become rulers and servants in turn? Is there any true ruler other than themselves?[24]

Manfred Porkert describes the ideas of connectedness and correspondence in terms of 'induction', using the word as in magnetism and electricity, where there may be interaction between two bodies in proximity but without there being any direct physical contact.

Chinese medicine, like the other Chinese sciences, defines data on the basis of the inductive and synthetic mode of cognition. Inductivity corresponds to a logical link between two effective positions [i.e. objects, events, circumstances] existing at the same time in different places in space. (Conversely, causality is the logical link between two effective positions given at different times based on positions that are separate in space.)[25]

The notion of connectedness and correspondence, in place of a sequence of cause and effect, led naturally to a system of relatedness between the individual and the cosmos; and there is in Chinese thought an almost exact parallel with the macrocosm-microcosm analogy[26] already mentioned in connection with early Greek thought, and with the writings of Paracelsus and Robert Fludd.

Qualitative and quantitative. Western science could never have made such progress since the sixteenth century without accurate techniques of measurement, and an adherence to a highly effective and universally recognized standard of measurement, for example, the centimetre-gram-second system. The Western way also involves classification, dissection and analysis of structure with a view to reducing everything to its ultimate components, and in the expectation that these will be expressible in numerical terms.

All this represents the ascendancy of the quantitative over the qualitative, and it has reached such a degree in the West that only quantitative data are really 'safe' in the scientific community. No one would offer research for publication in a scientific journal unless the descriptive material (qualitative) was stiffened up with some statistics.

Numerical information about blood pressure, the levels of oxygen and carbon dioxide in the blood, liver enzymes, exercise tolerance, and so on, is recognized as valuable quantitative data for understanding the function of a person's heart. Details about an individual's diet, habits, exercise, personal relationships, hopes and disappointments, questions about meaning in illness and the consequences of illness, are qualitative and are commonly disregarded – despite evidence of their importance – partly because they cannot be expressed in a numerical form.

From the patient's point of view, this emphasis on the quantitative can be distressing – the seemingly endless investigations, complicated drug regimens, and doctors who appear to be interested only in disease processes. The satisfaction of patients depends to a great extent on the attention paid to the qualitative aspects.

It is really quite difficult for many of us in the West to empathize with a qualitative system, at least I find it difficult. Take an example from cardiology. A few clinical virtuosos up until the 1960s could make astonishingly accurate statements about the structure and function of the heart using only an ordinary stethoscope. Since then techniques have been introduced (and not all of them are invasive or potentially dangerous) which can provide anyone with more accurate information than any clinical examination could ever reveal, and all are expressed in numerical terms. The virtuoso clinician is operating at an essentially qualitative level, while the investigatory techniques are quantitative. I prefer to have data in a quantitative form, wherever that is possible without distorting the reality too much. However, I would not want to be without my qualitative data, which at times can be more vivid and illuminating than the quantitative.

One of the most valuable lessons we could learn from classical Chinese medicine would be how to use qualitative data more systematically than is customary in the West, and also how to amalgamate the quantitative and qualitative into a coherent whole.

Quantitative statements (i.e. measurements of universal significance) rest upon conventional standards which are universally agreed. Qualitative statements (i.e. evaluations of universal significance) rest upon similar standards. Quantitative statements in the West are highly developed; qualitative statements in the scientific community tend to be relatively crude – for example, north-south (poles of a magnet), positive-negative (charges) or left spin-right spin. Manfred Porkert has attempted to explain to Westerners the subtlety of the Chinese qualitative system in relation to medicine. He uses the basic standards of value common to all Chinese science: the yin-yang polarity, and the Five Evolutive Phases.

Basic concepts

Yin-yang theory gives Chinese thinking its distinctive quality and it permeates the whole of Chinese culture. Yin and yang represent the polar points of an inseparable duality. They are not opposing forces, nor material entities, and are best seen as a construct which defines reality in terms of polarities. Yin-yang is a label which describes how things function in relation to other things, and to the universe as a whole. In yin-yang theory nothing is conceived in isolation but always in relation to something else. Neither is anything conceived as unchanging because change is fundamental, as it is in the Dao.

Evidence that reality was perceived in polar terms goes back to the second millennium BC in the form of motifs depicted on cult bronzes of the Shang period. The earliest actual descriptions represent yin and yang respectively as the shady and sunny aspects of a mountain; and by the second century BC the duality was blended into the inseparable combination known as the yin-yang.[27]

Yin and yang are inseparable in the sense that the poles of a magnet are inseparable. If a magnet is divided into two we get two magnets, each with a north pole and a south pole.

Everything has a yin aspect and a yang aspect. Time can be divided into night (yin) and day (yang); species into female and male; temperature into cold and hot. Yin and yang depend on one another for definition. Yin and yang also control each other to maintain a balance, and can transform into each other.[28]

Although yin and yang may not function in isolation from one another, it is permissible to deal with them separately as they may at times operate as qualifiers or adjectives; for example, one could speak of the 'yin' or the 'yang' aspect of an event.

Yin refers to building up, nurturing, conserving, condensing, consolidating, completing, etc. Yang refers to setting in motion, moving, transforming, expanding, being aggressive, etc. The yin and yang aspects are difficult to define in terms of what they actually 'are', but they can be summarized and simplified as follows:

YIN corresponds to all that is	**YANG** corresponds to all that is
contractive	expansive
absorbing into or within the individual	bringing to surface
centripetal	centrifugal
responsive	aggressive
conservative	demanding
positive	negative

These abstract attributes correspond to various natural phenomena called Primary Correspondences:

YIN	**YANG**
earth	heaven
moon (major yin)	sun (major yang)
things female	things male
autumn, winter	spring, summer
cold, coolness	heat, warmth
moisture	dryness
the inside, interior	the outside, surface
darkness	brightness
things small and weak	things big and powerful
water, rain	fire
quiescence	movement
night	day

From these are derived Secondary Correspondences; and in the West certain others are often listed which correspond variously to the original yin-yang concept or to the current Western idea of the 'feminine-masculine' stereotypes.

synthesis	analysis
feeling and intuition	thinking and rationality
holistic approach	linear-causal approach
introversion	extraversion
right side of the brain	left side of the brain
cooperation and mutual support	competition

Yin-yang theory can be summarized as follows:

– Yin and yang have qualitative, never quantitative significance. They are sometimes represented by numbers, but the [main] issue remains relations of qualities.
– Yin and yang are relative, and never absolute designations; something is yang only in relation to something else being less yang (that is, yin). An old man is yang with respect to a woman, but is yin with respect to a young man.
– Yin and yang are labels for characteristics; yin and yang are not ontological types, agents or forces, although they may describe things, agents, or forces.
– Yin and yang refer to modes of function; a thing is either yin or yang because of what it does.[29]

I doubt if anyone in traditional China would ever have presumed to evaluate a concept as all-pervasive as yin-yang. It is only we in the West, with our very different way of thinking, who would ever ask if it was worth while trying to imagine reality in polar terms. It may be an empirical fact that no creature is one hundred per cent male or one hundred per cent female, but need that concern us in our clinical dealing with men and women? True, we cannot conceive night without some concept of day, but can anything be gained by asserting this obvious point? I think it can, and part of the next chapter will be devoted to viewing the doctor and the patient in polar terms. Health and illness likewise lend themselves to this conceptualization, so that we may speak of health-illness as a continuum along which people may move, rather than two totally distinct states.

Five Evolutive Phases.[30] At first sight an explanatory model involving wood, fire, metal, water, and earth will seem like a Chinese version of elemental theory, comparable to the four elements of the ancient Greeks, and the three *dosas* in the Ayurveda. The Chinese model may once have been comparable with these, but since about the third century BC basic differences have been apparent.

The Phases – wood, fire, metal, water, and earth – each have correspondences, some of which have been listed already through their relationship to yin-yang. Fire corresponds with summer, noon, the direction south, and major yang (i.e. fully developed yang); Water corresponds with winter, midnight, north, and major yin; Wood with spring, east, and minor yang (i.e. developing yang); and metal with autumn, west and minor yin. Earth is seen as located in a neutral position at the centre of an imaginary circle created by the other four, which are placed at the cardinal points.

There are many other correspondences besides these, with such a wide range of possible combinations that meaningful relationships could be seen everywhere; and herein lies a great difficulty. If everything is somehow related to everything else, every connection, association or conjunction is meaningful: so how can one discriminate intelligently? This is the position of primitive peoples who see significance in everything that happens. Porkert, however, finds the concept satisfactory at the highly theoretical level at which he is working, as it is reasonably consistent, and it helps to organize the complicated inter-relationships that arise when one tries to comprehend the whole. Needham is more sceptical, saying that the concept of phases (or 'elements' as he calls them) was useful early on, and at least 'no worse than the Aristotelian theory of the elements which dominated European medieval thinking'.[31] Needham gives a table of twenty-nine correspondences for the five 'elements': each 'element' relating to a season, cardinal point on the compass (earth being at the centre), taste, smell, animal, number, musical note, heavenly body, individual planet, type of weather, style of government, colour, internal organ, sense organ, affective state, and so on.[32] Ted Kaptchuk writes as a practitioner of Chinese medicine, as opposed to a theorist, and he finds the concept less than satisfactory, regarding it as 'rigid metaphysical overlay on the practical and flexible observations of Chinese medicine'.[33]

We must take serious note of any schema which is designed to integrate the great range of phenomena that relate directly or indirectly to a sick person. We have nothing comparable in the West. When we talk about attending to the whole person, we usually mean that we have taken note of social and psychological factors. That enhances the quality of our appraisal but it merely means looking at more and more aspects of the person – at more and more of the parts – without any way of conceiving the person as a whole. The traditional Chinese doctors, we are told, were able to comprehend the whole. In Chapter 16, a method will be described for integrating the wide range of phenomena needed to make a proper clinical assessment into a model which should be acceptable to Westerners.

Japanese synthesis

Clinical medicine has not featured in this chapter, because my interest has been in the basic ideas and the Chinese approach to the whole, and how these ideas can help us in the West. Usually, our point of contact with Chinese practice is in connection with acupuncture, gymnastics, massage and herbalism; and too often these are promoted as practical and empirical activities devoid of an underlying theory. This is doubly unfortunate, since not only is their clinical value likely to be diminished when the underlying principles are omitted, but the general insights of the Chinese world view are lost as well.

Nevertheless, there is the question of the practical use of the traditional Chinese system, and what lessons it has for us, beyond being a rich philosophy of nature. Some kind of answer to that question can be found in modern Japan, as the Japanese are simultaneously exposed to both traditional Chinese and cosmopolitan medicine.

Traditional Chinese medicine was brought to Japan in the sixth century AD. It became firmly established there, with its background of Daoism, Confucianism, and Buddhism (which reached China in the second century AD); and was successfully amalgamated with the indigenous medical practices and with Shinto religion. The result is a medical system which, while essentially traditional Chinese, has been modified by the Japanese to suit their practical approach to health care, as many of the Japanese felt that the proponents of Chinese medicine were more interested in the theoretical niceties of the system than its practical applications.

There is a widespread use of herbalism, acupuncture and moxibustion, and massage in Japan; and a good many medically qualified practitioners also use them alongside their cosmopolitan approach. It is a particularly interesting aspect of contemporary Japanese medicine that there are around a thousand medical doctors[34] who practise a blend of traditional and cosmopolitan medicine. They are called *kanpo* doctors, the word meaning 'Chinese method'.[35]

The practice of *kanpo* medicine has been described most interestingly by Margaret Lock in a book with the unpromising title of *East Asian Medicine in Urban Japan*.[36,37] 'East Asian medicine' is really the proper descriptive term for what I have referred to hitherto as 'traditional Chinese medicine', as the system is spread around the Far East to Japan, Korea, Taiwan,[38] Hong Kong and parts of South-East Asia.

Margaret Lock surveyed the practice of East Asian medicine in Kyoto, a former capital of Japan which has a population of 1.4 million. She described the practice in the *kanpo* clinics which are private, and to which patients mainly refer themselves. At one *kanpo* clinic, for example, there are five doctors, graduates of Kyoto medical school, and mostly related to the senior doctor. In addition to the doctors, there are six nurses, two dietitians, three pharmacists, two laboratory technicians, an X-ray technician, and one licensed acupuncturist. All the doctors themselves practise acupuncture and moxibustion. There is a well-equipped laboratory and an X-ray machine in the building.[39]

The patients are subjected to an intriguing mixture of cosmopolitan and East Asian history-taking and examination, followed by whatever laboratory tests and X-rays are judged necessary. In addition to a conventional Western physical examination, the skin is examined – especially the face and palms – to determine dietary deficiency or excess, water retention and nervousness. The tongue is inspected to see if it is in a yin or yang state. The pulses are taken in the East Asian style;[40] and the abdomen, after routine palpation, is examined for areas of increased or decreased muscle tension and fluid retention. All this helps the doctors in deciding whether overall the patient is in a yin or yang state.[41]

The records are kept on diagnostic forms printed partly in German[42] (where the 'cosmopolitan' data were recorded) and partly in Japanese (for the 'East Asian' data).

The *kanpo* doctors spend more time with their patients than is usual in cosmopolitan medicine in Japan. They look for single causes of disease, and are also interested in the state of balance within the individual and in relation to the environment. They hold cosmopolitan beliefs about the cellular level of disease causation, use both cosmopolitan and East Asian methods of diagnosis, and a totally traditional system of therapy.[43]

Their philosophy is essentially Daoist, denying the possibility of a state of perfect health, since the body is constantly changing in its dynamic relationship with the environment. The best that can be hoped for is a dynamic equilibrium, and the doctor's task is to try to correct small imbalances as they occur.

Since man is a microcosm, all the compounds found in humans exist also in the rest of nature (the macrocosm). The *kanpo* doctor tries to preserve or restore the harmony and balance, or, as is said in the West, the homeostasis; and he does this by methods which are as gentle and as 'natural' as possible. Hence the importance placed on diet and the judicious use of herbs. What the *kanpo* doctors deplore is the use of strong agents in the form of purified extracts of herbs or the synthetic chemicals which are the normal medicaments in the West.[44]

Having said that, the *kanpo* doctors will be the first to advise surgery where necessary, or the treatment of acute infections by antibiotics. They are very conscious of what cosmopolitan medicine has to offer, and also what their East Asian system has to offer. Broadly speaking, cosmopolitan medicine is best for acute, and what might be called mechanical, conditions (injuries, hernias, varicose veins, mechanical blockages); and East Asian medicine best for incipient conditions, that is, when the system is running out of balance but has not yet manifested symptoms or signs. The East Asian diagnostic processes are claimed to be able to detect these fine imbalances which are beyond the capability of cosmopolitan clinical techniques or diagnostic machines. East Asian medicine also has a great deal to offer those with chronic conditions, and it is of course the chronic conditions which are the great challenge to medicine in the industrialized world today.

One *kanpo* doctor likened the different approaches to the differences between the European knight and the samurai.

A knight must never retreat, he attacks with all his might until the enemy is destroyed. A samurai, on the other hand, learns to bend before an opponent, he allows the opponent to advance, but he is watching for a 'weak' point. He then induces the opponent to destroy himself by luring him off balance, and in his weak position one small blow from the samurai is all that is needed to finish the contest.[45]

The *kanpo* doctors have clearly taken from traditional Chinese medicine what has suited them, and what they can incorporate into their interesting hybrid system. They seem to have achieved a realistic compromise between treating the whole person, and the inevitable demands of people for the relief of symptoms, even though these doctors appeared unwilling to deal with psychological and social issues in relation to illness. This is more reasonable than it might seem at first sight, because the patients are steeped in the Daoist-Confucian-Buddhist-Shinto tradition, and possess a world-view that easily connects physical, psychological, social and any other influences. Furthermore, there is a gentleness in child-rearing, and a preparedness to look after and nurture one another at times of personal need,[46] that really allows the doctor to concentrate on the purely medical aspects. Thus the Japanese *kanpo* system is not only offering the benefits of traditional and cosmopolitan medicine but is taking place in a culture well adapted to receive it.

By contrast, in the West there is excellent mechanistic medicine taking place in a fragmented and aggressive society in which displays of a need for caring are generally not appreciated. Our culture matches our medical system, and does not value people who are ill. Perhaps this means that more is expected of the professionals looking after the sick person. In case I seem to be idealizing the Japanese approach, their caring seems to be mainly for adult males: women are not expected to fall ill, and consequently they pay more attention to preventive measures.[47]

Back in modern China, cosmopolitan medicine was repudiated as a capitalist invention in the early years after the communist revolution, and even more strongly during the Cultural Revolution in the 1960s. Now there seems to be a happier relationship between the traditional and the cosmopolitan, and visitors to China in the 1980s describe a mingling of the two systems, comparable with *kanpo* medicine in Japan.

The value of the Chinese approach

I would like, finally, to summarize some of the aspects of the original Chinese theory which can enhance the way we think about illness in the West – and about the whole of existence, for that matter.

Yin-yang theory defines the world in terms of polarities, and the desirable state is a balance of complementary forces. There is no such state as one hundred per cent health, rather we can seek a point of equilibrium between the polarities – health-illness. The fulcrum will shift back and forth throughout a person's life, and so a person's general state will fluctuate.

Yin-yang theory can be acceptable to the mechanistically minded in terms of cybernetics systems. These will maintain the mechanism in a state of harmony or satisfactory functioning; and positive and negative feedbacks will be activated when any parameter deviates too far from a predetermined norm. The concept is of course a good deal richer than that, as it concerns essentially how we imagine reality, but the cybernetic analogy is a starting point.

The five evolutive phases combine with yin–yang to provide a comprehensive and complicated design for integrating a person's illness with a wide range of phenomena, and, in a general way, for linking everything that happens. As it stands, I find it is too loose to use (so did the *kanpo* doctors), since everything can be seen as relevant somehow to everything else. This may be how it is in reality but it expands the clinical appraisal beyond my grasp, since I cannot handle all the variables or components of this gigantic system. In practice I do not think it is necessary even to try to take account of everything; and anyway this model does not imply causal connections between the components, merely that there are correspondences. The parts stand in a meaningful relationship to one another, as in Needham's analogy with a group of dancers;[23] and of course their relationship to each other is also always changing.

A common example of these processes in action can be seen in a family where, for example, there are teenage children. The members stand in a meaningful relation to one another, but the daughter staying out late cannot be said to *cause* her father to become angry. Rather, the daughter's action has to be viewed as one action in a constantly changing network of interactions within her family; and including perhaps her boy-friend, and his family as well. The father's response owes something to his general state of well-being and satisfaction with life, his other relationships within the family and maybe his own experiences when young; and while the father's response may have been *precipitated* by the daughter's action it cannot be said to have been *caused* by it. To claim that the father's anger was caused by his daughter staying out late denies the possible significance of other members of the family, the father's general state, and the boy-friend's contribution. The possible associations, when one looks at a family as a dynamic system, are limitless, yet they can be reduced by experience that comes from a knowledge of family dynamics and from having worked with families.

The Chinese system is entirely qualitative, and if explanations are offered, they will be in terms of value. In the West, and especially in the medical profession, there is a desire to have explanations expressed in numerical terms, so that the *quality* is reduced to a *quantity* – the quality of sound, colour and radiation is reduced to vibrational frequencies. Then, doctors feel they have understood the object of their interest. They have become accustomed to expect all statements, including those about people, to be expressed statistically – with indications of significance – if they are to take them seriously. They have allowed themselves to believe that statistics can lead them to the truth, whereas statistics can at best only give a probability, and an answer about the average.

To return to the family: we want to know what is going on in *this* family, not what goes on in families in general, although such knowledge of the general enables us to create hypotheses about the particular. But that is the limit of the possible value of quantitative, statistical information. The family is about relationships, and these are described in terms of value – warm, secure, threatening. It *is* possible to rate relationships in some numerical manner, which can be useful in research, but only a description in qualitative terms – in terms of value – is likely to catch the essence of what happens in a given family.

The qualitative approach involves the use of images, symbols and metaphor. Arguments are developed by use of analogy and what is condescendingly called 'anecdote'. Anecdote, which is one person's experience, is conventionally treated with disdain compared to the average experience of a large number of people; yet one person's life story does have value, even if a numerical value cannot be assigned to it. There is some sign of movement in the West. Attitudes among editors of medical journals have become more tolerant of qualitative data than they were in the 1960s and 1970s, although, quite rightly, they will not accept easy generalizations emanating from the study of a single example.

The objective of the qualitative approach is to provide internal consistency, not to relate the conclusions to numerical or other values. This is a difficult issue. I have uncertainties about many qualitative conclusions, because, although I may feel I have reached the correct conclusions, say, about a family, which can lead to useful progress in the treatment, with resolution of the difficulties, how can I know that I know? What criteria determine the selection of one item of information and the discarding of another? How do I know that I have made a proper analysis (or should I say 'synthesis'?) of the available data when the outcome does not happen to be satisfactory? Reference to external bodies of knowledge and to numerical values, to some wise person or even to the accepted clinical opinion of the day, can all be reassuring, yet it should be possible to stay within the experience of the patient.

The interpretation of the patient's story has to be sought from within the story, and not from outside points of reference. There are no absolute external criteria because the patient's story is unique and no external data can characterize it precisely. The external data can help in that they can point the investigator in the correct direction and help with sifting bits of information, but they cannot answer the wider questions, especially those dealing with the psychological aspects and meaning of illness.

Cartesian-Newtonian science depends on external reference points, such as numerical values: literary criticism and the investigation of dreams, myths and fairy tales proceed in a different way, and the objective here is to elicit an internally consistent explanation, carrying its own validity. Each person's life also has a validity of its own, and cannot be understood exclusively in terms of outside values. It is worth noting that physicists concerned with very small particles aim for the same internal consistency with their theories, since there are no completely satisfactory external reference points for them either. Such internally consistent explanations are not to be regarded as second-best. Certainly external reference points would be useful, but the fact remains that the system under consideration, be it a sick person, a family or an atom, is there in its own right and not just in terms of something outside.

15

The Wounded Healer

The idea that a modern doctor could benefit from being wounded in some way stands rather ironically beside the contemporary image of medical practice in which superbly well-trained men and women are using the latest technologies to cure the diseases of their patients.

Yet there is the ancient maxim from myth, that 'only the wounded physician heals'. Whatever does this mean? Where did the idea originate and what is its relevance, if any, for the contemporary doctor?

I once saw a priest who had stolen some gramophone records from a shop. It had not been an impulsive act but one carefully premeditated. He was immediately apprehended, and later brought to court. The fine was nominal, but much more painful for him was the publicity, having to face his wife, teenage children and of course his congregation. It was one thing a priest simply should not do. Certain people have trust vested in them, and to break this trust betrays their special position.

The priest was shattered at the prospect of returning to work and felt that no one henceforward could possibly have any respect for him.

When he did finally face his congregation the result was the reverse of what he had expected. People warmed to him, and came forward with an openness he had not experienced from them before.

'Oh, I could never talk to you before . . .,' someone said.

And another, 'I had been wanting to tell you this for a long time but couldn't. I feel I can now.'

Jan Morris, describing how people reacted to her after her sex change, said in an interview, 'Because I've had this particular and curious life, it means that I am alien to nobody really. Nobody's frightened of me and everybody in a way feels that part of me is part of them.'[1]

Many people, after devastating reverses in their lives in which their previous ambitions and achievements have crumbled, have found new satisfactions, often through improved relationships with others. After a life-threatening illness, a cantankerous person can mellow.

Colleagues of mine who have been divorced are generally better therapists for the experience. Naturally it enhances their awareness of adversity and of the pain of relationships. More importantly, the experience alters their standpoint: no longer, even if they want to, or feel they ought to, can they maintain a show of being immaculate and competent citizens. Their new status re-positions them. It frees them of a particular burden, and it enables them, provided they seize the opportunity, to meet their patients on a more equal footing.

The wound, as the term will be used in this chapter, is essentially the awareness that can flow from the experience. It is also a challenge, and one that can be taken up or ignored. Some people are sensitive to the implications of challenges and setbacks in their lives, and respond by asking basic questions about themselves and where they are going. Others require a catastrophic event to shift them to another level of awareness. Many, of course, suffer desperate experiences which crush them beyond recovery, and either lack, or lose, whatever ability they may have had to respond to the challenge. However, this chapter is about doctors, who, as a group, are not likely to be crushed by external circumstances, and for whom renewal after misfortune should be a possibility.

The idea of the wound

In the dualistic philosophy of Descartes, the observer could stand back from the object being observed: the subject was separated from the object. The investigator might be studying the workings of a clock or the human body but was in no sense connected with them. Such separateness was welcome, and indeed necessary in seventeenth-century Europe, where until that time the world-view was of unity in nature and the interconnectedness of all things.

The Cartesian separation of observer from observed is best regarded as a heuristic device. A century before Descartes, Paracelsus could separate himself from the sick people he was treating with chemical agents, and regard their diseases as real and distinct entities; yet he held to the idea of essential unity in nature through the correspondence between human-kind (the microcosm) and the rest of the world and the universe (the macrocosm). Perhaps we can do something similar.

In Western culture, the idea of polarities is implicit, and, as was discussed in the previous chapter, no being is *totally* male or *totally* female, there can be no concept of night without a concept of day, and so on. But there is less readiness in the West to accept a description of the *whole* of nature in polar terms, where something can only be defined in terms of its opposite. Then, for example, the concept of doctor would be meaningless without the concept of patient, and vice versa; and also the idea of the role of the doctor would be inseparable from that of the role of the patient. In orthodox medical circles, such an idea would certainly not be acceptable, and it is customary to behave as though the observer (the doctor) is quite unconnected with the observed (the patient).

Even though the idea of polarities has lapsed in the West, it can be useful in thinking about the processes which occur between doctors and patients. Doctors and patients are inseparable, so why should we not conceive them as a duality, like the yin-yang duality? We can apply this to doctor and patient in their personal capacities and in their social/professional roles, and achieve the duality of doctor-patient.

How, then, does the idea of the wound fit in? If we are to imagine everything in polar terms, with what is the idea of a wound paired? I hope the answer to that question will gradually become apparent, but the idea of a 'wound' – and hence the wounded healer – does not feature, as far as I know, in traditional Chinese thought. This account of the wounded healer, therefore, is something Western; and I would like to develop it in Western terms from its Western origins.

Polarities can be seen in medical and psychotherapeutic practice because of the contrasting, yet complementary, roles of doctor and patient. It is not possible to imagine the role of 'doctor', or 'healer', without the existence of patients, and no one can become a patient until there is a doctor in the vicinity. Within the 'doctor-patient' continuum, then, the doctor represents power, knowledge and skill, while the patient represents weakness, fear and helplessness; and the two roles are never completely separated.

The idea of polarities is straightforward enough where a practical role is concerned, since the two parties are acting in a reciprocal and complementary manner towards a specified end. The idea, however, can be extended beyond individual behaviour into the person and image of the doctor, and into the person and image of the patient. Hence no doctor is one hundred per cent 'doctor' and no patient is one hundred per cent 'patient'. Rather, 'doctor' and 'patient' are polarities, so instead of thinking about 'doctors' and 'patients' we should think of the 'doctor-patient'; and, for completeness, the converse, 'patient-doctor'.

The doctor contains within him an element which is 'patient', and the patient an element which is 'doctor'. In other words, in addition to his expertise and experience, the doctor also possesses the weakness and helplessness inherent in the patient role. For the practising doctor, the 'doctor' pole of the continuum is manifest and dominant, while the 'patient' pole is latent. But the latent weakness and helplessness is there, and, if it can be consciously accepted, it is what is meant for the contemporary doctor by the term 'wound'.

Wounds

There are frequent references in Greek mythology to the single figure who both wounds and heals, and also to the idea of the healer who bears wounds. There are other figures who simply carried wounds with them as an essential part of their being. Odysseus was such a one. He had a wound in his thigh early in his life; it enabled his nurse to recognize him when he returned in disguise to Ithaca, and it is said to be the origin of the Latin form of his name.[2]

The story of Philoctetes, as told by Sophocles in his play *Philoctetes*, and by Edmund Wilson, in his book *The Wound and the Bow*,[3] exemplifies the idea of the wound and its connection with healing.

As Heracles (Hercules) was dying, he gave to Philoctetes the bow Apollo had given him, a bow from which arrows never missed their mark. It was a reward to Philoctetes for lighting Heracles' funeral pyre.[4]

Later Philoctetes went to the Trojan wars with Agamemnon and Menelaus. He stopped to make a sacrifice to the nymph Chryse at a small island of the same name in the northern Aegean. Only Philoctetes could find the way to the shrine, and when he was there he was bitten on the foot by 'a malignant water snake'.[5,6] Philoctetes' wound was intensely painful and his loud groans interfered with the rituals his companions wanted to observe at the shrine. The wound went on to suppurate, and the smell was so offensive that his companions put him ashore on the nearby island of Lemnos, where he remained for ten years.

At Troy the Greeks were making poor progress in the war, especially after the deaths of Achilles and Ajax. They captured Helenus, soothsayer of the Trojans, and forced him to reveal why the war was going so badly from their point of view. He told them that they would never win until they had brought to Neoptolemus, son of the slain Achilles, his father's armour, and, especially, until they had brought Philoctetes and his bow.

Odysseus went with Neoptolemus to the island of Lemnos, with the intention of stealing the bow, but Neoptolemus objected to the deceit. They had to bring the bow *and* Philoctetes to Troy.

In Troy Philoctetes' wound was healed by Machaon, one of the sons of Asclepius; and in time the war against the Trojans was won.

One does not try to 'explain' myths, or even the plays of Sophocles: the images are what matter, and they communicate their own message. All I would say is that the invincible bow and its arrows had no power except in the hands of the rightful owner. Neoptolemus realized this although Odysseus did not.

Another example from the Trojan wars illustrates the interconnectedness of the apparently opposite processes of wounding and healing. It concerns the story of Telephus, a warrior and son of Heracles, who was wounded by the spear of Achilles. The wound would not heal and so Telephus consulted an oracle. Apollo advised that the wound could only be healed by the weapon which had caused it. Telephus went to the Greek camp and asked Achilles to cure him. Rust from Achilles' spear was then applied to the wound which duly healed.

Apollo is the Greek god concerned, amongst other things, with archery and medicine. He is 'the god who kills, yet purifies and heals'.[7] He illustrates perfectly the commingling of wounding and healing, the coincidence in one person of apparently incompatible elements but which add up to a whole that is only definable in terms of polarities, and yet is greater than the sum of the polar qualities.

The same attitude seems to have been held by the God of the Old Testament, and the idea of opposing functions appears in Deuteronomy[8] when Moses delivered God's advice and warning to the children of Israel: 'I kill and I make alive; I wound and I heal.'

Asclepius

Asclepius was an important figure throughout the whole span of ancient Greek medicine, and a complex one as he was regarded as part mortal and part divine. The best known early accounts are in Homer, writing around 800 BC, and there are frequent references in the *Iliad* to Asclepius and his two sons, Machaon and Podalirius, who were both warriors and surgeons in the Trojan wars. At the other end of the classical era, in the second century AD, Asclepius was the guiding spirit for Galen who wrote of his debt to 'the ancestral god Asclepius of whom I declared myself to be a servant since he saved me when I had the deadly condition of an abscess'.[9]

Asclepius' father was Apollo and his mother a mortal woman called Coronis. Perhaps because she felt neglected by Apollo, she decided to take a mortal man as her husband, but Apollo was jealous at such an independent act and struck her dead for this offence. The unborn Asclepius was removed from his mother's womb while she was burning on the funeral pyre and was sent to be brought up by Chiron, the centaur, who taught him the healing arts. The centaur, combining the wisdom of man with the instinctive power of the horse, had himself been wounded from the poisoned arrow of Heracles. Chiron's wound never healed in his immortal state, and he eventually forfeited the prospect of immortality for mortal death which would deliver him from the pain of the wound. Chiron was also expert in the arts of war, and taught Achilles the skills which he later used to such effect in the Trojan wars.

Asclepius became a great physician but over-reached himself in the end by raising a slain victim from the dead by the use (or misuse) of Gorgon's blood. Zeus resented this act of hubris and killed Asclepius with a thunderbolt, but he subsequently allowed him to be deified.

The daughters of Asclepius, as well as his sons, became physicians, and two of his daughters, Hygieia and Panacea, feature, along with Asclepius himself, in the Hippocratic Oath.

The Hippocratic Oath, which probably owes more to the Pythagoreans in the sixth century BC than to the Hippocratic writers in the fourth,[10] indicates nevertheless how the historical Hippocrates related to the mythical Asclepius – or more correctly to the healing cult of Asclepius,[7,11,12] which thrived in many parts of Greece and what is now western Turkey, although mainly at Epidaurus.

There was an Asclepian temple on the island of Cos, where Hippocrates (460–377 BC) was established. Members of the Hippocratic school were interested in the natural processes of disease, and in restoring the harmony and balance that was assumed to have been disturbed. The Asclepians concentrated on helping their patients to activate their own healing potential by means of their healing rituals.[12] These two approaches flourished comfortably side-by-side on the island of Cos twenty-three centuries ago.

Shamanism and Christianity

The Western doctor is expected to have medical knowledge and skill but little beyond that. In tribal and non–literate societies, past and present, there are healers who have medical knowledge to a greater or lesser degree, and who discharge priestly functions as well. They are expected to be skilled in the arts of medicine and to possess special powers which enable them to reach higher levels of awareness or to make contact with the spirit world.[13–16] These people go by a variety of names, according to their particular bias, medical or spiritual, but the term 'shaman' will be used here in a generic sense to describe them. Certainly shamans can be regarded as primordial psychotherapists; and in societies where all illness is conceived in terms of the activities of supernatural forces requiring intervention at a spiritual level (rather than as a natural process to be dealt with on a practical level), shamans can be regarded as the primordial physicians also.

The shamanistic conception of illness depends on the belief that human beings are part of a larger cosmic order, and that illness is due to some disturbance of this larger system. The shaman's efforts, in part, are directed towards restoring the balance, even though the immediate illness was the result of divine or malevolent intervention. The shamans usually hold a primitive world view, which means essentially that everything that happens or exists in the world is somehow connected with everything else. It is easy therefore to find meanings behind events; and this was the case in the earliest Chinese philosophies, before they were subjected to the rigours (such as they were) of Daoist and Confucian thinkers.

My interest in shamans and the reason for discussing their activities here lies in the special role they have in their societies. This position is attained through their own psychological journey, involving a symbolic death and rebirth: in other words, it is a journey into the spirit world. They may also validate their position as people who have the ability to communicate with the spirits by going into trances, and by possessing an affliction, such as epilepsy with convulsions, which could be taken as direct evidence of the presence of supernatural power within them. A number of shamans have been known to have had, or to have described themselves as having had, psychological symptoms and difficulties in the past. This has naturally led some sceptical observers, trying to understand their bizarre activities, to argue that all shamans are crazy. Certainly there have been examples of shamans who were psychologically seriously disturbed but these are generally agreed to represent a small minority. A far greater number, in Ioan Lewis' words, have 'endured the experience of elemental power and emerged, not merely unscathed, but strengthened and empowered to help others who suffer affliction'.[17]

The essential feature of the shaman's experience is not merely the spiritual or psychological confrontation, or a physical or psychological affliction, but that the shaman has been able to assimilate the experience into his (or her) own being. In the case of an affliction, he may have recovered from it or have learned to live with it: in either event he will have related to his wound (to use the Western term) in a creative way, so that through it he can relieve others in need. Where the initiating experience has been a psychological or a spiritual one, the idea of the wound still holds, as such a person is transformed by the experience. A direct experience of the unconscious, or of the Spirit, is itself a wound.

In the Christian culture the principle of a healer who carries a wound is exemplified in the person of Jesus. Nothing is known of whatever travails he may have experienced early in his life, although after his baptism by John the Baptist he endured forty days and nights of fasting in the wilderness, during which he met the temptations of the Devil.[18] What is clearer is how his style changed after the critical scene in the Garden of Gethsemane. According to W. H. Vanstone,[19] the text of Mark's gospel indicates that Jesus was constantly active and, in grammatical terms, the subject of almost all the verbs referring to events in which he was involved. In other words, Jesus was very much in charge of what was going on around him. After the events in the Garden of Gethsemane, his position changed entirely. He was no longer active and initiating but passive and accepting. The biblical text shows him then as the recipient; things henceforward were to be done to him. In the remainder of his life, Jesus made no effort to control events, and allowed himself to be carried along towards the predictable end; through public humiliation, chastisement and, finally, crucifixion.

After Jesus' seizure in the Garden of Gethsemane, he moved from an active state into a 'wounded' state. His weakness was manifest as he entered the stage of his passion. In a sense Jesus was always a weak and wounded figure, in that he had no power or position in society. Even so he effected cures and influenced those around him. Yet it was in the time of his ultimate weakness that he bestowed his greatest gift. In his passion, Jesus was helpless as a patient in hospital is helpless.[20]

Some time after Jesus' death, in words attributed to St Peter, we can read: 'By his wounds you have been healed.'[21] At the time of Jesus' seizure by the authorities, Peter was to acquire his own wound. He had denied even having known Jesus, and he had to live with the knowledge of that betrayal throughout his subsequent ministry, as an everlasting reminder of his human weakness and fallibility.

St Paul wrote in his second letter to the Corinthians that God had said to him: 'My grace is all you need; power comes to its full strength in weakness.' Paul went on to say:

> I shall therefore prefer to find my joy and pride in the very things that are my weakness; and then the power of Christ will come and rest upon me. Hence I am well content, for Christ's sake, with weakness, contempt, persecution, hardship, and frustration; for when I am weak, then I am strong.[22]

The doctor-patient

The term 'archetype' can be used to describe the inborn potential for a particular kind of behaviour.[23] The concept is rather elusive but for practical purposes archetypes can be thought of in much the same terms as one thinks of instincts in animals. For example, birds build their nests when the time is ripe for mating and the production of offspring. The potential for building nests is present all along but it requires the mating season to activate it. Some people may prefer to think of archetypes as computer programs which are put into operation in response to appropriate commands. At least this analogy highlights the functional aspect as opposed to the structural, with software rather than with hardware. Jung tended to personalize the archetypes for descriptive purposes; and if we do the same and speak, say, of 'the healer within', we must not forget that we are describing an idea and not a demonstrable part of the human psyche. I stress this point because the concept of archetypes is weakened by people giving them a false substance.

The mother-child archetype refers to the intense reciprocal relationship which is activated once a woman has given birth to a child. The potential for this type of relationship is present in all women but it is not activated until there is an actual child.

The doctor-patient relationship can also be expressed in archetypal terms, and the potential is present in all people, healthy and sick. When the person happens to be a *doctor*, then the 'doctor' aspects are brought to the fore and concentrated, or, to use Jung's term, 'constellated'.[24] For the person who falls ill, it is the 'patient' aspects which are constellated. Someone might ask what would happen when a doctor falls ill. That would depend on which role the sick doctor was occupying at the time – the doctor/healer role or the patient role. If the ailing doctor had fallen seriously ill, he would clearly fall into the patient role. During recovery, or if he had suffered only a mild illness in the first place, then the precise role he was adopting might be more ambiguous.

These two polarities exist in the same integral relationship as in the examples already given from myth. The 'doctor' component, or the 'doctor' pole of the archetype, is knowledgeable and confident and well able to cope with any crisis. The 'patient' component is frightened and dependent. When someone falls ill, this doctor component is constellated in the doctor with all the attendant expertise. Simultaneously, the patient slips into the expected patient role, and the patient component is being constellated.[25]

The manifest, conscious or dominant pole of the archetype is obvious enough as that is what we regularly observe and experience, but the main point of the concept of a bi-polar archetype revolves round the function of the covert, unconscious and passive pole. It is an important principle in Jung's psychology that whatever is manifest in consciousness has its opposite (or converse) in the unconscious. Thus, a man has his traditional masculine attributes (to do with thinking and rationality) manifest in his consciousness; while in the unconscious are represented certain feminine attributes (again, to use sexual stereotypes, the feeling, empathic and intuitive functions). The point here is not that men necessarily utilize mainly their rational functions and women their feeling functions, although it may be a fair generalization, but that whatever functions are dominant in the conscious, their converse is represented in the unconscious. Furthermore, the more highly the conscious attributes are developed, the poorer may be the unconscious development, with consequent imbalance.

As the doctor prepares to treat a sick person, his medical consciousness is activated, and the patient experiences, we hope, a capable and confident doctor. Simultaneously the other pole is activated within the doctor, that is the patient pole of the archetype; and it represents the traditional patient attributes of fear, helplessness and a desire to be looked after.

The archetypal approach to the relationship between healer and patient gives us a model, or a language, for thinking about the problems that can occur in this relationship, with the hope that it will lead to a means of dealing with them.

I will describe some of the adverse reactions which occur when the patient pole of the doctor-patient archetype is not accepted consciously by the doctor; and then go on to the way in which the whole issue can be managed constructively, with the patient pole acknowledged and incorporated into the doctor's practice.

If the patient pole of the archetype is suppressed from consciousness altogether, we have the familiar, brash, all-knowing doctor, who dispenses treatments, advises and carries out surgical operations, without ever acknowledging that there is any more to illness than pathology requiring attention. The patient's experience is disregarded because the doctor's sensitivity is suppressed. He is acting as though illness were devoid of emotional significance. He has shut off from consciousness his awareness of experiences which are the converse of those of a rational doctor, and therefore he cannot, or will not, recognize any feeling in the patient.

Another undesirable way of dealing with the patient pole of the archetype within the doctor is to project it on to the patient. Projection, by definition, can only involve aspects of which an individual is not conscious. The doctor cannot project his conscious doctor pole, only the unconscious patient pole where there are represented attributes which he cannot acknowledge consciously: such as his need for intimacy and dependancy, his need to care, his need for respect and admiration – nearly all of which would lead him to bind patients to him in a dependent way. He shifts the dimly perceived weakness within himself on to his patients, who therefore carry a double burden of weakness – their own and the doctor's. This type of doctor is dominating and all-powerful, and he pushes his patients into the utterly supine and helpless position familiar to so many sick people today. The doctor has all the information and the patient knows nothing. Such a doctor requires helpless and uninformed patients to carry his unacknowledged weakness for him; and the more highly technological the medical practice the less the patient can participate constructively unless the doctor permits it.

Turning now to the *patient*, we have the converse archetypal pattern: what might be called the patient-doctor. When someone falls ill, the patient–doctor archetype is activated, with the patient pole manifest. The doctor pole is covert and latent. Since in orthodox medicine the initiative lies with the doctor, the patient's only opportunity for participation is in responding to the doctor's lead; so to a great extent it is the doctor who determines how the sick person will cope with illness. In archetypal terms, the crucial aspect of this process from the patient's point of view is not the patient pole, which is obvious, but the doctor pole (perhaps more realistically called the healer pole), for it carries the patient's potential for self-healing.

Albert Schweitzer made the same point, when explaining to a sceptical visitor to his hospital at Lambarene, in what is now called Gabon, about the way the local witch doctor worked. 'The witch doctor succeeds,' said Schweitzer, 'for the same reason all the rest of us succeed. Each patient carries his own doctor inside him. They come to us not knowing that truth. We are at our best when we give this doctor who resides within each patient a chance to go to work.'[26]

The doctor has great power, either to activate the patient's own potential for healing, or else, because of the need to deny his own weakness, to suppress this potential in the patient who is thereby condemned to a helpless state.

Jung makes the same points even more strongly, with regard to psychotherapy.

By no device can the treatment be anything but the product of mutual influence, in which the whole being of the doctor as well as that of his patient plays its part. In the treatment there is an encounter between two irrational factors, that is to say, between two persons who are not fixed and determinable quantities but who bring with them, besides their more or less clearly defined fields of consciousness, an indefinitely extended sphere of non-consciousness. Hence the personalities of doctor and patient are often infinitely more important for the outcome of the treatment than what the doctor says and thinks (although what

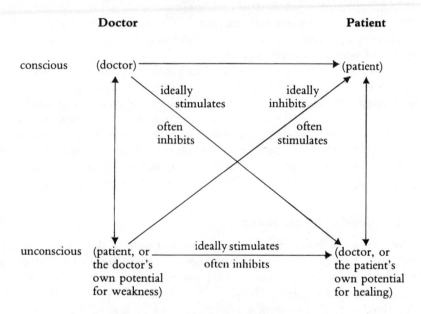

he says and thinks may be a disturbing or a healing factor not to be underestimated). For two personalities to meet is like mixing two different chemical substances: if there is any combination at all, both are transformed. In any effective psychological treatment the doctor is bound to influence the patient; but this influence can only take place if the patient has a reciprocal influence on the doctor. You can exert no influence if you are not susceptible to influence.[27]

At the risk of over-simplifying a subtle idea, I will try to give an impression of the complex interactions between doctor and patient at a conscious and unconscious level by means of a schema, adapted from Gerhard Adler[28] who in turn adapted his schema from Jung[29] (see diagram).

The interactions between doctor and patient are represented schematically. They involve interactions at a conscious and unconscious level, which can assist and impede the communications.

The general idea here is that there is a two-way interaction between the conscious and unconscious aspects of the doctor, and those same aspects of the patient. Ideally in this schema the doctor's conscious would be interacting with the patient's conscious, and at the same time stimulating the patient's unconscious – in this context the patient's own healing potential. The doctor's unconscious, or the potential patient in him, is

217

engaging with the patient's conscious and unconscious, implicitly acknowledging his own wounds or weakness, and thereby facilitating the healing potential in the patient.

What happens so often in practice is that the doctor makes a powerful conscious contact with the patient. At the same time the doctor's conscious and unconscious are inhibiting the healing potential in the patient by making him feel helpless and incompetent.

This kind of figurative formulation can be irritating to certain people because untestable assumptions are used, such as the theoretical construct of an unconscious mind. Nevertheless, it is a useful model for thinking about the complicated interaction between doctor and patient, just as Jung's ideas about archetypal behaviour are also useful in this respect. David Zigmond, a psychiatrist, has approached the same question using the model of transactional analysis.[30] Certain models have greater explanatory power under particular conditions, or may suit the temperaments of particular investigators.

Throughout this section on the doctor-patient archetype, there have been similarities with yin-yang theory. Both are polar conceptualizations, but yin-yang theory is all-embracing and defines the whole of nature. The archetypal examples given may be part of a grand theory of nature and reality but they are not offered here as such. They are no more than models which can be useful in trying to understand what goes on in the interaction between doctor and patient, and which can indicate how things may be improved.

The wounded healer today

Within the psyche of the doctor, the patient pole of the doctor-patient archetype describes the part of the doctor which is vulnerable and weak. It is this part which, in contemporary formulation, can be related to the wound. In ancient myths the wounds were described as actual wounds sustained in combats of various kinds, although it is always clear that it is the symbolic aspect of the wound which really matters. The wounded healer was one who had suffered some affliction, physical or psychological, and had assimilated the experience of it into his being in such a way that his experience could help in the healing of others.

The wound creates a new state of affairs for an individual after which nothing can ever be quite the same. In the example, given earlier, of the priest who stole some records, the wound involved a severe blow to his self-esteem and the concept he had of himself. He had, henceforth, to discover himself anew, and as someone different from the person he had been before.

218

All wounds affect an individual's self-concept in some degree, and they may (and certainly should) also increase his sensitivity.

In ordinary life, a wound may come from the experience of suffering, particularly of loss, material or personal. Examples are the loss of the integrity of one's body through the losing of a limb or a faculty; or from the development of a condition, such as diabetes, which involves life-long dependence on an outside agent. The loss might be from the death of a close friend or relative, or through the break-up of a relationship; or the loss of a job or of one's home.

The wound could be a profound personal experience: being close to death in an accident; being taken prisoner by terrorists or the agents of an unscrupulous regime; or in the course of an adventure in a hostile environment, such as getting into serious difficulties in a small boat on the ocean. It could come from the experience of love; from the experience of the essential unity of all things; or through a recognition of the world of the spirit.

A wound may derive from a personal failure. In a medical setting this could involve a clinical error, misjudgement or neglect, as when a surgeon cuts the common bile duct when removing the gall bladder, and everyone in theatre knows that he has cut it. It could involve a general practitioner wrongly diagnosing a child as suffering from influenza who later dies from meningitis; or an overworked hospital doctor who fails to get out of bed to see a man brought in with a head injury, and instead gives advice over the telephone which leads to the patient's death. Such events are of course deplorable in themselves, and the fact that some good may come from a tragedy is not a mitigating factor.

A positive response to the wound can lead to new consciousness and a development and deepening of the personality; and this has to happen if it is to become a creative force in the doctor's life and enhance his ability as a healer. Healers will often turn out to be people who have been wounded in some degree. But sadly the converse does not apply, as by no means all people who have had the kinds of experience mentioned are healers or even people of empathy and understanding.

The practical outcome of the wounded state is that people acknowledge within themselves their vulnerability, their potential for being wounded. This means accepting in full consciousness one's human frailty and weaknesses. Many doctors may admit as much in private: few will live their professional lives with the humility that comes from owning tacitly that they bear some blemishes.

The doctor can facilitate the patient's self-healing by consciously recognizing his own vulnerability. This seemingly simple step can halt the disabling of patients which is too often characteristic of medical practice. Yet it would be wrong to make it all sound easy. The first realization of vulnerability can come as an unpleasant shock, and especially to a doctor who has just completed his full professional training and is beginning to feel the agreeable sense of mastery that comes from being able to do a difficult job effectively.

In the case of the doctor, the experience which leads to new awareness – for example, a serious accident or personal tragedy – may cause him to withdraw for a while from ordinary life. The new awareness can be a disturbing business. This confrontation with another dimension of existence, that is to say, with the wound, may lead to a period of disillusionment and depression, such as may accompany any fundamental change of direction in life, when old ways have to be abandoned and the new path has not yet been found. Then, according to how this potentially creative period is handled, the doctor moves forward psychologically, or he remains stagnant. He accepts the reality and assimilates it into his being, or he rejects it and suppresses it from consciousness.

The doctor's wound, now, corresponds to the patient pole of the doctor-patient archetype, the doctor bearing the *potential* for pain and suffering which is explicit in the patient. Acknowledging honestly the patient pole of the archetype enables the doctor to allow the actual patient to be other than the passive recipient of medical care. The doctor helps the patient to mobilize whatever healing potential lies within, that is, in the present model, the doctor pole of that doctor-patient archetype which is within the patient.

Three ideas have been linked here: the idea that the doctor acknowledges a wound or at any rate a sense of vulnerability; that every doctor can see himself as part patient as well as being healer; and that each patient has a potential for self-healing provided the doctor concedes it. They derive from ancient concepts yet are as fresh today as they ever were, although reformulated here in psychological language.

Although the passage to the 'wounded' state may not be easy, there can be great relief from having arrived there, or even from having taken the first step away from the notion of the assured, detached, objective and self-controlled doctor inculcated into students in medical schools. The ideal of being the exemplary citizen, possessed of special medical wisdom and skill, is bound to lead to disappointment later in life when the realities of practice show it to be false. The doctor who openly admits that he is not all-powerful and all-knowing relieves himself of an impossible burden. He can then allow patients to participate in the healing process which leads not only to more effective practice but also to a much more satisfactory life for the doctor.

220

Part V

Re-Visioning Medicine

16

The Whole, Health and Systems

'Re-visioning' is a word I have borrowed[1] to describe looking afresh: doctors looking afresh at illness, at their clinical practice, at their social role, and at themselves. The purpose of this last part of the book is not to provide answers, so much as to resolve difficulties and ask better questions; rather in the spirit of Bertrand Russell, summing up his views about the value of philosophy:

> Philosophy is to be studied, not for the sake of any definite answers to its questions, since no definite answers can, as a rule, be known to be true, but rather for the sake of the questions themselves; because these questions enlarge our conception of what is possible, enrich our intellectual imagination, and diminish the dogmatic assurance which closes the mind against speculation.[2]

We are always being told to look at the whole person, but what is a *whole* person? What should be the range of our interest? Clearly we need to extend our vision beyond the level of individual organ or system pathology, but how far are we to go?

Where the traditional Chinese practitioner seeks out correspondences, a Westerner deals with variables. The word 'correspondence' implies connection between phenomena and events, as these are all different aspects of one reality; a variable, by contrast, is a term used in statistics as part of the process of discovering (in the Western view) whether a 'significant association' or 'causal connection' really exists. Thus, the moment we in the West try to focus on the whole, we can fall into a trap because our language is liable to be analytic and reductive: we try to talk about the whole using concepts and language devised for the study of the parts.

223

In this chapter I would like to explore this business of looking at the whole, and to suggest a way through it or, perhaps, round it.

The earliest medical practitioners held the unitary world-view that was universal among primitive people. The world was one, and everything within it was interconnected. Whatever happened in one part affected the rest, and every event was, or could be, seen to be connected with every other event. Only the deity (or deities) stood outside, yet even so he (or she, or they) penetrated every aspect of reality. This was a unified conception of the world. It was the norm in Europe until the sixteenth century, and in many parts of the world it still prevails.

Since then, the European success has encouraged people in other cultures to think of the world in Cartesian-Newtonian terms, that is, in terms of the parts. This is a practical requirement for most contemporary scientific and medical activity; and only in the twentieth century has there been a serious attempt in secular language to reconstruct the idea of the whole.

The notion of the whole

It is interesting that the very scientific tradition that led the West towards fragmentation is now active in the movement to reconsider the whole. Niels Bohr (1885–1962) and Werner Heisenberg[3] (1901–76), both major figures in the development of physics in this century, were keenly aware of the need for synthesis and taking account of the whole; and they both noted parallels between their work and the philosophical and mystical traditions of Asia. Bohr even incorporated the yin-yang symbol as the central motif of his coat of arms.[4]

This new move towards the whole has come for purely practical reasons: because the mechanistic models based on structure rather than on function, and the general assumption that a study of structure was the way to full understanding, failed to interpret what was being observed.

In particular, it was the discoveries of relativity and quantum mechanics that stimulated this new development in the scientific community. The utter impossibility of making direct observations of sub-atomic particles, and the ineffectiveness of thinking about them in mechanistic terms, prompted particle physicists, especially, to challenge the mechanistic world-order. Certain philosophically-minded physicists have now taken the matter beyond their immediate needs and have in effect constructed new models of the universe. David Bohm is one of these. He is a physicist, sharing some of the ideas of Krishnamurti,[5] and has taken up the idea of the whole at its most extensive; that is, thinking of everything in the world, material and psychological, as an unbroken whole. He asks: 'How are we to think coherently of a single, unbroken, flowing actuality of existence as a whole, containing both thought (consciousness) and external reality as we experience it?'[6] Bohm, like Heraclitus and the Daoists, sees reality, not as something static, but something always moving. He uses the image of 'the flowing stream, whose substance is never the same. On this stream, one may see an ever-changing pattern of vortices, ripples, waves, splashes, etc., which evidently have no independent existence as such. Rather, they are abstracted from the flowing movement, arising and vanishing in the total process of the flow.'[7]

The stream is an example of the whole, the true reality; the vortices, ripples, waves and splashes are merely epiphenomena which in the ordinary way are taken for reality. This conception of an all-embracing reality creates enormous difficulties, as even observing or thinking about external events or phenomena implies that one's thought is somehow imagined to be separate from that which one is contemplating.[8]

For ordinary practical purposes (like clinical medicine) I do not think this point matters too much, beyond recognizing that the observer and the observed are bound together in a network of some kind. At a theoretical level and when dealing with sub-atomic particles, such considerations become much more important; although using two modes of thinking – one for the ordinary, and one for the very large or very small – suggests that there may be something lacking in both approaches. In fact, Bohm feels that we may be at the beginning of a new conceptual era, entering a new paradigm; rather in the position of Galileo when he began his enquiries. Galileo saw the shortcomings of the old order – the cosmology of the ancient Greeks and Ptolemy – but could not formulate a new order. The new order was discovered by Newton. Bohm suggests that there are new ideas (it is implied that they deal with how we imagine wholeness) which 'may ultimately carry us as far beyond quantum theory and relativity as Newton's ideas went beyond those of Copernicus'.[9]

A practical example of Bohm's ideas of wholes can be found in the hologram. This is a picture produced by a special optical process which causes each part of the picture to contain information about every other part. For example, if the picture is of a horse, and part of this picture is broken off, the broken fragment will be found to contain the image of the entire horse. The hologram can be contrasted with an ordinary photograph, in which the camera lens produces a point-to-point representation of the subject on the film. Break off part of the photographic print, then only the part of the picture broken off will be visible.

The hologram is an example of Bohm's 'implicate order' (derived from the Latin, *implicare*, to enfold or fold inward) in which 'everything is enfolded into everything'[10] – every part is found in every other part. However, the hologram is static, whereas reality is constantly changing. Bohm therefore uses the term 'holomovement' to describe the perpetual change, and to emphasize the importance of movement in his conception of reality.

I have described Bohm's ideas as they can form a kind of contemporary base line for thinking about the whole. He is a physicist and has presented his theory in scientific terms. At the same time he realizes that mathematics cannot tell the whole story, and that there is a great deal that has to be expressed 'intuitively, in images, feelings [and] poetic use of language'.[11]

In a sense we have come full circle. Some cultures have held on to the awareness of the whole that they always had. Westerners are beginning to learn about it all over again, helped in no small measure by writers such as Fritjof Capra,[12,13] who has developed in a most interesting manner the parallels between Eastern philosophy and mysticism and Western atomic physics noted by Bohr and Heisenberg.

There is a much more general awareness of and interest in the notion of the whole in the latter part of the twentieth century, now that people are coming to see the Earth as one great biological system which remains in balance, provided humans do not interfere with it too destructively.[14,15] This awareness has taken a long time to appear, because in the three hundred years up to the twentieth century, the question of the whole was largely ignored in the West.[16]

Bohm suggested that even thinking about phenomena implied a separateness from them,[8] so that if one was really to be true to the notion of the unbroken whole, it would be impossible to describe anything. In practice, the dilemma is that one must separate things in order to define them, and then connect with them (or otherwise influence them) in order to observe them.

In the holistic view there is an assumption of connectedness, just as in the mechanistic view there is an assumption of separateness – that is, that the structure or organism under study can be broken down into ultimate units which are separate. The assumption in holism is that the world cannot be broken down into ultimate units: the ultimates will only be connections. As Heisenberg put it with regard to quantum theory:

When one compares this order with older classifications that belong to earlier stages of natural science one sees that one has now divided the world not into different groups of objects but into different groups of connections. In an earlier period of science one distinguished, for instance, as different groups, minerals, plants, animals, men . . . Now we know that it is always the same matter, the same various chemical compounds that may belong to any object, to minerals as well as animals or plants, also the forces that act between the different parts of matter are ultimately the same in every kind of object. What can be distinguished is the kind of connection which is primarily important in a certain phenomenon. For instance, when we speak about the action of chemical forces we mean a kind of connection which is more complicated or in any case different from that expressed in Newtonian mechanics. The world thus appears as a complicated tissue of events, in which connections of different kinds alternate or overlap or combine and thereby determine the texture of the whole.[17]

Holism and holistic medicine

In 1926 came the first work in this century, as far as I know, explicitly devoted to the whole, and from which we have acquired the word 'holism'. This was J. C. Smuts' *Holism and Evolution*.[18]

The word 'holism' comes from the Greek, *olos*, meaning 'whole', and the J. C. Smuts who coined it is the man better remembered as Field-Marshal Jan Christian Smuts (1870–1950), variously a guerrilla leader, fighting soldier, lawyer, prime minister and international statesman. He was also something of a philosopher, and his book, *Holism and Evolution*, is about what he regarded as an inherent tendency in nature towards the formation of 'wholes'. To begin with, atoms, molecules and chemical compounds form 'limited wholes'.[19] At a more advanced level there are whole plants and animals; human organizations;[20] works of art;[21] and 'finally, there emerge the ideal wholes, . . . or absolute Values'.[20] This reads rather like a version of the stratified order of systems (to be discussed later), and it was contemporary with some of the early writing about systems in biology.[22] For Smuts, however, this ladder represented a natural line of human progress, and he argued that humans have an innate tendency to develop their higher faculties, beyond whatever may be required for survival of the species. He was writing in the tradition of 'creative evolution', and was influenced by Henri Bergson (1859–1941), A. N. Whitehead (1861–1947), and the theory of relativity. Today, the main interest of the book stems from the word Smuts gave us, and the fact that this remarkable man, who was so involved in military and political affairs, ever found time to write it.

The word 'holism' is now well established in the language and has accumulated a number of meanings. It can refer to any approach to a unified view of existence such as David Bohm sets out, or be used as an adjective to describe a healthy and balanced way of living. The word may thus describe an approach to reality and at the same time be value-laden to describe various attitudes assumed to be good. Just as in the society of mechanistically-minded people the word 'scientific' is regarded as laudatory, so among those who favour alternative or 'new age' life-styles the word 'holistic' is a compliment and an indication of a shared world view. This creates difficulties when it comes to trying to understand its principal usage at the present time which is in connection with what is called 'holistic medicine'.

Holistic medicine is a good thing, we are told, but what is it? No one has successfully defined it; and formal definition may be impossible since to a great extent it involves a certain attitude of mind. I will therefore say what I understand by the term 'holistic medicine' and hope that it will be acceptable to a reasonable number of people.

There are three main parts to holistic medicine: (a) conceptual, (b) practical and (c) personal.

(a) *Conceptual*. The holistic model of illness assumes that the doctor will take account, not only of the body, but of the mind and the spirit as well; and there is a further assumption that everything is interconnected, that all events affect one another, and that the organism is in constant interaction with the environment. Plainly this model requires the doctor to handle a broad range of information but not an excessive range. It is not the same as a statistician juggling an array of (possibly) discrete bits of information to see if there are significant connections: it is rather that the significance of the connections is assumed, even though the precise significance may be obscure.

Now, with the diffidence already expressed, I would like to describe three aspects of the holistic concept – body, mind and spirit.

The sick *body* is more or less self-evident. It corresponds to everything that comes under the heading of orthodox or cosmopolitan medicine, and involves pathological structural or functional change of any kind, temporary or permanent.

The *mind* refers to the psychological reactions to illness: what the sick person feels about being ill (worries about lost income, job security, fear of mutilation, etc.); also a variety of circumstances which can affect someone's state of mind, such as problems in relationships (intimate, family, with dependants), loss of any kind, personal or material, or difficult environmental conditions.

Other psychological processes – some conscious but the more

228

important ones unconscious – involve all that passes between doctor and patient in the course of their encounters with each other, as described in the previous chapter.

The *spirit* is altogether more difficult to describe, if indeed it can be described at all.

The spiritual aspect of illness refers to what goes on in the deeper levels of the psyche, and in the relationship between the psyche and whatever lies beyond. These are the levels experienced in dreams, and sought in meditation and prayer; and from which a person communicates with the ultimate or with God.[23]

The spiritual aspect has to do with meaning, with the special significance the illness may have in the course of a person's life. The illness is not being said specifically to mean this or that; rather, when it is viewed against the person's life as a whole, connections can appear between the illness and other events which give the impression that there is a pattern behind it all. It is a statement, containing a message – possibly a warning – and it must be waited upon with respect. Thus the illness may have a purpose, and needs to be accepted by the sick person.[24]

To some, this may seem like subjectivism and rationalization, but I hope that this qualitative way of looking at events will come to be seen as legitimate, and of practical value.

In the West there is more appreciation than there used to be of psychological and social factors affecting the aetiology and of course of illness, especially since a married person's death has been shown to be associated statistically with a higher than expected morbidity and mortality in a surviving spouse. But there is little general interest, on the part of doctors, in any aspects of illness beyond the physical, except for certain correlations with life events.

In the Daoist system, there are such close correspondences between all aspects of life that the body-mind-spirit triad is more or less meaningless; and all the more so since, as Joseph Needham says, 'in the Chinese philosophic tradition the need for a Supreme Being had never been felt'.[25] Ayurvedic medicine is closer to us in the West in this respect as there are deities in the Hindu religion. For that reason, this aspect of the Ayurvedic system deserves our attention: the Ayurvedic practitioners seem more explicitly than others (i.e. traditional Chinese and contemporary Westerners) to think in terms of the body, the mind and the spirit.

Another difference between orthodox and holistic medicine at a theoretical level relates to the placing of the origins of illness. In orthodox medicine, origins are usually seen in terms of toxic agents, invading micro-organisms, or diseased organs or systems. In holistic medicine the search for origins goes further back, so to speak. What goes for the 'cause' in orthodox medicine, from a holistic standpoint, is usually regarded merely as the pathological process which mediates the illness. An understanding of the origin of the illness would be sought more in the circumstances of the person's life, often in answer to the questions: why this person? why now? why in this form? The answers will seldom be simple or single, indicating that a particular event or time was significant. That would be mechanistic cause-and-effect thinking which holistic medicine is trying to transcend. Instead, an examination of the background to someone's illness can reveal a network of influences, a set of correspondences in the Chinese sense, which are related to one another yet not causally connected. This can be quite a novel idea for Westerners – that there may be a significant association between phenomena without any causal connection.

(b) *Practical*. From the practical point of view, the holistic practitioner should seek the best treatment available, regardless of the philosophy underlying it. Thus, in practice, holistic medicine should be pragmatic. However, the practical aim of holistic practice is not only to remove symptoms, but to help sick people take stock of their lives, to consider how they may have pressed their adaptive resources too far, and how in the future they can better maintain a balance in their lives.

Some of the complementary or alternative therapies – notably homeopathy, acupuncture, herbalism – have in common a broad approach to the sick person, even though the conceptualizations of the illness are different in each of them, and each approach has its strengths and weaknesses. Orthodox Western medicine also has its strengths and weaknesses: it is conspicuously good with acute conditions, injuries and other mechanical conditions; it is less good with chronic ailments and where there are psycho-physical interactions.

The holistic doctor should be sufficiently familiar with orthodox medicine and with the complementary and alternative systems to be able to make an informed judgement about what is best for a given patient. Holistic medicine should not become synonymous with complementary and alternative medicine, nor should it describe merely a gentle and caring approach to patients.

Deciding what is best for a given patient from the repertoire of orthodox medicine and the alternative and complementary therapies can be difficult; and it is doubtful if any doctor, however well informed, can make a truly detached judgement. A greater range of information is sought than is usual in the practice of orthodox medicine, enquiries being made concerning life events, relationships, attitudes to illness, and so on. The diagnostic formulations are the same as in orthodox medicine, and there will be riders concerning the actual person who is ill and that person's feelings and experience.

The choice of treatment depends to a great extent on the patient's wishes: some prefer to receive herbal preparations rather than chemical drugs. Some favour techniques which will allow their own bodily responses to illness to function at their maximum. The sick person's wishes are respected, and the holistic doctor tries to give responsible advice, which, apart from anything else, does not conflict sharply with sensible conventional Western practice. For example, a modern doctor would be regarded as acting irresponsibly in agreeing to someone's request for herbal treatment once acute appendicitis had been diagnosed. For many other infections, the judgement can be less clear. If someone with lobar pneumonia desires homeopathic treatment, the doctor taking a holistic viewpoint has to balance the advantages of orthodox antibiotic treatment, which would probably knock out the infecting micro-organisms, against the homeopathic remedies, which might stimulate the person's own immune system. The latter of course is nice in theory, the question the doctor has to answer is: which approach on this occasion is in this person's best interest? It is altogether easier to decide where chronic conditions are concerned, especially as the patient will probably have experienced various unsuccessful orthodox attempts at cure.

Holistic doctors are likely to make use of some complementary and alternative techniques, and some may have undergone formal training in one or more of these disciplines. Thus the holistic doctor, in addition to caring for the whole person, has to make a pragmatic and, as far as possible, unprejudiced judgement about the best line of treatment for the particular patient.

(c) *Personal*. The ideas and practice of holistic medicine make personal demands on the doctor and the patient in a way which orthodox medicine does not. Both doctor and patient have obligations to live sensibly and not to abuse their systems with harmful foodstuffs or hectic life-styles. Orthodox medicine is engaged in a small way in what is called 'health education', but nowhere is any serious attempt made to *oblige* people to look after themselves and do all they can to keep their bodies in good order. The main thrust of orthodox medicine is to treat diseases, not to maintain health.

Holistic doctors encourage patients to mobilize whatever healing potential they have within themselves. Patients are expected to play an active part in the process of getting well or adapting to illness, to be involved in making informed decisions and not simply be passive recipients of medical care. However, all people at certain times need to be looked after and nurtured, and this need must be respected. Margaret Lock has described how this need is recognized explicitly in Japan; in fact she says there is a special word for it – *amaeru*, meaning 'a desire to presume on another's love'.[26] People need at times to be allowed to be passive, and sometimes doctors have to make decisions for them. For example, a woman who has just had a malignant breast lump diagnosed which requires urgent treatment may not be in a position to grasp and evaluate all the possible treatments, involving various permutations of surgery, radiotherapy and chemotherapy. At such times the doctor has to be decisive, even when he would rather share the decision-making with the patient. To do otherwise would be avoiding responsibility and placing an unfair burden on a worried person.

This section on wholes arose out of a desire to find a way of serving people better by relating the diseased organ to the person, and placing the person in some kind of social or cosmic context. Clearly it is no longer acceptable or satisfactory to think only at the level of organ or system pathology, and to take the whole of reality into account is impossible. So where is one to begin?

It is unlikely that Westerners, however dedicated, are going to be able to think synthetically or holistically as the Chinese and Indian practitioners do, or at any rate used to do. We are committed to our quantitative approach, as opposed to their qualitative approach, and it is equally unlikely that we will change at such a fundamental level without a good deal of effort.

Therefore an approach is needed that can enable us to expand the range of phenomena that we can handle, yet at the same time not demand too much of a conceptual revolution.

A model of illness is required which can enable a sick person to make some sense of the event and the experience in its totality. This involves not merely elucidating the processes by which the illness came about, important as these are, but the relationship of the illness to the person's life looked at as a whole, with a past, a present and a future.

A satisfactory model of illness takes account, not only of the presenting complaint and its ramifications, but also of the person's attitudes to the illness and general attitude to life, ways of coping with adversity, the quality of relationships, and the physical setting of the illness, at home or in hospital. The model has to allow for worries more or less directly connected with the ailment, such as income while ill, job security, relationships with employers and subordinates, and also general worries about children and family, living conditions and the immediate physical environment.

The doctor is integrally involved in the patient's network of relationships. The pre-existing relationship between patient and doctor, and its fluctuations throughout the illness, will be incorporated as important factors affecting progress for better or worse.

The fundamental and elusive issue of the meaning of the illness for the individual may begin to emerge once the person's life is regarded as a whole. That involves considering not just a solitary patient who has an illness, but a sick person who is part of a network of relationships; who has values from the culture and the family; who has genes and a certain constitutional make-up. Reflection on these matters may begin to give some insight into the question 'Why?' Why this person? Why now? Why in this form? And what consequences will flow from the illness? It is a matter of reflection, or even meditation, on these questions.

There is no single answer. One cannot ask the question, 'Why did this person fall ill now?' and expect a direct answer, 'This person fell ill because . . .' This is a cause-and-effect answer which disregards the complexity of the issues. It is more illuminating to think in terms of the Zen *koan*, which is a paradoxical question that cannot be answered directly, but merely resolved. The question, 'Who am I?' does not have a direct answer, except at a superficial level. However, the question can be resolved and made to give up some meaning by means of concentration and meditation upon it. Many sick people ponder in this way upon their afflictions. They are often apologetic about it when they talk to doctors, feeling that it is rather morbid and unhealthy. Doctors usually agree with them and even state that thinking about your illness is a mistake; but how is anyone to gain insights into an illness unless attention is focused upon it?

The Cancer Help Centre in Bristol was founded to help people with cancer become more aware of themselves and their bodies, and better able to mobilize whatever resources they have to meet the invader. It shows what well-motivated people with cancer can do to help themselves. In addition to establishing a good diet and a positive attitude towards their cancer, there is a particular technique, called imaging, which involves focusing on the condition. In this the sufferer concentrates attention on the malignant tissues and visualizes the immune system attacking the malignant cells which are then carried off by the body's white cells. This is the technique evolved by Carl Simonton, an immunologist, and his wife, a psychotherapist.[27] These and similar techniques[28] can strike the robust doctor as dangerous fantasies which have no place in the repertoire of responsible practitioners, yet they are based on logical principles (that one can influence one's own immune system) and they bring satisfaction to many sick people; and there are many claims of cures, even though these would not stand up to hostile statistical analysis.

A systems view

A model well-equipped to fulfil the requirements set out for an explanatory model is that of systems theory. It can accommodate a great range of disparate information, taking account of relationships, feelings and questions of meaning. It also has the great advantage of making few conceptual demands on the observer. In fact, it is basically common sense, and scarcely requires the title of 'theory'.

Any conglomeration of parts which interact to perform some function can be called a system.[29,30] It might be a mechanical device, such as a traditional clock, where a great many parts have to move together in an unvarying manner to measure time accurately. It also might be a family whose members are interacting with constantly changing and evolving relationships, yet remaining cohesive and outwardly stable. These are examples, respectively, of what can be called mechanical systems and natural systems, [31,32] and they provide the two important explanatory models for understanding illness, although in orthodox medicine the mechanical-system model is used almost exclusively.

In no sense is one type of system better than the other. Natural systems are the more complicated and have a broader scope; their study involves synthesis and viewing the organism at several different levels of complexity. Mechanical systems, by contrast, are generally simpler, and their study is analytic and reductionist. Bodily function can be understood in terms of both types of system. It is useful at times to think of the heart in terms of a pump or the kidney in terms of a filter. At other times these organs are more meaningfully regarded as part of a larger network of function. The mechanical (or biomedical) model has been the one favoured over the past three hundred years, so this account will concentrate on the model of natural systems to see what it has to offer.

Natural systems are those systems which do not owe their existence to conscious human planning and execution.[33] A basic system is the atom, comprising electrons, neutrons and protons. (Smaller systems have not so far proved amenable to precise study.) The next system, in terms of complexity of organization, is the molecule, and clusters of these combine to form a cell. Cells then combine to form organs, and the organs (in the case of humans) together make up the human body. Humans make up family systems, and groups of families form communities, which together form nations, eventually involving the whole of the

234

human race, and ultimately the biosphere of all living things. Each system is a component of the system above. The person, however, occupies a special position in this discussion, being at the same time at the top of the organ hierarchy and at the bottom of the social hierarchy, as depicted in the diagram.[34]

Stratified Order of Natural Systems

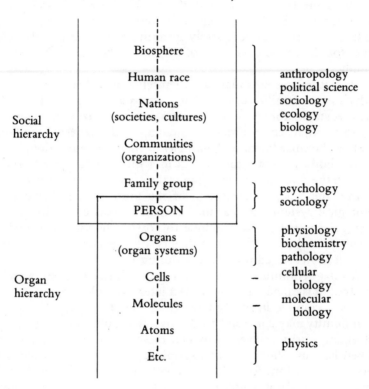

Each level of the system functions according to different principles, and each is contained within the level above it. The PERSON is top of the organ hierarchy and bottom of the social hierarchy. Each level has to be studied in its own right, using suitable concepts, as indicated by the disciplines in the right-hand column. Orthodox medicine can only make sense of problems at the organ level and below. Other approaches are needed to understand the higher-level systems.

235

Natural systems have certain qualitative properties, and I draw here on Ervin Laszlo's analysis.[31] (1) Natural systems are wholes with irreducible properties. If something (such as a virus) is added to a cell, it becomes qualitatively different. By contrast, if another bottle is added to a pile of rubbish, it makes only a quantitative difference – it becomes a bigger pile of rubbish, since the pile is nothing more than the sum of its parts. The cell, by contrast, would change its very nature. Two lovers coming together create a relationship which is something different from the sum of the same two people in isolation. They form a system which is irreducible. If they are split apart the system ceases to exist, nor can the system be described adequately in terms of the individuals. The same goes for the constituent parts of the human body or the members of a family.

(2) Natural systems maintain themselves in a changing environment, which is the familiar principle of homeostasis, expressed in a different way. A stable atom is a closed system, meaning that it does not exchange energy with its environment, though it could be affected fundamentally by heat, bombardment with particles or chemical interaction. The tissues of the body maintain themselves in a more-or-less steady state, even though the constituent parts change through the normal turnover of cells within the body. This is one of the more extraordinary aspects of biological systems, in that the function persists even though the parts change repeatedly. We continue to possess the same personalities and intellects although the constituents of the cells in our brains are completely changed many times during life.[35]

A village community is an open system which continues as a whole and evolves. It is called 'open' because it interacts with its environment, with supplies coming in and goods going out for sale. Members of the community may come and go, yet overall the unit continues, adapting to changing circumstances, provided these do not become too extreme. There is, thus, a high level of determinacy for the system taken as a whole but great freedom for the constituent parts, in this case, the villagers. Indeed, it does not matter much what the 'parts' do, within limits. In a closed sub-atomic system it does not matter at all what the constituents do, since the movements of electrons are (supposedly) random and unique events of no definable significance. It does not matter how the individual molecules of a gas behave, provided they maintain a suitable pressure, volume and temperature for the gas as a whole. It does not matter in a healing wound *which* cells multiply, provided that the correct number multiply at the right time and to the right extent.

The relationship of the parts to the whole exemplifies the fundamental difference between natural and mechanical systems, as here defined. The mechanical system is no more than the sum of its parts, each of which has a prescribed function. The elaborate clocks which were Descartes' examples of mechanisms (or, in twentieth-century language, mechanical systems) would cease to function if any one part failed because each component is precisely determined: nothing, for example, could take the place of the mainspring. These mechanisms are best understood by a detailed consideration of their parts, which are unchanging and in no way self-renewing. Of course one's ideas about mechanical systems may be upset by the new generation of computers which, it is claimed, will possess intelligence and so be able to make decisions as opposed merely to carrying out commands. When these come into operation they will provide an interesting borderland between natural and mechanical systems.

In natural systems, the relationships between the constituent parts are sometimes more interesting than the parts themselves, at least as far as the function of the whole is concerned. In the case of a family or a community (or any other natural system) the experience of any one member affects the experience of the whole unit. This is the central tenet of family therapy, for example, where the system is studied rather than the constituent members. A referral to a family therapist is usually made because one member, perhaps a teenage son, has a symptom – stealing at school, for example. The family therapist pays him little attention, possibly none at all to begin with, but concentrates on the processes within the family; and out of this exploration will emerge information which makes the boy's behaviour intelligible, and thus open to modification.

The stratification of systems involves all living structures, down to the smallest identifiable units. These also involve the whole range of natural and social sciences in an array of different disciplines. Just as each system is an irreducible whole with its own properties, so each requires its own methods of study according to its special principles. Methods of study suitable for molecules can be, at best, of limited value in trying to study people, still less when trying to make sense of family processes or whole communities. It is axiomatic that the methods of investigation are matched with the object under study, and herein is one of the greatest weaknesses of orthodox medicine.

The success of modern medicine has been in investigating systems from the organ level downwards, and here the traditional physical sciences provide satisfactory models. For the higher-level systems, concepts are needed which can encompass human development, human aspirations and relationships, marriage, parenthood, loss and death; and at a higher level still, the organization of society, national and international politics. In other words, the accepted medical disciplines of molecular biology, physiology, biochemistry and biophysics suffice very well when considering organs and below. Psychological, sociological, political and anthropological concepts have to be invoked to make proper sense of the whole person and above – that is, people in groups and in society, and the whole question of the meaning of illness for the individual.

We live in a world of natural systems from the single atom to the Earth taken as a whole. Although every level of system is extensively interconnected with every other, each is independent and has, so to speak, its own language. If we are studying molecules, we use the language of molecules – molecular biology. With cells, we use cell language – cellular biology; for organs, we use the language and methods of biochemistry and physiology; for whole people, psychology; and on up the scale, to sociology, political science and anthropology.

It sounds simple, reasonable and rather obvious to use methods of investigation appropriate to the object under study. In clinical practice, doctors who wish to concentrate their efforts on organs rather than people can devolve the management of problems concerning the higher-level systems to para-medical workers such as social workers, community nurses and psychologists, who are well versed in the psychological and sociological concepts and the clinical techniques pertaining to them.

It often happens that clinical presentations which baffle doctors thinking only at an organ level or below turn out to be quite intelligible when viewed with concepts appropriate to the level concerned. An example is a woman in her twenties who was referred by a specialist in internal medicine because she had intractable pelvic pain and diarrhoea, for which no cause had been found after careful physical investigation. Shifting attention to the person and her experiences, and then again to the network of relationships in which she lived, the symptoms became meaningful and closely connected with the origin of her difficulties.

Her parents had divorced when she was twelve, and she felt somehow responsible for this, at least her mother used to blame her for it. Her father later died, and she continued in a close and acrimonious relationship with her mother. At the time she was seen, she had been living for two years with a man. The liaison had temporarily broken up a year or so before they began living together, and during the time they were apart she found she had become pregnant by him, and had the pregnancy terminated without his knowledge. From the time they started living together again, she complained of pelvic pain, particularly during love-making.

Drawing these different threads together, we had, in addition to the complaint of pain and diarrhoea, a woman who felt guilty about the break-up of her parents' marriage and the termination of her pregnancy, who had unresolved feelings towards her dead father, and who had a difficult relationship with her mother as well as with the man with whom she was living. An awareness of all these wider issues did not lead to an immediate cure of her pain and diarrhoea, although the symptoms improved. The main achievement was that the therapeutic dialogue was at last focusing on issues which were intensely important to the patient, the pressure was reduced on the general medical services, and there was every chance that she would resolve some of her many problems and move on to a more fulfilling life.

There is no essential conflict between the reductionist approach, which deals with people as though they were mechanical systems, and the holistic approach, where the model of natural systems is used. One is not better, or more 'scientific' than the other, merely different and complementary. There are times when the reductionist approach works best, and times when the holistic approach is best.

Doctors are actually much more familiar with the idiom of natural systems than they think they are, and are all accustomed to talking in the language of natural systems at a physiological level without even realizing it. The endocrine system is a natural system *par excellence*. The balance and interplay of hormones of various kinds, involving loops of negative feedback (restoring the system to its ordinary state, as after exertion) and positive feedback (moving the system on to a new state, such as pregnancy), is an example of a natural system in action; the principles are generally acceptable physiological principles described in the standard textbooks of physiology.[36]

Claude Bernard (1813–78) was thinking in terms of natural systems when he advanced the concept of the *milieu interieur*.[37] Temperature, blood pressure, concentrations of various substances in the body fluids, the volumes of fluids in body compartments, and the density of red cells in the blood, for example, are all maintained in balance to preserve the quality of the internal environment. The values for these can only vary within narrow limits, and if the dynamic equilibrium is upset, reactions take place to restore the balance. In the early years of this century W. B. Cannon (1871–1945) took Bernard's ideas further by demonstrating the mechanisms by which this control is maintained, and he coined the term 'homeostasis'.[38]

Claude Bernard's concept of balance in the internal environment was treated in the nineteenth century as something entirely new. Certainly it was new, formulated in terms of Western physiology, but ideas about harmony and balance within the organism have been current for millennia. In Bernard's words:

> The ancient emblem representing life as a closed circle, formed by a serpent biting its own tail,[39] gives a fairly accurate picture of things. In complex organisms the organism of life actually forms a closed circle, but a circle which has a head and a tail in this sense, that vital phenomema are not all of equal importance, though each in succession completes the vital circle. Thus the muscular and nervous organs sustain the activity of the organs preparing the blood; but the blood in its turn nourishes the organs which produce it. Here is an organic or social interdependence which sustains a sort of perpetual motion, until some disorder or stoppage of a necessary vital unit upsets the equilibrium, or leads to a disturbance or stoppage in the play of the animal machine.[40]

Bernard tells physiologists that

> [We] must take account of the harmony of the whole, even while trying to get inside, so as to understand the mechanism of every part. . . . We really must learn, then, that if we break up a living organism by isolating its different parts, it is only for the sake of ease in experimental analysis, and by no means in order to conceive them separately. Indeed when we wish to ascribe to a physiological quality its value and true significance, we must always refer it to this whole, and draw our final conclusion only in relation to its effects in the whole.[41]

Bernard, who greatly admired Descartes, certainly made major contributions to the detail of physiology (the discovery of vasomotor nerves; the nature and action of curare and other poisons on neuro-muscular transmission; the functions of pancreatic juice in digestion; and the elucidation of the glycogenic function of the liver),[42] but his most important contribution was his concept of the organism functioning as a whole to maintain its internal environment.

A great advantage of the stratified order of systems is that it enables us to hold on to familiar explanatory models. Valuable as the Chinese system of correspondences is as an indication of the interrelationship of everything in the world, it is asking too much of us in the West to abandon altogether our quantitative and analytic approach on which our very effective mechanistic medicine depends. And there is certainly no evidence to suggest that traditional Chinese medicine is superior to Western medicine over the broad span of illnesses.

The systems approach leaves mechanistic medicine as it is and adds to it. The disciplines of psychology and sociology are there to make sense of phenomena at the level of the whole person and family groups, and so on up the scale, as already mentioned. Each of the disciplines from biophysics to anthropology may be superficially quite reductionist and mechanistic within its own domain. 'Superficially' is the operative word, because the more one goes into detail the more the systemic connections become apparent. Nevertheless, for practical purposes the mechanistic approach will do, and all that is asked of clinicians is that they recognize the existence of other systems and accommodate to their particular concepts and languages. When doctors are dealing with whole people or with families, they should use concepts developed for studying whole people and families. The principle is readily intelligible. The doctor needs to raise his sights above the level of the individual organ, and also to deal with whatever anxieties and prejudices may be operating within him, and which cause him to narrow his vision and dehumanize people.

There still remain the bridges between the different levels of system, and the interactions between each level and the environment. Strictly speaking, the biosphere represents the environment, but it is too vast an idea for practical purposes: the physical and social environment is more immediate, and as the adjacent system it is more relevant.

The links between systems have formed the subject matter of psychosomatic medicine and the more physiologically based work on psycho-physical interactions. Generally speaking, correlations have been sought between a life event or a personality trait and the onset of a specific disease. For example, the loss by death of a close relative of a person who has an obsessional personality may be correlated with that person subsequently developing ulcerative colitis. At a more physiological level the association may be sought between emotional arousal – from driving a car in heavy traffic, or giving a lecture – and pulse rate and blood pressure.

A vast amount of work of this kind has been done since the Second World War, and it has been very important, although for good experimental reasons the correlations have tended to be one-to-one: one life event (e.g. bereavement) with one response (e.g. ulcerative colitis). More recent work has involved a number of possible causative factors, and statistical tests have been employed to discover which factors are the most important in the causation of the illness. This trend is desirable but it is merely an extension of the Cartesian 'A causes B' approach. A is regarded as separate from B, and the person who experiences the illness

241

is separate again. Needless to say, the observer is also outside the objects and events under scrutiny.

How are we to work – let alone research – in a setting where everything is connected somehow with everything else? We could find correlations everywhere: between the divorce rate and the consumption of bananas, between the weather and the number of satellites orbiting the earth. Statistical tests, which we are accustomed to look to, to tell us what is 'significant', can be disappointing; and anyway they are concerned with populations or groups of people, not with an individual's experience.

In clinical practice it is quite possible to think organically (or holistically) about the system in which a person exists, and this is most easily illustrated by an example. A woman in her mid-forties is referred because she is depressed and has headaches. She has been fully investigated by her general practitioner whom she has visited on so many occasions that he is desperate, as nothing that he does has any affect at all.

The woman's situation looks less hopeless when her position in her system is worked out. Her husband is out of work and rather distant from her. She has a son of twenty-four who is in work, and is an irritant to her when he is in the house. Her daughter is married and has to work, so the patient is given the two-year-old grandson to look after three days a week. The house is comfortable, there are no problems in the neighbourhood, and relations with other people in the street are good. Money is short but not critically so.

The woman, who is the patient, is living in a network of relationships in a particular physical environment. It is assumed that she is involved with all those around her, with her physical environment, and, now, those members of the helping professions who are trying to assist her. It would be impossible meaningfully to formulate or describe her system in statistical terms, that is to say, to express all the people with whom she is involved and the physical environment in terms of factors which carried a certain weighting according to their importance. It would also be impossible to make any predictions, in terms of probability, about what was going to happen next in a system of this kind. Yet family therapists and community health workers every day see people in such circumstances, and they manage to bring about worthwhile changes.

By taking the family system as the unit of reference, it emerged, in this case, that the woman felt very uncomfortable and uncertain about her role, particularly with regard to the grandchild. She felt she was being pushed back into the role of mother, with all the expectations that come from it, and she felt she had already had enough of that role, but could not make her feelings felt. In the setting of a family interview, she was able to explain her position, and it proved possible by working with the dynamics of the family system to bring about changes to everyone's benefit, and the woman lost her headaches.

The key difference between the statistical approach, which tends in our culture to stamp respectability on any enquiry or activity, and the work with a family, such as I have described, is the difference between the quantitative and the qualitative. The statistical approach is quantitative, even when tests concerning value are being employed, because the answers will always come out – how many of this, how many of that, and so on. The direct work with the family is qualitative, analogy and metaphor are used in place of numbers, and what transpires relates to that family and to that family alone. It is an approach which should recommend itself to the traditional Chinese, as the point of reference all along is the whole – in this case, the whole system, the whole family. The components of the system interact and change, and the system continues. Helpers come into the system for a while and modify it, then they withdraw.

Family workers certainly are dealing with wholes, or at any rate at higher levels in the stratified order of systems than is usual in clinical medicine, yet many of their concepts are derived from the very kinds of statistically controlled quantitative surveys that they might feel they had left behind them. It is an example in the West of researchers starting off in the reductionist mould and moving on to employ broader concepts.

A family system is described because it is common and relatively straightforward. Many people do not have families but everyone inhabits some kind of network in which fortunes fluctuate. There is no clinical presentation of a patient which cannot be illuminated by considering the system in which the sick person lives. The requirements for employing this approach are the assumptions that every aspect of the person's life is potentially relevant and that concepts are used appropriate to the level of system under consideration.

17
Personal Reorientations

Throughout this book the focus of interest has been the doctor and how the doctor determines the style and quality of health care. Although health services are no longer run by the medical profession to the extent they once were, doctors still wield great influence – to facilitate improvement or perpetuate stagnation, to open up the provision of health care or to try and keep it as the exclusive preserve of doctors.

In this chapter, I describe ways in which doctors can deal with some of the undesirable traits and habits referred to in earlier chapters. Examples of these are: the tendency of the medical profession as a whole, and of doctors individually, to seek power over others; the way doctors try to deal with their personal needs and problems by an excessive involvement in their clinical work; the habit of doctors to behave as though they are somehow invulnerable to the effects of fatigue from long hours of work, and to the emotional pressures of working with distress and suffering.

Most of the discussion of these issues will be about the degree to which an aspect or a habit is apparent. For instance, it is good for a doctor to be supportive and to shield a sick person from difficult decisions at a time of crisis. It is not good for a doctor (nor for the patient) for this kind of parenting to become a permanent feature. The balance between being supportive yet not over-controlling, and the judgement about when to take over completely and when to let the patient make decisions, is subtle and cannot be defined precisely. There are polarities here as with everything else. A balance must be sought, and if one aspect is promoted too much, the work becomes distorted.

The benign, liberal doctor and the over-controlling doctor can be seen as polarities. Neither represents the proper style all the time for every doctor in all clinical circumstances. The proper style for the doctor to adopt depends on all the considerations which make the encounter between doctor and patient unique: that is to say, the personality of the patient; the presenting complaint; the various somatic, psychological and spiritual aspects; social and environmental aspects; the quality of the

244

relationship with the doctor. Then there is the doctor's agenda: his general state of well-being and satisfaction with life; pressure of work; feelings towards the patient; attitudes towards and experience of the patient's presenting complaint.

Since the doctor is in the controlling position in the encounter, he will determine its style, and that will depend on his general mental and physical state at the time of the encounter. He can be represented as occupying positions on a series of continua between polar points. He will fall somewhere between being the benign, liberal doctor and the over-controlling doctor; between being relaxed and tense; happy and sad; rested and fatigued; warm and hostile; clinically confident and unsure of himself; comfortable about his personal life and worried about personal matters; and so on.

In all these continua there is a positive aspect and a negative aspect, and most of the time, though not always, these will correspond to desirable and undesirable qualities.

The doctor has already been discussed in polar terms in connection with the doctor-patient archetype, whereby there is a valuable patient component, so to speak, in the unconscious of the doctor, provided he does not suppress it. Another polar or archetypal pattern is seen in the activity of the doctor, whereby the doctor is the one who heals and also kills. The god Apollo exemplifies this as 'the god who kills, yet purifies and heals'.[1]

The first archetypal pattern – the doctor-patient – refers to the person of the doctor, the second – the healer-destroyer – more to what the doctor actually does. The other polarities described earlier refer to further aspects of the doctor's behaviour in the clinical setting.

This may seem a complicated way of saying 'moderation in everything', but it is more than that. The doctor has great power to affect the course of the patient's life, and the whole interaction between doctor and patient is highly charged emotionally because of the archetypal forces involved; and also of course because of the potentially serious nature of their business.

Another reason for presenting the issue in this way is to remind doctors how readily they can suppress the 'patient' aspects of themselves, and also how they can slip from being the healer to being the destroyer or, in its milder form, the charlatan. The eminent and able doctors described in Chapter 8 revealed how they could be taken over by false ideas, with their ordinary critical faculties suspended. In Chapter 9, examples were given of doctors who could act quite literally as destroyers, often for reasons which are understandable when viewed in their social and political context.

This shadow aspect of medical practice is always there, and doctors are liable to slip into these dangerous ways unless they learn to watch themselves and maintain an ever-critical view of their work. One way especially in which they fall victim is by denying the reality of death. Doctors who deny the inevitability of death and the fact that we are all actually in the process of dying, create an unreal world for themselves in which it is assumed that we have the capacity to enter an epoch of unbroken health, provided a few more fundamental discoveries are made. It then becomes possible for doctors to imagine that they can offer a golden age of health,[2] along with an elimination of death. It is a crazy and potentially harmful fantasy which merely soothes some doctors' anxieties concerning mortality. Such people should listen to Alfred Ziegler, a Swiss psychiatrist and analyst, who takes an opposite position to those who believe that perfect health is achievable. Ziegler says that 'human beings are healthier when they are a little bit sick . . . We are all chronic patients who from time to time get better.'[3]

The bare descriptions in the earlier chapters of doctors' problems often implied the solutions, even though these were not pursued at the time. Some of these solutions will now be taken up under headings relating to the kinds of action involved. This leads inevitably to repetition, which I have tried to keep to a minimum by taking a direct line about what can be done to improve the human aspects of clinical doctors' work.

Individual needs

Personal needs of the doctor may be met by the practice of medicine, through over-involvement with patients and excessive busyness.

It is altogether good when someone's emotional energy, or libido, flows into the work. All successful people are investing a good deal of themselves in their enterprises. They have more energy and more enthusiasm than those who are just serving time, and they are likely to be more creative and inspire others. However, enthusiasm for the work can pass beyond the point where the doctor is solely meeting the patient's needs, or, in a comfortable way, those of both doctor and patient.

The classical example is the middle-aged doctor who is consulted by a sensitive, sympathetic and often younger woman. The doctor behaves quite properly, according to the dictates of the Hippocratic Oath and the General Medical Council, but he happens to give the patient in question longer appointments, and later in the day than usual. An intense interaction is quickly set up which engages a disproportionate amount of the doctor's time

246

and emotional energy. It may do the woman some good, to begin with, and the doctor will feel revived as if he was beginning a love-affair.

Such beguiling encounters take the doctor's energies away from his main relationships, which may be less soothing, yet in the long run are likely to be more fulfilling, and certainly better for the doctor's own development.

Especially at times of personal difficulty and at the stage in life when the main outward goals have been achieved, doctors need to be sensitive about undue feeling and energy flowing into their relationships with patients. It is important at times of crisis that emotions flow in directions that can lead to some resolution of the problems, rather than towards the patients, when underlying difficulties are avoided and so cannot be resolved.

Doctors can make themselves extremely busy. Clinical work of any kind can meet various needs in the doctor. The interminable busyness may simply distract him from personal difficulties that he is not ready or prepared to face. Being busy, and so in constant demand, is reassuring of his worth and popularity. Busyness may be a manifestation of a compulsive need to care.

It is quite easy for a doctor to scrutinize his routines if he wants to. It is even easier for his colleagues, partner and family – and patients – to do so, if he will let them. Many doctors act as though every call has to be answered at once, although few are real emergencies. For far too many doctors the fire-brigade mentality endures because it gives them an emotional boost. They can take a critical look at each day's clinical contacts, pause before rushing off to a call, and ask the question: 'Why am I hurrying to this person?' Doctors can contribute to disabling their patients by coming in to take over in every crisis. As a potential patient, it is reassuring to know that the doctors are there: as a doctor, I should be clear that I am responding to the patient's need and not to my own.

Personal limitations

The doctor is an ordinary and vulnerable human being, whose professional competence and psychological state can be affected adversely by long hours of duty, and by distressing events at work or at home.

The robust and elitist streak in many doctors inveigles them into thinking that they are more durable than in fact they are; more durable indeed than anyone could reasonably expect to be. Many doctors almost need to be given permission to rest, and reassured that they will not be regarded as layabouts or weaklings, or worse still as 'neurotics', if they ask for time out to restore themselves after a taxing period of work or during a difficult period in their private lives. They need to be convinced that there really is no great virtue in trying to act as though they possess superhuman constitutions.

Examples have been given of how doctors could make errors of observation and judgement when fatigued from long hours of duty or when preoccupied by personal worries. Doctors do not generally think much about their cognitive processes, because not only is such reflection alien to the orthodox medical ethos but the doctors concerned are not likely to be faced with the consequences of errors made while fatigued. By contrast, the singlehanded transatlantic yachtsmen I studied[4] were very sensitive indeed to their state of alertness and to the likely quality of their powers of judgement; and the more experienced the sailor the better developed was this awareness. The same applies to all experienced adventurers, and of course their own lives depend on the reliability of their observations and decision-making.

Doctors who accept that their physical endurance has limits and that their perceptual processes are not flawless can learn to monitor the quality of their functioning by becoming sensitive to what their bodies (and minds) are doing. They can teach themselves to watch out for early signs of fatigue, so that at times when they suspect that they are functioning at a poor level (and have no chance of resting) they can at least reduce the risk of errors. I can best describe what is required at such times by using quite specific and didactic language.

Know how long you have been awake, know when you last ate. Make sure you rest, eat regularly and adequately, and do not feel that there is anything shameful about insisting on this (even though senior doctors will often humiliate juniors who want to maintain themselves in a proper state for efficient working).

When the pressure is on, and you simply have to keep going: recognize when a familiar job is taking longer than usual or seeming to be extra burdensome – slowing down is usually the first sign of fatigue. Notice negative feelings about tasks which are ordinarily done automatically. Check observations even more thoroughly than usual, and write everything down. Keep asking yourself questions. 'Am I observing the whole clinical picture or narrowing down on to simple details with which I feel comfortable? Am I making the proper clinical decision or the one that allows me the least further effort? Could I defend in a court of law the treatment I have just prescribed? What would so-and-so (a respected teacher) do in similar circumstances?'

Be sensitive also about the general state of your personal and professional life – worries about relationships, money, career, etc. If you know that in addition to being tired you are in a period of personal difficulty, this can be allowed for as well.

The tough attitude towards physical endurance in the doctor is also seen in relation to emotional distress among patients. The same kind of denial is used, and this time it amounts to ignoring that sick people may be afraid and distressed. This distress that the doctor fails to acknowledge in the patient he is also denying in himself; and he has the doctor's persona which protects him from the impact of any behaviour or feeling in the patient that he does not like. In time this persona can obscure the real person altogether, so that the doctor becomes a kind of caricature.

The twin denials of physical limitation and emotional vulnerability impose an intolerable and unnecessary strain on the doctor; while to admit their existence merely means accepting himself as an ordinary human being. And that, most of the time, is what patients long for – a doctor who will meet them on equal terms and not as an authoritarian figure who hands down judgements and instructions.

It is really all right to cry with a patient. When I was a surgical junior such an idea would have been inconceivable, and regarded by the other doctors as a sign of incipient breakdown. It would have been seen as behaviour incompatible with the standards expected of a responsible member of the medical profession. I now know that, far from being a sign of weakness, it can be a sign of strength; an indication that the doctor's feelings are not split off from his rational functions. Assuming that overall the doctor is in control, tears will indicate to the patient that the doctor cares.

The crucial requirement is the tacit acknowledgement, by the doctor, that he is like other people, is vulnerable and has weaknesses like the rest of humanity.

Shedding authoritarian attitudes

Doctors need to modify some of the untherapeutic attitudes acquired during medical training, particularly those relating to power.

Sad to say, the better students please their teachers in medical schools, the less well equipped they will be for a satisfying and satisfactory life in ordinary medical practice. Medical school teachers like to produce doctors 'in their own image', and their ideal product will be male, someone who sees himself as a member of a superior group in society, who should be handsomely rewarded and privileged for involving himself in that delightfully interesting intellectual activity known as clinical medicine.

It can take years for some doctors to overcome the disappointment that the realities of medical life do not conform with the expectations generated in medical schools, especially when their choice to study medicine was connected with aspirations for a powerful place in society. Those of a defensive and authoritarian disposition are often attracted to the traditional major specialties of surgery and internal medicine, in which their conservative attitudes can find expression. If these same doctors happen to obtain posts at teaching hospitals, then these undesirable attitudes are liable to be passed on to the next generation of student doctors.

By contrast, those doctors who have never introjected authoritarian attitudes move away from the hospital circuit as soon as they can after qualifying, and seek work in the community where they find the values more congenial. With the growth of holistic medicine and the complementary and alternative therapies, there are now more opportunities for doctors to meet colleagues who take a broad view of the essence of medical work.

The complementary and alternative practitioners charge fees for their services, unlike the great majority of doctors, in Britain at any rate, who are paid by the state. Private medicine is represented by some as a social evil, but regardless of its effect on the overall quality of medical care, it does mean that the patient's wishes become of some account, and so the balance of power between doctor and patient is potentially shifted. The patients may not always receive better personal care because many of the eminent doctors engaged in private practice are trading on their reputations as technical experts, and such charm as they can register may be determined by the fee they anticipate, and will not necessarily spread over into their 'public' work. Private medicine at its best is very good indeed from the patient's point of view (and it is completely confidential), and all doctors can benefit from some experience of the more equal relationship that occurs in the private contract.

Many of the untherapeutic attitudes referred to are related to the tendency of professional groups to organize themselves into powerful positions which have little to do with their original ideals. Medical organizations are active in maintaining the advantages of particular groups, and, wherever possible, securing new advantages. They are also fighting for what they regard as the 'rights' of the profession in relation to salaries and the provision of resources. All this is essentially politics at a trade-union level – obtaining the best conditions for a particular group. A great deal of passion is expended on these activities, and doctors can easily be led to suppose that the best interests of the patients are ultimately served by such manoeuvrings, but of course they are not. Even if doctors collectively benefit from the negotiations, they must remember that the negotiators are embroiled in a medico-political process which, in its nature, has no end: nor do the doctors committed to such entanglements want it to end.

Many doctors like to avoid political issues and concentrate on the work they were trained to do. They can avoid medical politics or even party politics, but they cannot avoid politics in the wider sense, because the circumstances of most people's lives are determined by political decisions. The amount of money spent on housing, on education, on health services, is all as a result of political decisions; and no doctor working with ordinary people can disregard this fact.

The doctor prescribes tranquillizers to a young mother living in a damp and dilapidated house, to help her keep going and cope with her children. He knows she needs rehousing rather than tranquillizing. He should hold in the forefront of his mind an awareness of the interdependence of housing, education, social benefits and the provision of health care.

The political decisions that lead to these provisions are made largely as a result of pressure put upon the government of the day. As it happens, the medical profession is in a better position to put pressure on the government and to raise public sympathy for its favourite causes than, say, those in need of proper housing. The result is that the housing stays the same and more personal medical services are provided.

The doctor needs to be clear about what is happening. He has better medical resources, yet millions of patients – like the woman with the children – continue to be unhealthy. Left-wing doctors agitate about such matters because the issues are set out in their social theories, and this may inhibit the politically more moderate doctors, but the interconnection of housing, education and health transcends political ideologies. Everybody knows that most of the improvements in health in modern times are due to social and environmental measures, not to medical discoveries,[5] so observations about the effects of poor housing should come as no surprise. All doctors should think politically when it comes to the provision of resources. If nothing else, it will stop them becoming frustrated when their medicines fail to create healthy citizens out of the inhabitants of slums.

Professional limitations

Doctors have to accept the limitations of medical expertise.
Doctors in training are taught only about curing diseases. They are implicitly given to understand that they have the answer to all human ills,

251

therefore they are liable to construe all human behaviour and maladies in terms of organic pathology. The effects of this 'medi-think' are two-fold. First, patients coming to see their doctor feel that they have to formulate their problems in terms of bodily symptoms if they want to be taken seriously. Secondly, doctors feel that their medical expertise should enable them to solve all the problems that are brought to them.

This medi-think can lead to peculiar dialogues between doctors and patients about medical symptoms when the real problems are social, psychological and spiritual, and neither party feels able to be explicit: the patient does not want to offend the doctor, and the doctor has not learned how to deal with psycho-social-spiritual issues. From the doctor's point of view (and the patient's too), the medicalizing of every-thing is in the long run profoundly frustrating and depressing. Social, psychological and spiritual problems will not be solved by a medical dialogue.

When a patient dies of a predictably fatal condition, the doctor can feel depressed and a failure because of a nagging suspicion that if he had tried harder and used superior skill the patient would not have died. Such feelings afflict especially recently qualified doctors and are a direct consequence of the ideology that curing diseases or correcting pathology is the proper occupation for a doctor, mere caring and supporting being regarded as a second-class activity. The practical doctor in the real world has to learn afresh that attending people and giving comfort is often the most important part of any doctor's work, and the part that patients may value more than any amount of medical skill.

It is absurd for doctors to imagine that they can control the natural processes of life and death; and the sooner they become conscious that they may be cherishing illusions of superhuman powers the happier they will be. Doctors are too ready to take total responsibility for the patient. This feeds their sense of self-worth and allows the patient to regress. It should be resisted: the doctor cultivating a role which encourages the patient to take some measure of responsibility.

Medicine has plenty to offer at a simple and practical level. Everybody who has access to good medical services is, or should be, profoundly grateful for them. There is no need for doctors to imagine that they should be offering exceptional medical services, or creating an impression that they can solve the social, psychological, and spiritual problems that oppress people in our society. It would be much better for them to concentrate their efforts on the unspectacular chronic conditions which demand the broadest approach in terms of ideas and practice.

Unfortunately, deciding on the limits of a doctor's responsibility can be far from simple. The doctor-knows-best philosophy implies that each doctor, on the basis of having been exposed to a medical education and having a certain amount of clinical experience, will simply *know* what is right for a given patient. Once upon a time, when much less could be done for sick people, medical practice was often a private and discreet transaction between doctor and patient. The doctor may have had a close knowledge of the patient and the family over years, and may in fact have known what was best. Nowadays, despite the advent of more professional family practice, illness more frequently involves large numbers of staff, expensive life-support equipment, and well-informed patients and relatives. Thus decisions about life and death become immensely complicated. The limits of medical responsibility are now open to public debate, and one day we may have a code of medical conduct to tell us what we must do, what we must not do, and what we do not have to do.

My reason for touching on questions of medical responsibility is to separate the real issues from the spurious ones, such as arise from the doctor blaming himself when he cannot save someone dying from widespread malignancy; or when he cannot solve the medical problems arising as a result of insanitary housing; or restore the faith in someone whose life has lost its meaning.

Doctors must be clear about what is within the range of medical expertise. They must be equally clear when a condition is beyond cure or a problem is not strictly medical at all, and then give whatever comfort is possible or whatever advice is relevant. They must be careful not to confuse the categories.

Taking care of the doctor

Doctors should apply to themselves the good advice they dispense to others.
At times of illness, the permission to let go and accept help comes from another doctor, but too often it is expressed in tentative terms, as though the doctor who is in need of advice really knows best and it would be discourteous for one doctor (the advisor) to tell another doctor (the patient) about how to eat, rest, exercise, and so on. Doctors advising other doctors must be definite, and on such occasions they can be as authoritarian as they like.

Most of the time doctors do not seek professional advice from colleagues, and in general they are improving in the way they treat their bodies, in that they smoke less, take more exercise and eat better food; but there is little evidence that doctors are organizing their lives any better.

The processes of fatigue are of relatively short duration, lasting only for hours or days as a rule. In addition to those transient crises is the continuous task of preserving an equilibrium between the professional and personal demands and the restorative powers of the human system. When this equilibrium is disturbed, the effects are less of simple tiredness than of disillusionment and a sense of futility.

I like the image of the mountain lake.[6] Pure bright water fills it from the melted snows above, and it gives out water to nourish the land below. If there is no inflow the lake dries up, without an outflow it becomes stagnant.

Doctors need to maintain themselves in a state of equilibrium in which all the parts of the body and the psyche are working as a harmonious whole. To achieve this they must be able to monitor themselves, and learn to detect small movements away from the point of balance. Not, let me repeat, to detect pathological change but rather movement away from harmony, such as was described in relation to East Asian medicine. One of the most important aspects of the East Asian system for Westerners is how small degrees of imbalance can be detected. In fact the main role of the East Asian practitioner is to assess an individual's equilibrium and bring about corrections before the imbalance reaches a point where actual symptoms appear: the point, of course, where cosmopolitan medicine can be said to begin.

Some technique is needed to enable doctors – and everyone else, for that matter – to acquire an awareness of themselves and their bodies. Not perhaps with the subtlety of an East Asian practitioner but with sufficient sensitivity to be able to recognize the effects of the pressures of a busy life.

There are many techniques currently available in the West for achieving this. Most of the popular systems of relaxation and meditation begin with a stage of quiet reflection in which the subjects, in a relaxed posture, become aware of the state of their bodies – the tense muscles around the neck and shoulder girdle, around the jaw, down the back, in the perineum. This physical awareness and taking stock of the state of the body is a prelude to developing psychological awareness.

Psychological awareness involves focusing on one's life and evaluating it. It means asking basic questions about one's relationship to other people, to the world and to the cosmos; and asking the basic questions about meaning.

The middle years. Doctors are good at striving, building careers and concentrating energies in the pursuit of goals. They are less good, in general, at simply being in a harmonious relationship with their environment, in which the different parts of life are integrated, so that, while they may work hard, they retain a rhythm and equilibrium in their lives. Such a balanced state is the antithesis of the professional race for personal distinction and advancement, which depends on objectives

254

which are passionately sought yet which cannot be clearly defined, because they are, in essence, illusory. The busy doctor is thus always in pursuit. He does not stop, or try to take account of where he is, and therefore he never understands what he is really achieving or where he is going. Unless you know where you are, you cannot know where you are going.

Techniques of self-awareness or meditation enable people to discover where they are and how they are. So far so good, but that leads on to the question, 'What is it for? What is the purpose of my career and my life?' These are the great questions of existence. They are *koans*, and even though they do not lead to answers (but rather to resolution) they must be asked. They are the vital questions which arise in the later thirties and beyond after the building-up has been done. Anyone of middle years who is disinclined to ask such questions probably has his energies too much outside of himself. It has much to do with the issue of meaning. It is not that one asks questions and discovers the 'meaning' in life, but that one asks the questions and lives with the uncertainty. Most people do manage to find some kind of meaning in their lives. It may be in terms of their work, their family relationships, their religious observance. Many people actually live in this harmonious state without ever thinking about it explicitly, and to them these words will seem obvious.

Many people, including doctors, do not feel their lives to be harmonious, and they are dissatisfied despite material affluence. Often doctors are disillusioned with the way their careers have turned out. They have achieved positions of influence yet they are unfulfilled, and their professional and personal relationships are unrewarding. Their energies have flowed outward in the extraverted tradition of the West, and at the point when they reach the pinnacle, they feel cheated.

The yearning most people have for a sense of meaning in their lives may require at some stage a change of direction. The energies which in the past have flowed so successfully out into the world need to be redirected inwards. The choice to change the direction of one's energies is hard for many people. To begin with, the actual idea may be incomprehensible. For many, the very thought of looking inwards is a disturbing business.

Most people trying to reflect seriously on their lives and take stock of where they are are likely to find the experience disturbing, just as the early phase of psychological analysis is likely to be negative. This is to be expected. Indeed, an initial feeling of depression usually indicates that a person is facing the real issues and is likely to make progress. The feeling of being in the wilderness at this stage is healthy, because one *is* in a

255

wilderness: the previous signposts are no longer accurate, and new ones have not yet been found. So one waits in the empty space.

> wait without hope
> For hope would be hope for the wrong thing; wait
> without love
> For love would be love of the wrong thing; there
> is yet faith
> But the faith and the love and the hope are all
> in the waiting.[7]

There are many who cannot stop their hectic striving because any deflection from these outward activities leaves them in this empty space which they cannot tolerate. Such people perceive intuitively that any slowing down in the race threatens their fantasy of control and may pitch them into an ocean of uncertainty. Thus they keep driving onwards when they ought to stop and ask questions. They push ahead even though they have achieved their early objectives and the daily round is beginning to lose its meaning. These people avoid the eternal and painful questions. Instead they become depressed, indulge in middle-aged fancies, or redirect their energies for better or worse. The redirection may happen to lead to new and creative activities, or to a more positive approach to life. Too often the spectacle is of a doctor who is unable to find fulfilment in his routine work once he is established, and directs his passions instead into making money, achieving respectability, and playing the interminable administrative chess game. Many of the undesirable practices, described earlier, represent the unhappy methods doctors have employed to resolve the need for meaning in their lives.

I have developed this theme at some length because the issue of the redirection of energies in mid-life is so fundamental. I am suggesting that the point in life when the doctor is confronted, however ambiguously, by the crisis of meaning is the crucial point. The habits and values which once sustained him have lost their substance. This was the position of Dante at the opening of the *Inferno*, when he wrote:

> In the middle of the journey of our life
> I came to myself in a dark wood,
> Where the straight way was lost.[8]

Dante, at the age of thirty-five, had lost his way in a dark wood. His medieval image enriches our twentieth-century formulations: we speak of a period of disillusionment brought about by the failure of past values and sources of sustenance, and the apparent lack of any alternatives.

This experience is a 'wound', in the sense that the word was used in connection with the idea of the wounded healer. It is a challenge, and as such it can be met in different ways. A number of different challenges were described in Chapter 15; the challenge of ageing is discussed here because everybody has to meet it who lives sufficiently long. To connect this experience with an actual age, or to talk about a 'mid-life crisis', is to over-simplify the concept. It is preferable to speak of a crisis of meaning – a time when one is challenged to take stock of life thus far, and life ahead.

Two of the doctors' responses to this challenge are of especial importance. There is the way forward simply through denying the challenge of meaning and continuing to direct the energies outward, and so building ever greater edifices of prestige and power. Also there is the way of the wounded healer, who can accept uncertainty and the vulnerability of the human condition, and who realizes that strength lies in acknowledging one's weakness.

18

Partnership and Participation

If doctors are to make any fundamental changes in the way they work, they will need to reappraise their relationships with their medical colleagues, with health professionals of various kinds, and with their patients.

Doctors helping one another

The 'problem' of the 'sick doctor' has interested the medical profession since the late 1970s,[1] and is part of the larger issue known as 'professional burn-out'.[2,3]

The notional 'sick doctor' is an elusive character, and I am not at all sure what kind of person my colleagues have in mind when they debate the 'problem'. It might be a doctor who is under personal pressure and desires an outside counsellor, one who is failing in his work and does not realize it, one who forgets his appointments and smells of alcohol, or an anaesthetist who sniffs the narcotic gas before administering it to the patient.

Apart from heavy-drinking colleagues, these 'sick doctors' are vaguely evocative of the lonely, disillusioned doctors who used in Britain to be arraigned by the General Medical Council and struck off the Medical Register for 'infamous conduct in a professional respect'. It was as though certain members of the tribe stumbled in a way which rendered them unacceptable, so that they had to be eliminated. The General Medical Council is well placed to do this, since it functions both as a policing body and a court, and the ordinary procedures regarding appeal do not apply.[4]

Against such a background, the various schemes for helping doctors before they get into serious difficulties are welcome. Certain of the Royal Colleges and other professional organizations, and even the General Medical Council itself, now somewhat reformed, have been active in this direction.[5] Some of the schemes are primarily directed towards protecting

258

patients, and others towards providing support for doctors in personal difficulties.[6]

People have a right to take their personal problems to whom they will, and often there are good reasons for consulting someone outside the domestic or professional circle. Many will on principle avoid any discussion of personal matters with family, friends and colleagues. They say that 'one should try to make the best of things', that 'life is tough and there is no good crying on people's shoulders', that 'that is the way to lose your friends', and so on. However, a fair proportion of doctors adopting these attitudes do so on account of their own difficulties with the whole question of the expression and flow of feeling, of sexuality, and the acknowledgement of their human vulnerability. Doctors who have such difficulties are not likely to be at ease in the company of people who are expressing feelings,[7] and are likely to inhibit displays of distress, frustration or anger among their patients.

When there is a crisis in the doctor's personal life, and he realizes at last that he requires some outside help, he probably consults a medical colleague. The doctor whom he consults is quite likely to have the same anxieties about feeling, and so the personal problem – as a personal problem – may be denied, almost collusively, and reinterpreted as a medical problem.

This is how it can go. A doctor has been living in a distant relationship with his wife. Lately their differences have become more acute, with open rows in front of the children, to the extent that a continuing life together seems almost impossible. The doctor becomes despondent and depressed at the implications either of parting or battling it out together. (His wife feels the same and has the same depressing realizations.) The doctor is ashamed of the emotions which assail him, and all the more so as he is conscious that his attention is not focused properly at work, and he is avoiding tasks that formerly he threw himself into with alacrity. He begins to sleep badly, and wakes in the small hours of the morning. He loses some weight. He consults his general practitioner and offers symptoms that can be seen as those of depressive illness.

The general practitioner is in a crucial position at this point. He can respond to the medical 'offerings' in the form of symptoms of depression, or he can look beyond them. For most patients, this general practitioner would look beyond the presenting complaint, and would quickly uncover manifest personal distress. But will he do the same for a fellow doctor?

Problems about feelings, sexuality and relationships are threatening to the doctor who is being consulted if he is out of touch with these aspects of himself. In that case he can avoid the real issues, reach for his prescription pad and prescribe anti-depressant drugs. Both doctors can be relieved: one has avoided an embarrassing dialogue about feelings; the other can go home with the new 'insight' that he is ill and needs treatment, and that his wife will have to be more understanding of him in future. Both doctors have denied their vulnerability.

Those who cannot accept their own vulnerability, or the wounds within themselves, will not be able to respond to the vulnerability or wounds in others: their vision will be distorted by their need to protect themselves.

Doctors are in implicit competition with one other. Specialists compete for resources and staff, general practitioners are locked into complicated partnerships which produce discord. This simmering professional rivalry is not a good starting point for a discussion about one's own difficulties and anxieties, or for acknowledging one's wounds. St Paul's words, 'for when I am weak, then I am strong',[8] may be true, but it would be a denial of the realities of professional politics to suggest that doctors will be able to talk easily about painful personal matters with their immediate colleagues.

This is a reflection on the profession. Doctors may be able to support people within the well defined limits of a medical consultation, which is conducted according to strict, unspoken rules. When the person in need is a fellow doctor it becomes more complicated.

For a great many over-intellectualized people – and that includes a large proportion of doctors – warm feelings are fully expressed only in love-making (if then), and anger is only allowed to burst forth at their children, or their subordinates. The feeling functions in such people are in a sense undifferentiated, that is, they are rather primitive and infantile. There is no easy flow of laughter and warmth, and alternatively of frustration and anger. Instead, there is a generally austere demeanour, and then, without warning, an outburst of anger or some uncontrollable laughter, which is quite inappropriate to the occasion and quite incongruent with the persona.

People who are not in touch with their feelings tend not to think about feelings at all. The subject is uncomfortable, just as the prospect of a mountain torrent liable to burst forth at any moment is uncomfortable.

Very considerable demands are placed on doctors who try to make warm and supportive relationships with patients, and at the same time preserve the intellectual detachment which enables them to make rational and reliable judgements.

This difficult task may be facilitated by appreciating the differences between a personal relationship and a professional one. In a personal relationship, especially an intimate one, there are no limits or conditions, generally speaking. Embarking on a love affair is a journey into an emotional unknown, and there is very little control over feelings and actions. In a more gentle friendship there may be unspoken boundaries, say, regarding physical intimacy, but no clear limits to the demands which each might make on the other.

The professional relationship is different because there are clear boundaries and – most important – a definite control. This means that the relationship can be entered into and withdrawn from at will. While the doctor is with the patient there is total involvement; when the encounter is over, the empathy is set aside. For the duration of the session there is real closeness, as close as in any other non-physical relationship, but it does not continue afterwards.

It is hard to describe this process without making the doctor sound calculating or even cynical: that the emotion is produced to order and then withdrawn. The good doctor does not switch on and off like that, rather there is an awareness of what is happening, such as there has to be in an artistic performance. The artist must be true to the essence of the work, and a reliable and faithful performance is founded on technique, which is consciously acquired and which involves rational processes rather than feeling. Only when the technique has been mastered can the feeling be used effectively and consistently.

There are two aspects here: the feeling or empathic aspect and the thinking or rational. No worthwhile relationship can exist between people unless there is empathy between them. The rational element comes in during a professional relationship to enable the doctor to be conscious of the feelings that are flowing and to be, to some extent, in control of them.

Doctors seldom need any help with their thinking or rational functions, since these have been developed to a high degree in their training. Where feeling and empathy are concerned, most doctors have a good deal to learn. However, doctors qualifying after the mid-1970s, generally speaking, have a more open attitude towards feelings and relationships than their older colleagues. It is a feature of the changing culture, and the change is welcome.

Doctors who want to learn about the expression of feeling can discover a tremendous amount through participating in groups which are designed to help people communicate at an empathic level, as opposed to the rational-intellectual level. There are many varieties of such groups: encounter, sensitivity, co-counselling, gestalt; as well as a number specifically organized for doctors.

It can come as a surprise to some highly educated doctors that useful work can actually be done on *feelings*, that feeling is a function of the mind, just like the intellect, and accessible to training and development. Of course, feelings are not all sweet and positive. In any close relationship there will be negative feelings, and it is a mark of a good relationship when anger can be tolerated as well as love. Therefore improving the flow of feeling between people will permit the easy and direct expression of resentment – something which medical colleagues seldom manage in a relaxed way. It is quite possible for apparently hostile remarks to be passed between colleagues, not as aggressive utterances from one person to another, but as statements about how the speaker happens to feel; about the speaker's private response to what the other person has said or done. This distinction is crucial, and examples are: 'I resent having to do your clinical work while you go off to attend conferences'; or 'I get angry at some of the things you say when you are chairing our staff meetings'; or 'I feel uncomfortable when I see you with so many people in attendance on your ward rounds'. The sting is taken out when the emphasis is placed on the speaker and how the speaker is feeling, and not upon the person who is being addressed. The speaker is letting out the emotion directly, instead of holding it in or complaining privately to people who will agree with him, which of course resolves nothing. But he is not laying bad feelings on the other person.

It can be a very moving discovery for people attending these groups, especially gestalt groups, that the direct expression of feelings, even apparently hostile ones, provided they are direct and authentic and coming 'straight from the guts', far from dividing people, actually brings them closer together. There even develops a kind of camaraderie among people who have become used to the style of such groups, because there is a sense of closeness and relaxedness which stems from knowing that any direct expression of distress will be accepted, and a blast of anger will merely indicate how the speaker happens to feel, and so need cause no offence.

This, of course, is merely the subjective aspect of anger, but once it is brought out into the open it no longer causes smouldering resentment, and the objective issues, such as they may be, can then be dealt with on a rational basis.

Although schemes for sick doctors are to be welcomed, we must never lose sight of the fact that ultimately we are talking about ourselves, and not about a particular category of person whom we can describe, package and consign to experts for treatment. Sick doctors are not some qualitatively different kind of medical graduate: they are right here within us. The problems lie within our psyches. If we accept our humanity wholeheartedly, then we can allow ourselves to be more open to the frustrations, humiliations, disappointments and compromises inherent in clinical work – and perhaps in other aspects of our lives as well. If we are going to try to accept our human frailty, then we must also accept the shadow side of things: that nothing is entirely good, and that there is always a dark aspect. We have to accept that there is a shadow side to the way we deal with patients, that we are always in danger of trying to become omnipotent and omniscient, and prone to take control of patients to meet our own needs. We have to accept the shadow aspect of our own relationships, how we can hurt those we love, and manipulate our families for our own ends.

Although experienced doctors should learn to look into themselves, the same cannot be expected automatically of junior doctors, still less of medical students. All those who have the privilege of teaching aspiring doctors, and who are therefore in a position to influence the future of medical care, need to be especially careful not to pass on traditional and undesirable attitudes that are still prevalent in the circles of medical power. Particularly to be avoided are the attitudes of elitism and robustness; that is, that doctors are superior persons, not subject to ordinary human limitations.

Helping students and junior doctors requires established doctors to set an example along the lines sketched out in the last chapter: to recognize their personal needs and their personal and professional limitations, and to shed whatever undesirable attitudes they may have acquired in medical schools. Then students and young doctors can cope with the considerable pressures of learning and working, without the additional burden of feeling that there must be something the matter with them because from time to time they feel exhausted, or become distressed by all the suffering around them.

Partnership with health professionals

Doctors complain that they are overworked, that too many people come to them with minor conditions or emotional problems, and that they can never give people the time they need. Doctors continue to make these complaints even though they are surrounded by a growing number and range of capable, interested and well-trained health professionals.

In the medical network in Britain there are health visitors and community nurses of various kinds. There are also a very few nurse practitioners, although in North America there are many more.[9-11] There are social workers and practice counsellors, and a large army of volunteers who have plenty to contribute when encouraged and effectively organized.[12]

If doctors take full advantage of all the skilled help that is at hand, they can transform their work. They can give patients the time they feel they need; and they will not have to syringe ears, take blood and do other routine tasks. Where emotional problems are concerned (and they seem to account for about 30 per cent of primary-care consultations), the doctor will probably continue to be the person who identifies the problem, and then will be able to refer the patient to someone better placed to give the skilled and time-consuming care which is required. The advantages of this are two-fold: the doctor is freed for activities which make more direct use of medical expertise, and the people seeking help for personal problems will not need to present themselves as needing medical care.

Health professionals can work well in the medical arena, making clinical judgements and coping with medical emergencies. For example, community psychiatric nurses can deal with most of the acute psychiatric crises which erupt, and, in the ordinary way, frustrate general practitioners, taking up time which they could better employ in their main base. Many other calls to visit people in their homes can be answered, in the first instance at any rate, by community nurses, many of whom have special experience in the care of babies, children and the elderly.

Why then are many doctors reluctant to work with these non-medically qualified professionals? The reasons given are quite clear on the surface, and somewhat less clear when examined critically. It is therefore worth while looking below the surface for the origins of the doctors' reluctance, because if the difficulties can be overcome, the way opens towards a different kind of medical practice.

The main objection offered concerning non-medically qualified workers is that they may miss serious pathology. Associated worries are that the question of clinical responsibility is unclear, and that the patients may be unhappy about not seeing a 'real' doctor. In my own field of psychiatry, I have found these objections to be surmountable with regard to the work of community psychiatric nurses and social workers. Indeed I now see these as expressions of scepticism or anxiety on the part of certain consultants and general practitioners, and once these doctors realize what a great deal these competent people have to offer they become their staunch advocates. This is not just a generalization from psychiatry: nurses can equally well be involved in the management of general medical conditions, such as hypertension,[13] diabetes[14] and childhood asthma.[15] The more I see of the work of competent community nurses, the more aware I am of how few clinical conditions cannot be managed by them.

There are some more deep-seated difficulties, however, which relate to the intractable issue of power within the medical profession, and for that reason can provoke passionate and powerful reactions from certain doctors.

Community workers see themselves as serving the community and not the doctors. They work with the doctors, and are happy to do so up to a point, but, not having gone through a medical training, they do not have any allegiance to the medical profession. Nor do they share the doctors' concept of patients (or clients) as 'theirs', or accept that the doctor has some kind of proprietorial right over what happens to 'his' patient. Furthermore, the community workers have often had personal experiences which make them aware of what people actually need, and how much distress can be relieved by giving time and seeing people in their homes. Personal experiences may have led community workers into this kind of work in the first place, but such experiences are seldom given by doctors as a reason for deciding to study medicine.

The non-medical workers also have a totally different point of view from doctors. Community workers are primarily interested in health while doctors are primarily concerned with illness. Needless to say, people with such diametrically opposed viewpoints define problems in different ways. Doctors are very good when it comes to coping with illnesses, but they are not much interested in health or how to maintain it. The non-medical workers do not have a training in pathology, bacteriology and disturbed physiology, so they do not become absorbed by the subtleties of diagnosis. That is not to suggest that these workers are not capable of making diagnoses or of dealing with diseases and their consequences, merely that diseases are not their main interest. This different viewpoint can lead to clashes with doctors, as a primary interest in the maintenance of health presupposes an awareness of the interdependence of health, housing, economics and education. The ideologies connected with this wider view of health care tend to be slightly leftish and liberal, and they can conflict with the generally more conservative ideologies of doctors.

Any discussion of non-medically qualified health workers raises the issue of the 'barefoot doctors' in China or *feldschers* in the Soviet Union – that is, people with a limited medical training who work on their own in small communities, or else alongside fully qualified medical practitioners. Western doctors are quite right if they perceive these as a threat to their status. In China, they were part of the movement during the Cultural Revolution of the 1960s and 1970s to destroy the power of the medical profession. To a great extent they were successful, although the Chinese seem now to be rebuilding a medical profession with a structure familiar to us in the West,[16] yet with provision for the practice of traditional Chinese medicine. There is no question in any developed country now of

265

creating a new grade of medical worker with a limited medical training. There are, after all, plenty of workers, such as those already mentioned, in existing professions who have all the necessary skills.

I think the doctors' fears of being displaced are unfounded. There will always be a place for them if they are any good, and they will have an opportunity – although not automatically – to coordinate a team of health professionals who will work with them but will not necessarily be answerable to them. This team approach is potentially more rewarding, although more challenging, for the doctors, because skilled and articulate people from different disciplines bring to bear on each problem quite different kinds of expertise and assumptions about people and society. The doctors, however, have a singular advantage from their extensive theoretical training, which places them in a favourable position to understand and assimilate technological advances as they come along.

At the same time, if doctors are to be acceptable as coordinators of health teams in the community, or of more specialized teams in hospital, they will have to be prepared to justify their position by their medical expertise, administrative skills, and a practical knowledge of the work of all the members of the team.

In Britain the General Medical Council is slowly becoming more liberal in its style but its guide to professional conduct still has hard words for any doctor who wants to associate with non-medically qualified workers.

> The Council recognises and welcomes the growing contribution made to health care by nurses and other persons who have been trained to perform specialised functions . . . [but] the doctor should retain ultimate responsibility for the management of his patients because only the doctor has received the necessary training to undertake this responsibility.
>
> For this reason a doctor who improperly delegates to a person who is not a registered medical practitioner functions requiring the knowledge and skill of a medical practitioner is liable to disciplinary proceedings.[17]

Any doctor working, as I do, with community nurses will regularly trangress this edict, which sadly fails to recognize that many community nurses develop skills beyond those which can be expected of most doctors. For example, community psychiatric nurses are nowadays the most expert group in the management, in the community, of the long-term medication used for the people described as chronically psychotic. They administer the drugs, are in regular contact with the patients, have a more subtle grasp of the unwanted effects of the drugs, and also a greater interest in such work, than most doctors. Yet a completely inexperienced house officer, say, in orthopedic surgery, has a standing in this field which the experienced community nurse does not have.

When the work of community nurses is put to the test the results can be impressive.[13] A recent randomized controlled trial of the work of psychiatric nurse therapists in the treatment of people with phobic and obsessive-compulsive conditions showed that patients did better with behavioural treatment from the nurses than with what was called 'routine non-behavioural management by the general practitioner'. The patients also much preferred being treated in their own homes or on the general practitioner's premises, rather than in a hospital outpatient department.[18]

Further, many novel and informal ways of running clinics and delivering health care can be developed once nurses and others are given scope. To some extent this is an example of women organizing things for women, since most of the health workers in the community are women and three-quarters of those who use the services are women. The male domination of all medical services for so long has caused them to be arranged in a way which does not suit the convenience of women. The informal style often looks to men like chaos but it works: for example, having a clinic for pregnant mothers and mothers with their babies at the same time. They are all mixed up in the same waiting room, with infants of various ages crawling around on the floor. The women there can be supportive to one another, and they can at the same time get the specialist advice they need.

There is a great deal of therapeutic talent and goodwill in our communities. There are people keen to help others and, because of their various backgrounds, to explore different ways of giving care. In the mid-1980s these people still look to the doctors to take up their offers and generally to take a lead, although with the burgeoning of self-help groups and of complementary and alternative therapies the doctors are in danger of losing credibility as people who are interested in serving the population. It is important that doctors deal with their anxieties and move with the current of events, thus helping themselves and their patients at the same time.[19]

Partnership with patients

Patient participation groups are multiplying at an exponential rate in Britain. There was one in 1972; there were two in 1973, three in 1974, thirteen in 1981,[20] and sixty-seven by the end of 1983.[21] There were about 9,000 practices in Britain when the figure of sixty-seven groups was recorded, and that gives a ratio of one group for every 135 practices (0.7 per cent). They are concentrated mainly in urban areas and involve patients in all social groups. Their objectives are all broadly similar and they share a fundamental aim of trying to improve the quality of the dialogue between the providers and the consumers of health care, so that each can become properly aware of the objectives, aspirations, and difficulties of the other.

Patient groups can draw attention to unmet needs, such as those of immigrants or the housebound; to shortcomings, such as excessively long waiting lists for appointments at hospitals; and to personal difficulties that can arise with staff at clinics and health centres, or in relation to individual doctors. Education is also a prominent feature, and it is designed to show people how they can maintain and improve their own health, or how they can cope with their personal problems or chronic afflictions.[22–28]

My aim in this section is to see how far real partnership between doctor and patient can actually go. In two practices there have been specific attempts to achieve such a partnership, and these have both involved doctors with fairly radical political views.

The first is that of Alastair Wilson (1914–81) in Aberdare, South Wales. The practice was in an industrial town and had 'a tradition of social commitment by the doctors' dating back to 1849.[29] Wilson's father, brother, sister and brother-in-law all worked in the practice.[30] The philosophy of the Aberdare Patients' Committee was essentially democratic, and it was all the more radical for trying to be just that. As Wilson put it:

> The service is a national one; it does not belong to the doctors – it belongs to the people. So it is natural that the people should take part in running it. . .
>
> Our practice maintains that the general public should not only participate, by elections, in running the services but they should also be told about how to ensure the highest levels of care that modern medicine can provide. . .
>
> The elected patients' committee . . . is an example of local democracy and accountability from the health team to the people. Doctors have to be accountable. Why not to our patients who we know?[29]

Another practice run on unusual lines was that at Limes Grove, in Lewisham, south-east London. The Limes Grove Management

Collective was set up in 1976, and was an attempt to break down professional barriers. The doctors were all women working on a sessional basis, and they also employed a psychotherapist and a medically qualified acupuncturist. The staff were all paid the same, and most had other jobs as well. There were weekly workers' meetings, and monthly meetings of the management collective for staff and patients, where policy was decided. These meetings were informal, and since the patients' role was not clear, the staff tended to take the initiative. In the waiting room, there was evidently a notice inviting patients to inspect their own notes. The guide to the practice suggested that the practice staff were 'against the kind of control that doctors usually have over their patients'; and the staff hoped that by discussing problems 'people will learn about health and how to maintain it'.[31]

These two practice groups were the creations of doctors with left-wing sympathies, although there is no essential reason why their objectives of accountability, equality as far as possible between doctor and patient, and the practice of 'open medicine' should have political associations of any particular shade. These groups took on explicitly three of the most pressing issues in contemporary medical practice. No doubt doctors in other groups are trying to cope with these issues, perhaps in a more discreet manner in keeping with their local needs and circumstances; and perhaps they will be more successful than those who have taken up the struggle head-on.

Unfortunately, the good intentions of the two radical practices were not sustained. Alastair Wilson was a dedicated and charismatic figure, and when he died in 1981, much of the special character of his practice – which was really a benign paternalism – died with him. The Limes Grove practice ran into difficulties over the bourgeois question of salaries. It was a brave idea for all the workers at the practice to take home the same pay; but after a while the prime mover, Dr Barbara Jacob, found it difficult to interest doctors, in effect, in taking home the same pay as the cleaner; so the Limes Grove practice has had to modify its ideals.[32]

Throughout the literature of patient participation it is clear that it is the doctors who are in charge. Indeed the very term 'patient participation' suggests that the patients are being let in on something. There are murmurings about 'patient power'[33] but virtually everywhere in the Western world doctors are so well organized that when sickness strikes, patients are in no position to make demands. In other words, the only time when most people have contact with doctors is when they are in need, and that is not the moment to agitate for change. So, for the time being, the doctors remain firmly in control.

My interest in the process of participation between doctor and patient is less at the organizational level than at the point where the two meet each other in consultation, and there is an exchange between the two people.

The patient is sick and the doctor has the skill to bring relief. The patient also has the capacity for self help, and that capacity the doctor must foster, even though all Western medical education and the whole ethos of the medical profession encourage the doctor to be omniscient and to render the patient helpless. So, what does the doctor have to do to encourage a positive attitude in the patient?

Patients who are going to make use of the potential for healing that they have within themselves, and so participate in the healing process, require a world view which can accept some responsibility for the origin of the illness. The insights which are necessary for coming to terms with one's illness cannot be separated from the processes that may have led to its occurrence in the first place. It may be satisfactory for someone to accept a heart attack as a random event, and then work constructively to adapt to it. It would be better if the heart attack could be viewed in relation to the overall pattern of the person's life – habits of diet and exercise, emotional balance, pace of living, beliefs, anxieties and aspirations. Thus, participation at the deepest level starts by making demands on the patients. It is not enough to have lectures and group discussions: a clear measure of responsibility must be borne.

Self-help groups are a constructive step. Not only do they have practical objectives, they inculcate the idea that there is a great deal that people can do to help themselves;[34–39] and this is the object of the College of Health formed in Britain in 1983.[40]

The principle of 'open medicine' is good. It involves sharing information, and so reduces the power of the one who used to hold it exclusively. Yet there should be sufficient trust between doctor and patient for some secrets to be allowed, just as some secrets are acceptable between two people who have a close regard for one another. Perhaps this looks like paternalism again, and perhaps it is. Whenever the capacity is there, patients should be expected to take an informed interest in their malfunctions, and should not be allowed to adopt the passive attitude of 'doctor knows best'. But there are times when everyone needs to be allowed to be helpless, and the doctor should recognize that.

It is hard, therefore, to envisage a partnership between doctor and patient involving total equality. The patient will almost always initiate the transaction; it will be because of personal need, and the doctor is in a position to offer help.

Doctors should hold in their minds the idea, and the ideal, of partnership. They should remember that they have the knowledge and power to help people only in virtue of the training they have been given. Otherwise they have no special gifts, and they are vulnerable and fearful like everybody else. They should remember that they can give advice, administer treatments and relieve pain and distress. Doctors do not heal people. That healing comes from within the sick person and from beyond.

Notes and References

Introduction   Medicine lost

1   See Chapter 2
2   Bennet, G. (1979) *Patients and their Doctors: The Journey Through Medical Care*. London: Baillière Tindall, Chapters 3 and 4
3   Huxley, A. (1949) *Grey Eminence: A Study in Religion and Politics*. London: Chatto and Windus, p. 112
4   I touch on the question of what led me to study medicine in the first place, at the beginning of Chapter 6
5   Goffman, E. (1961) *Asylums: Essays on the Social Situation of Mental Patients and Other Inmates*. New York: Doubleday–Anchor. Harmondsworth: Penguin, 1968
6   Stockwell, F. (1972) *The Unpopular Patient*. London: Royal College of Nursing

Chapter 1   How doctors work

1   Berger, J. (1967) *A Fortunate Man* London: Allen Lane (Penguin, 1969. Also illustrated edition, London: Writers and Readers Publishing Cooperative, 1976). Romanticized medical fiction in books and on television is now a major industry
2   Bennet, G. (1983) *Beyond Endurance: Survival at the Extremes*. London: Secker and Warburg. New York: St Martin's Press
3   Clark. R. (Chairman) (1983) *Review Body on Doctors' and Dentists' Remuneration: Thirteenth Report, 1983*. Cmnd 8878. London: Her Majesty's Stationery Office
4   Lowe, M. (1985) Are doctors working harder? *British Medical Association News Review*, **12** (January), 13. See also *British Medical Journal* (1986) **292**, 1540–41
5   Bennet, G. (1983) Ref. 2 above, Chapters 8 and 9
6   Consumers' Association (1980) Should the 'chronic appendix' be removed? *Drug and Therapeutics Bulletin*, **18**, pp. 7,8
7   Bennet, G. (1983) Ref. 2 above, p.78
8   Friedman, R. C., Bigger, J. T. and Kornfeld, D. S. (1971) The intern and sleep loss, *New England Journal of Medicine*, **285**, 201–3

9   Friedman, R. C., Kornfeld, D. S. and Bigger, T. J. (1973) Psychological problems associated with sleep deprivation in interns, *Journal of Medical Education*, **48**, 436–41
10 Poulton, E. C., Hunt, G. M., Carpenter, A. and Edwards, R. S. (1978) The performance of junior hospital doctors following reduced sleep and long hours of work, *Ergonomics*, **21**, 279–95
11 Poulton, E. C. (1970) *Environment and Human Efficiency*. Springfield, Illinois: C.C.Thomas
12 Bennet, G. (1983) Ref. 2 above, p. 101
13 ibid. p. 119
14 Davis, D. Russell and Cullen, J. H. (1958) Disorganisation of perception in neurosis and psychosis, *American Journal of Psychology*, **71**, 229–38
15 Leighton, K. and Livingston, M. (1983) Fatigue in doctors, *Lancet*, **1**, 1280
16 Freudenberger, H. J. (1974) Staff burn-out, *Journal of Social Issues*, **30** (1), 159–65
17 Edelwich, J. and Brodsky, A. (1980) *Burn-Out: Stages of Disillusionment in the Helping Professions*. New York: Human Sciences Press
18 Cherniss, C. (1980) *Staff Burnout: Job Stress in the Human Services*. Sage Studies in Community Mental Health 2. Beverly Hills: Sage Publications
19 Paine, W. S. (ed.) (1982) *Job Stress and Burnout: Research, Theory, and Intervention Perspectives*. Beverly Hills: Sage Publications
20 Perlman, B. and Hartman, E. A. (1982) Burnout: Summary and future research, *Human Relations*, **35** (4), 283–305
21 Farber, B. A. (ed.) (1983) *Stress and Burnout in the Human Service Professions*. New York: Pergamon
22 Roberts, G. A. (1986) Burnout, *British Journal of Hospital Medicine*, **36**, 194–97
23 Edelwich and Brodsky (1980) Ref. 17 above, p. 28
24 Paine, W. S. (1982) Ref. 19 above, p. 37

Chapter 2   How doctors live and die

1   Registrar General (1978) *Decennial Supplement, England and Wales 1970–72, Occupational Mortality*. London: Her Majesty's Stationery Office. Only figures for male doctors are reported here
2   Williams, S. V., Munford, R. S., Colton, T., Murphy, D. A. and Poskanzer, D. C. (1971) Mortality among physicians: a cohort study, *Journal of Chronic Diseases*, **24**, 393–401
3   Ogle, W. (1886) Statistics of mortality in the medical profession, *Medico-Chirurgical Transactions*, **69**, 217–37
4   Registrar General (1958) *Decennial Supplement, England and Wales, 1951, Occupational Mortality (1951)*. London: Her Majesty's Stationery Office
5   Murray, R. M. (1978) The health of doctors: a review, *Journal of the Royal College of Physicians*, **12**, 403–15
6   Harrington, J. M. (1983) Cancer and the health industry, *Journal of the Society for Occupational Medicine*, **33**, 114–18
7   Doll, R. and Peto, R. (1976) Mortality in relation to smoking: 20 years' observations on male British doctors, *British Medical Journal*, **2**, 1525–36

8   Doll, R., Gray, R., Hafner, B. and Peto, R. (1980) Mortality in relation to smoking: 22 years' observations on female British doctors, *British Medical Journal*, **1**, 967–71

9   Doll, R. and Peto, R. (1977) Mortality among doctors in different occupations, *British Medical Journal*, **1**, 1433–36

10 Auld, P. (1959) *Honour a Physician*. London: Hollis and Carter

11 Mawardi, B. H. (1979) Satisfactions, dissatisfaction, and causes of stress in medical practice, *Journal of the American Medical Association*, **241**, 1483–86

12 a'Brook, M. F., Hailstone, J. D. and McLauchlan, I. E. J. (1967) Psychiatric illness in the medical profession, *British Journal of Psychiatry*, **113**, 1013–23

13 Vaillant, G. E., Sobowale, N. C. and McArthur, C. (1972) Some psychologic vulnerabilities of physicians, *New England Journal of Medicine*, **287**, 372–75

14 Krell, R. and Miles, J. E. (1976) Marital therapy of couples in which the husband is a physician, *American Journal of Psychotherapy*, **30**, 267–75

15 Shortt, S. E. D. (1979) Psychiatric illness in physicians, *Canadian Medical Association Journal*, **121**, 283–88

16 See Chapter 3, in particular, Refs. 5 to 10

17 Vaillant, G. E., Brighton, J. E. and McArthur, C. (1970) Physicians' use of mood-altering drugs: a 20-year follow-up report, *New England Journal of Medicine*, **282**, 365–70

18 Further details in Chapter 11

19 Murray, R. M. (1977) Psychiatric illness in male doctors and controls: an analysis of Scottish in-patient data, *British Journal of Psychiatry*, **131**, 1–10

20 The discharge rate is used here in place of first admission rate. It includes readmissions, which in this survey were commoner amongst the doctors than the controls, and also deaths in hospital

21 Welner, A., Marten, S., Wochnik, E., Davis, M. A., Fishman, R. and Clayton, P. J. (1979) Psychiatric disorders among professional women, *Archives of General Psychiatry*, **36**, 169–73

22 According to Bowman and Allen (ref. 37 below, pp. 63,64) these same data were interpreted differently by a similar group of authors (Clayton, P. J. *et al* (1980) Mood disorders in women professionals, *Journal of Affective Disorders*, **2**, 37–46), although with basically similar conclusions

23 Green, R. C., Carroll, G. J. and Buxton, W. D. (eds.) (1978) *The Care and Management of the Sick and Incompetent Physician*. Springfield: Charles C. Thomas

24 Scheiber, S. C. and Doyle, B. D. (1983) *The Impaired Physician*. New York and London: Plenum

25 Callan, J. P. (ed.) (1983) *The Physician: a Professional under Stress*. Norwalk, Connecticut: Appleton-Century-Crofts

26 McCue, J. D. (1982) The effects of stress on physicians and their medical practice, *New England Journal of Medicine*, **306**, 458–63

27 Stoudemire, A. and Rhoads, J. M. (1983) When a doctor needs a doctor: special considerations for the physician-patient, *Annals of Internal Medicine*, **98**, 654–59

28 Pond, D. A. (1969) Doctors' mental health, *New Zealand Medical Journal*, **69**, 131–35

29   Small, I. F., Small, J. G., Assue, C. M. and Moore, D. F. (1969) The fate of the mentally ill physician, *American Journal of Psychiatry*, **125**, 1333–42

30   Waring, E. M. (1974) Psychiatric illness in physicians: a review, *Comprehensive Psychiatry*, **15**, 519–30

31   Watterson, D. J. (1975) Psychiatric illness in the medical profession: incidence in relation to sex and field of practice, *Canadian Medical Association Journal*, **115**, 311–17

32   Franklin, R. A. (1977) One hundred doctors at the Retreat: a contribution to the subject of mental disorder in the medical profession, *British Journal of Psychiatry*, **131**, 11–14

33   Osmond, H. and Siegler, M. (1977) Doctors as patients, *The Practitioner*, **218**, 834–39

34   Jones, R. E. (1977) A study of 100 physician psychiatric inpatients, *American Journal of Psychiatry*, **134**, 1119–23

35   Martin, M. J. (1981) Psychiatric problems of physicians and their families, *Mayo Clinic Proceedings*, **56**, 35–44

36   Rucinski, J. and Cybulska, E. (1985) Mentally ill doctors, *British Journal of Hospital Medicine*, **33**, 90–93

37   Bowman, M. A. and Allen, D. I. (1985) *Stress and Women Physicians*. New York: Springer-Verlag

38   Thomas, C. B. (1976) What becomes of medical students: the dark side, *Johns Hopkins Medical Journal*, **138**, 185–95

39   Zigmond, D. (1984) Physician heal thyself: the paradox of the wounded healer, *British Journal of Holistic Medicine*, **1**, 63–71

40   Shapiro, E. T., Pinkser, H. and Shale, J. H. (1975) The mentally ill physician as practitioner, *Journal of the American Medical Association*, **232**, 725–27

41   Meissner, W. W. and Wohlauer, P. (1978) Treatment problems of the hospitalized physician, *International Journal of Psychoanalytic Psychotherapy*, **7**, 437–67

42   *Committee of Inquiry into the Regulation of the Medical Profession* (1975) Chairman: A. W. Merrison. London: Her Majesty's Stationery Office, p. 111

43   Bissell, L. and Jones, R. W. (1976) The alcoholic physician: a survey, *American Journal of Psychiatry*, **133**, 1142–46

44   Ruben, H.L. (1983) Substance Abuse and the Professional: How it Affects You, your Family, and your Colleagues. In Callan, J. P. (1983) ref. 25 above, p. 224. This estimate allowed for the fact that there are four times as many alcoholic men as women, and that college graduates are over-represented

45   Murray, R. M. (1976) Characteristics and prognosis of alcoholic doctors, *British Medical Journal*, **2**, 1537–39

46   Murray, R.M. (1977) The alcoholic doctor, *British Journal of Hospital Medicine*, **17**, 144–49

47   Lloyd, G. (1982) I am an alcoholic, *British Medical Journal*, **285**, 785–86

48   i.e. Member of the Royal College of Obstetricians and Gynaecologists

49   Lloyd, G. (1984) Professional self-help for alcoholism, *Bulletin of the Royal College of Psychiatrists*, **8**, No.1 (January), pp. 7–8

50   Strega, M. (pseudonym) (1978) Protecting the public, *World Medicine*, **13** (22 March), 47–48

51   Johnson, R. P. and Connelly, J. C. (1981) Addicted physicians: a closer look, *Journal of the American Medical Association*, **245**, 253–57

52 Moodlin, H. C. and Montes, A. (1964) Narcotics addiction in physicians, *American Journal of Psychiatry*, **121**, 358–65
53 Putnam, P. L. and Ellinwood, E. H. (1966) Narcotic addiction among physicians: a ten year follow-up, *American Journal of Psychiatry*, **122**, 745–48
54 Allibone, A., Oakes, D. and Shannon, H. S. (1981) The health and health care of doctors, *Journal of the Royal College of General Practitioners*, **31**, 728–34
55 'To ensure confidentiality, the questionnaires were identified only by a serial number which was linked to the name of the doctor through a register held by an independent body, the Royal College of General Practitioners'; ibid.
56 *Journal of the American Medical Association* (1903) Suicides by physicians and the reasons, **41**, 263–64 (an impressionistic leading article)
57 Friel, P. (1983) Physician Suicide, in *The Physician: a Professional under Stress*, ed. J. P. Callan (1983), see ref. 25 above, p. 180
58 Steppacher, R. C. and Mausner, J. S. (1974) Suicide in male and female physicians, *Journal of the American Medical Association*, **228**, 323–28
59 Bowman and Allen (1985) ref. 37 above, p 57. They question the assertion that women physicians have a higher sucide rate than male physicians
60 Rich, C. L. and Pitts, F. N. (1979) Suicide by male physicians during a five-year period, *American Journal of Psychiatry*, **136**, 1089–90
61 Pitts, F. N., Schuller, A. B., Rich, C. L. and Pitts, A. F. (1980) Suicide among US women physicians, 1967–1972. *American Journal of Psychiatry*, **136**, 694–96
62 Bruce, D. L., Eide, K. A., Smith, N. J., Seltzer, F. and Dykes, M.H.M. (1974) A prospective study of anesthesiologist mortality, 1967–1971, *Anesthesiology*, **41**, 71–74
63 Harrington, J. M. and Shannon, H. S. (1975) Mortality study of pathologists and laboratory technicians, *British Medical Journal*, **4**, 329–32
64 Brauchitsch, H. von (1976) The physician's suicide revisited, *Journal of Nervous and Mental Disease*, **162**, 40–45
65 Rich, C. L. and Pitts, F. N. (1980) Suicide by psychiatrists: a study of medical specialists among 18,730 consecutive physician deaths during a five-year period, 1967–72, *Journal of Clinical Psychiatry*, **41** (8), 261–63
66 Rose, K. D. and Rosow, I. (1973) Physicians who kill themselves, *Archives of General Psychiatry*, **29**, 800–805. (See also Richings, J. C., Khara, G. S. and McDowell, M. (1986) Suicide in young doctors, *British Journal of Psychiatry*, **149**, 475–78)
67 Epstein, L. C., Thomas, C. B., Shaffer, J. W. and Perlin, S. J. (1973) Clinical prediction of physician suicide based on medical student data, *Journal of Nervous and Mental Disease*, **156**, 19–29

Chapter 3 Doctors' marriages and families

1 Dalrymple-Champneys, W. (1959) Wives of some famous doctors, *Proceedings of the Royal Society of Medicine*, **52**, 937–46
2 Osler, W. (1908) The Student Life, in *Aequanimitas: with Other Addresses to Medical Students, Nurses and Practitioners of Medicine*, 2nd edn. London: H. K. Lewis, p. 435

3   Weber, M. (1905) *The Protestant Ethic and the Spirit of Capitalism*, trans. Talcott Parsons. London: George Allen and Unwin (1976)

4   Clapesattle, H. (1941) *The Mayo Brothers*. Minneapolis: University of Minnesota Press, p. 173

5   Scarlett, E. P. (1965) The doctor's wife, *Archives of Internal Medicine*, **115**, 351–57

6   Evans, J. L. (1965) Psychiatric illness in the physician's wife, *American Journal of Psychiatry*, **122**, 159–63

7   Lewis, J.M. (1965) The doctor and his marriage, *Texas State Journal of Medicine*, **61**, 615–19

8   Miles, J. E., Krell, R. and Lin, Tsung-Yi (1975) The doctor's wife: mental illness and marital pattern, *International Journal of Psychiatry in Medicine*, **6**, 481–87

9   Fine, C. (1981) *Married to Medicine: an Intimate Portrait of Doctors' Wives*. New York: Atheneum, p. 160

10 Elliot, F. R. (1979) Professional and family conflicts in hospital medicine, *Social Science and Medicine*, **13A**, 57–64. The numbers in this study were small (34 junior doctors and 16 dentists) but all the subjects and their wives were interviewed by the author, so the quality of the data makes up for the small sample

11 Elliot, F. R. (1978) The conflict between work and family in hospital medicine, *Health Trends*, **10**, 17–18

12 Elliot, F. R. (1978) Occupational commitments and paternal deprivation, *Child: care, health and development*, **4**, 305–15

13 Elliot, F. R. (1981) Mobility and the family in hospital medicine, *Health Trends*, **13**, 15–16

14 Bates, E. (1982) Doctors and their spouses speak: stress in medical practice, *Sociology of Health and Illness*, **4**, 25–39

15 Gerber, L. A. (1983) *Married to their Careers: Career and Family Dilemmas in Doctors' Lives*. London and New York: Tavistock

16 ibid. p. 103

17 ibid. p. 108

18 Nelson, E. G. and Henry, W. F. (1978) Psychosocial factors seen as problems by family-practice residents and their spouses, *Journal of Family Practice*, **6**, 581–89

19 Bates, E. M. and Carroll, P. J. (1975) Stress in hospitals: the married intern, vintage 1973, *Medical Journal of Australia*, **2**, 763–65

20 McClinton, J. B. (1942) The doctor's own wife: his fourth investment, *Canadian Medical Association Journal*, **47**, 472–76

21 Fine, C. (1981) Ref. 9 above

22 ibid. p. 104

23 ibid. p. 71

24 Garvey, M. and Tuason, V. B. (1979) Physician marriages, *Journal of Clinical Psychiatry*, **40**, 129–31

25 Heins, M., Smock, S., Martindale, L., Jacobs, J. and Stein, M. (1977) Comparison of the productivity of women and men physicians, *Journal of the American Medical Association*, **237**, 2514–17

26 Bowman, M. A. and Allen, D. I. (1985) *Stress and Women Physicians*. New York: Springer-Verlag, pp. 28–34. This is a general review of women in medicine

27 Heins, M., Smock, S., Jacobs, J. and Stein, M. (1976) Productivity of women physicians, *Journal of the American Medical Association*, **236**, 1961–64

28 Jussim, J. and Miller, C. (1975) Medical education for women: how good an investment? *Journal of Medical Education*, **50**, 571–81

29 Maynard, A. and Walker, A. (1978) *Doctor Manpower 1975–2000: Alternative Forecasts and their Resource Implications*. Research Paper Number 4, for Royal Commission on the National Health Service. London: Her Majesty's Stationery Office

30 Editorial (1979) *Journal of the Royal College of General Practitioners*, **29**, 195–99

31 Fine, C. (1981) Ref. 9 above, p. 216

32 Nadelson, C.C., Notman, M.T. and Lowenstein, P. (1979) The practice patterns, life styles, and stresses of women and men entering medicine: a follow-up study of Harvard Medical School graduates from 1967 to 1977, *Journal of the American Medical Women's Association*, **34**, 400–406

33 Rapoport, R. and R. N. (1971) *Dual-Career Families*. Harmondsworth, Middlesex: Penguin

34 Johnson, C. L. and Johnson, F. A. (1977) Attitudes toward parenting in dual-career families, *American Journal of Psychiatry*, **134**, 391–95

35 Lorber, J. (1984) *Women Physicians: Careers, Status, and Power*. New York and London: Tavistock

36 Bowman and Allen (1985) Ref. 26 above, Chapter 11

37 Zigmond, D. (1984) Physician heal thyself: the paradox of the wounded healer, *British Journal of Holistic Medicine*, **1**, 63–71

38 Vaillant, G. E., Sobowale, N. C. and McArthur, C. (1972) Some psychologic vulnerabilities of physicians, *New England Journal of Medicine*, **287**, 372–75. More details of this study in Chapters 2 and 11

39 Rosow, I. and Rose, K. D. (1972) Divorce among doctors, *Journal of Marriage and the Family*, **34**, 587–98

40 ibid. Timing of marital dissolution (mean years):

	Age at marriage	Years to separation	Age at complaint
All men	27.4	8.5	36.2
Managers, administrators*	28.2	10.1	38.4
Professionals*	28.9	10.3	39.6
Doctors*	30.3	12.2	43.1

*Men and women

41 Gerber, L. (1983) Ref. 15 above, p. 118

Chapter 4   Centuries of medical power

1 Sigerist, H. E. (1951) *A History of Medicine*, Vol. 1, *Primitive and Archaic Medicine*. New York: Oxford, p. 110

2 Gordon, B. L. (1949) *Medicine Throughout Antiquity*. Philadelphia: F. A. Davis, p. 109

3   Sigerist, H. E. (1951) Ref. 1 above, p. 320
4   Herodotus, *The Histories*, Book II, Chapter 84
5   For more details about this period, see Chapter 14
6   Phillips, E. D. (1973) *Greek Medicine*. London: Thames and Hudson
7   Allbutt, T. C. (1921) *Greek Medicine in Rome*. London: Macmillan (New York: Benjamin Blom, 1970)
8   Castiglioni, A. (1947) *A History of Medicine*. 2nd edn. New York: A. A. Knopf, p. 299
9   Clark, G. (1964) *A History of the Royal College of Physicians of London*, Vol. 1 (of three). Oxford: Clarendon Press, p. 6
10 ibid. p. 9
11 Dobson, J. and Milnes Walker, R. (1979) *Barbers and Barber-Surgeons of London: A History of the Barbers' and Barber-Surgeons' Companies*. Oxford: Blackwell, p. 9
12 ibid. p.18
13 ibid. p. 31
14 Clark, G. (1964) Ref. 9 above, pp. 15 and 17
15 Leeson, J. and Gray, J. (1978) *Women in Medicine*. London: Tavistock, Chapter 1
16 Clark, G. (1964) Ref. 9 above, pp. 54, 55
17 ibid. p. 58
18 Dobson, J. and Milnes Walker, R. (1979) Ref. 11 above, p. 32
19 Clark, G. (1964) Ref. 9 above, p. 84
20 ibid. p. 83
21 Dobson, J. and Milnes Walker, R. (1979) Ref. 11 above, p. 118
22 Clark, G. (1964) Ref. 9 above
23 Dobson, J. and Milnes Walker, R. (1979) Ref. 11 above
24 Cope, Z. (1959) *The Royal College of Surgeons of England: a History*. London: Anthony Blond
25 Wall, C., Cameron, H. C., and Underwood, E. A. (1963) *A History of the Worshipful Society of Apothecaries of London, 1617–1815*, Vol. 1. London: Oxford University Press
26 Copeman, W. S. C. (1967) *Apothecaries of London: a History, 1617–1967*. Oxford: Pergamon Press
27 Clark, G. (1964) Ref. 9 above, p. 332
28 Cook, R. I. (1980) *Sir Samuel Garth*. Boston: Twayne Publishers/G.K. Hall
29 Garth, S. (1975) *The Dispensary*. Facsimile reproduction with introduction by J. A. Bradham. Delmar, New York: Scholars' Facsimiles and Reprints Inc.
30 Clark, G. (1966) *A History of the Royal College of Physicians*, Vol. 2 (of three). Oxford: Clarendon Press, p. 472
31 Fraser, D. (1973) *The Evolution of the British Welfare State: A History of the Social Policy since the Industrial Revolution*. London: Macmillan
32 Conybeare, J. (1957) The crisis of 1911–13: Lloyd George and the doctors, *Lancet*, **1**, 1032–35
33 *British Medical Journal* (1983), **286**, 65–66
34 For further discussion of Paracelsus, see Chapter 12
35 Prince Charles (1985) *The Times*, 16 December

36 Hyde, D. R. *et al.* (1954) The American Medical Association: power, purpose and politics in organized medicine, *Yale Law Journal*, **60**, 938–1022 (May)

37 Berlant, J. L. (1975) *Profession and Monopoly: a Study of Medicine in the United States and Great Britain.* Berkeley: University of California Press

38 Raffel, M. W. (1980) *The U.S. Health System: Origins and Function.* New York: Wiley

39 Berlant, J. L. (1975) Ref. 37 above, p. 192

40 Bell, W. J. (1965) *John Morgan: Continental Doctor.* Philadelphia: University of Pennsylvania Press

41 Berlant, J. L. (1975) Ref. 37 above, p. 202

42 ibid. p. 209

43 ibid. pp. 234 *et seq.*

44 ibid. pp. 225 *et seq.*

45 Flexner, A. (1910) *Medical Education in the United States and Canada: A Report to the Carnegie Foundation for the Advancement of Teaching.* New York

46 Ehrenreich, B. and English, D. (1978) *For Her Own Good.* New York: Doubleday. London: Pluto Press, pp. 74–84. This passage contains accusations that the real effects of the Flexner report were to concentrate medical power in the hands of big business

47 Berlant, J. L. (1975) Ref. 37 above, p. 342

48 Carr-Saunders, A. M. and Wilson, P. A. (1933) *The Professions.* Oxford: Clarendon Press

49 Larson, M. S. (1977) *The Rise of Professionalism: a Sociological Analysis.* Berkeley: University of California Press

50 Parsons, T. (1951) *The Social System.* New York: The Free Press. London: Routledge and Kegan Paul

51 Freidson, E. (1970) *Professional Dominance: the Social Structure of Medical Care.* New York: Atherton Press

52 Freidson, E. (1975) *Profession of Medicine: a Study of the Sociology of Applied Knowledge.* New York: Dodd, Mead

53 Freidson, E. and Lorber, J. L. (eds.) (1972) *Medical Men and their Work: a Sociological Reader.* Chicago: Aldine

54 For further references, particularly to the socialization of doctors in training, see Chapter 6

55 Weber, M. (1968) *Economy and Society: an Outline of Interpretive Sociology,* Vol. 1, (ed.) G. Roth and C. Wittich. New York: Bedminster Press

56 Freidson, E. and Lorber, J.L. (1972) Ref. 53 above, p. 6

57 General Medical Council (1986) *Annual Report for 1985,* 44 Hallam Street, London, W1N 6AE, p. 16. Also *British Medical Journal,* **291**, 364

58 The populations Mrs Savage was serving were economically deprived; the kind shown in the Black Report (Townsend, P. and Davidson, N. (1982) *Inequalities in Health: the Black Report.* Harmondsworth: Penguin, p. 81) to have made least use of ante-natal services because they had difficulty getting to hospital clinics, although they were the social group most in need of such care

59 Documentation for these statements was produced at a meeting held at the Royal Society of Medicine on 22 March 1986; see the summary in the *Journal of the Royal Society of Medicine* late 1986. Also there is Mrs Savage's own

book, *A Savage Enquiry*. London: Virago, 1986. Other documentation comes from transcripts of the inquiry which appeared in *The Times* and the *Guardian* between 4 February 1986 and 10 March 1986. Reports and comments in the *British Medical Journal*, **292**, 476, 549, 613, 686, 753–54; and *Lancet*, **1**, 376, 434, 550, 594, 837, 864–65. Also background material from: *New Statesman* 31 May and 12 July 1985; and THS Health Summary (32 King Henry's Road, London, NW3 3RP), March 1986. For the point of view of Mrs Savage's main opponent, see interview with Professor Gedis Grudzinskas in *Hospital Doctor* (Update-Siebert Publications, 13/21 High Street, Guildford, Surrey), 11 September 1986, p.8

60 *Guardian*, 8 February 1986, p. 4
61 This kind of 'authoritarian' behaviour will be discussed further in Chapter six
62 Ferriman, A. and Leigh, D. (1985) Women's right go on trial in childbirth row, *The Observer*, 16 June

Chapter 5 Defensive medical attitudes

1 Jung, C. G. (1953) *Two Essays on Analytical Psychology*, Vol. 7 of *The Collected Works*. London: Routledge and Kegan Paul. New York: Bollingen/ Pantheon, para. 305
2 Jung, C. G. (1983) *Selected Writings*, ed. A. Storr. London: Fontana, p. 94
3 Gregory, J. (1772) *Lectures on the Duties and Qualifications of a Physician*. The Works of John Gregory, Vol. 3. London: Stahan and T. Cadell, p. 52
4 Nokes, P. (1967) *The Professional Task in Welfare Practice*. London: Routledge and Kegan Paul
5 Waitzkin, H. and Stoeckle, J. D. (1972) The communication of information about illness: clinical, sociological and methodological considerations, *Advances in Psychosomatic Medicine*, **8**, 180–215
6 Shenkin, B. N. and Warner, D. C. (1973) Giving the patient his medical record: a proposal to improve the system, *New England Journal of Medicine*, **289**, 688–91
7 Metcalfe, D. H. H. (1980) Why not let patients keep their own records? *Journal of the Royal College of General Practitioners*, **30**, 420
8 *Lancet* (1983) Confidentiality and accountability, **1**, 277–78
9 Northover, J. M. A. (1985) Filophilia, *Journal of the Royal Society of Medicine*, **78**, 93–95
10 Cohen, R. N. (1985) Whose file is it anyway? Discussion paper, *Journal of the Royal Society of Medicine*, **78**, 126–28
11 Bird, A. P. and Walji, M. T. I. (1986) Our patients have access to their medical records, *British Medical Journal*, **292**, 595–98
12 Short, D. (1986) Some consequences of granting patients access to consultants' records, *Lancet*, **1**, 1316–18
13 Guggenbühl-Craig, A. (1971) *Power in the Helping Professions*. Dallas: Spring Publications
14 Solzhenitsyn, A. (1971) *Cancer Ward*. London: The Bodley Head (Harmondsworth: Penguin), Part 2, Chapter 9
15 Lorber, J. (1984) *Women Physicians: Careers, Status, and Power*. New York and London: Tavistock, p. 42

16 Heims, M., Smock, S., Martindale, L., Jacobs, J. and Stein, M. (1977) Comparison of the productivity of women and men physicians, *Journal of the American Medical Association*, **237**, 2514–17

17 Bowman, M. A. and Allen D. I. (1985) *Stress and Women Physicians*. New York: Springer-Verlag, Chapter 6

18 Kent, A. (1985) The man power problem, *BMA News Review*, **11**, 16–17 (May)

19 Cooke, M. and Ronalds, C. (1985) Women doctors in urban general practice: the patients, and the doctors, *British Medical Journal*, **290**, 753–58

20 The work of the health professionals is described briefly in Chapter 18 under heading 'Partnership with health professionals'

21 Lorber, J. (1984) Ref. 15 above, pp. 21–29

22 Rosenthal, M. M. (1979) Perspectives on women physicians in the USA through cross-cultural comparison: England, Sweden, USSR, *International Journal of Women's Studies* (Montreal: Eden Press), **2**, 528–40

23 Roos, P. A. (1983) Marriage and women's occupational attainment in cross-cultural perspective, *American Sociological Review*, **48**, 852–64

24 Maguire, P. (1985) Barriers to psychological care of the dying, *British Medical Journal*, **291**, 1711–13

25 Robbins, G. F., Macdonald, M. C. and Pack, G. T. (1953) Delay in the diagnosis and treatment of physicians with cancer, *Cancer*, **6**, 624–26

26 Alvarez, W. C. (1931) How early do physicians diagnose cancer of the stomach in themselves? a study of the histories of forty-one cases, *Journal of the American Medical Association*, **97**, 77–83

27 Byrd, B. F. (1951) Fatal pause in diagnosis of neoplastic disease in physician-patient, *Journal of the American Medical Association*, **147**, 1219–1220

28 Rabin, D., P. L. and R. (1982) Compounding the ordeal of ALS: isolation from my fellow physicians, *New England Journal of Medicine*, **307**, 506–09, 1650–51. See also this paper and others by the Rabins in *To Provide Safe Passage: The Humanistic Aspects of Medicine*, ed. by P. L. and D. Rabin (1985). New York: Philosophical Library

Chapter 6 Doctors in the making

1 World Health Organization (1973) *The Selection of Students for Medical Education*. Report of a working group, Berne, 1971 (EURO 6203). Copenhagen: WHO, Regional Office for Europe

2 Barker, V. F. (1976) The selection of medical students: select bibliography, 1970–75, *Medical Education*, **10**, 514–16

3 In Chapter 4, also in Chapter 5

4 Adorno, T. W., Frenkel-Brunswik, E., Levinson, D. J. and Sanford, R. N. (1950) *The Authoritarian Personality*. New York: Harper and Row (New York: Norton Library, 1969)

5 Rokeach, M. (1960) *The Open and Closed Mind: Investigations into the Nature of Belief Systems and Personality Systems*. New York: Basic Books

6 Kohn, P. M. (1972) The authoritarianism-rebellion scale: a balanced F scale with left-wing reversals, *Sociometry*, **35**, No. 1, 176–89

7   Hare, R. T. (1972) Authoritarianism, creativity, success, and failure among adolescents, *Journal of Social Psychology*, **86**, 219–26

8   Dixon, N. F. (1976) *On the Psychology of Military Incompetence*. London: Jonathan Cape (London: Macdonald/Futura, 1979). Chapter 22 provides a good account of authoritarianism

9   Kline, P. and Cooper, C. (1984) A factorial analysis of the authoritarian personality, *British Journal of Psychology*, **75**, 171–76

10 Kline, P. and Cooper, C. (1985) Rigid personality and rigid thinking, *British Journal of Educational Psychology*, **55**, 24–27

11 Adorno, T. W. *et al* (1950) Ref. 4 above, p. 248 (1969 edition used)

12 Some workers question the association between rigid personality and rigid thinking, e.g. Kline and Cooper (1985), Ref. 10 above

13 Hudson, L. (1966) *Contrary Imaginations: a Psychological Study of the English Schoolboy*. London: Methuen (Harmondsworth: Penguin, 1967).

14 Hudson, L. (1968) *Frames of Mind: Ability, Perception and Self-Perception in the Arts and Sciences*. London: Methuen (Harmondsworth: Penguin, 1970).

15 Parlow, J. and Robinson, A. I. (1974) Personality traits of first year medical students: trends over a six-year period 1967–1972, *British Journal of Medical Education*, **8**, 8–12

16 Hudson, L. (1966) Selection and the Problem of Conformity, in *Genetic and Environmental Factors in Human Ability*, ed. J. E. Meade and A. S. Parkes. Edinburgh: Oliver and Boyd

17 Hudson, L. (1960) Degree class and attainment in scientific research, *British Journal of Psychology*, **51**, 67–73

18 Sheldrake, P. (1975) How should we select? – a sociologist's view, *British Journal of Medical Education*, **9**, 91–97. See also McManus, I. C. and Richards, P. (1986) Prospective survey of performance of medical students during preclinical years, *British Medical Journal*, **293**, 124–27

19 Fredericks, M. A. and Mundy, P. (1976) *The Making of a Physician: a Ten-Year Longitudinal Study of Social Class, Academic Achievement, and Changing Professional Attitudes of a Medical School Class*. Chicago: Loyola University Press

20 Merton, R. K., Reader, G. G. and Kendall, P. L. (eds.) (1957) *The Student Physician: Introductory Studies in the Sociology of Medical Education*. Cambridge, Mass.: Harvard University Press

21 Becker, H. S., Greer, B., Hughes, E. C. and Strauss, A. L. (1961) *Boys in White: Student Culture in Medical School*. Chicago: University of Chicago Press

22 Bloom, S. W. (1971) The medical school as a social system: a case study of faculty-student relations, *The Milbank Memorial Fund Quarterly*, **49**, No. 2, Part 2

23 Bucher, R. and Stelling, J.G. (1977) *Becoming Professional*. (Vol. 46, Sage Library of Social Research). Beverly Hills: Sage

24 Coombs, R. H. (1978) *Mastering Medicine: Professional Socialization in Medical School*. New York: The Free Press

25 Schwartz, A. H., Swartzburg, M., Leib, J. and Slaby, A. E. (1978) Medical school and the process of disillusionment, *Medical Education*, **12**, 182–85

26 Shuval, J. T. (1980) *Entering Medicine: the Dynamics of Transition. A Seven Year Study of Medical Education in In Israel.* Oxford: Pergamon
27 The concept of persona is discussed in Chapter 5

Chapter 7 Technology, drugs and people

1 Bennet, G. (1974) Scientific medicine? *Lancet*, **2**, 453–56
2 Saunders, C. (1976) The Challenge of Terminal Care, in *Scientific Foundations of Oncology*, ed. T. Symington and R. L. Carter. London: Heinemann Medical Books
3 Council for Science and Society (1982) *Expensive Medical Techniques: Report of a Working Party.* London (3 St Andrew's Hill, EC4V 5BY): Council for Science and Society.
4 Jennett, B. (1986) *High Technology Medicine: Benefits and Burdens* (1983 Rock Carling Fellowship). 2nd edn. London: Nuffield Provincial Hospitals Trust
5 ibid. p. 133
6 McKeown, T. (1979), *The Role of Medicine: Dream, Mirage or Nemesis?*, 2nd edn. Oxford: Blackwell, Chapter 8. See also critical review by G. E. Godber (1980) *British Medical Journal*, **1**, 102
7 Townsend, P. and Davidson, N. (1982) *Inequalities in Health: the Black Report.* Harmondsworth: Penguin. See also Smith, R. (1986) Whatever happened to the Black report?, *British Medical Journal*, **293**, 91–92; and Marmot, M. G. and McDowall, M. E. (1986) Mortality decline and widening social inequalities, *Lancet*, **2**, 274–76
8 ibid. p. 206
9 Hart, J. T. (1982), The Black Report: a challenge to politicians, *Lancet*, **1**, 35–37
10 Hart, J. T. (1971). The inverse care law, *Lancet*, **1**, 405–12
11 Charlton, J. R. H., Hartley, R. M., Silver, R. and Holland, W. W. (1983), Geographical variation in mortality from conditions amenable to medical intervention in England and Wales, *Lancet*, **1**, 691–96
12 Gardner, M. J., Winter, P. D. and Barker, D. J. P. (1984) *Atlas of Mortality from Selected Diseases in England and Wales 1968–1978.* Chichester: Wiley
13 Doyal, L. (1979), *The Political Economy of Health.* London: Pluto Press
14 Cochrane, A. L. (1972), *Effectiveness and Efficiency: Random Reflections on the Health Services.* London: Nuffield Provincial Hospitals Trust
15 Illich, I. (1976), *Limits to Medicine. Medical Nemesis: the Expropriation of Health.* London: Marion Boyars. See also critical review by D. F. Horrobin (1978) *Medical Hubris: a Reply to Ivan Illich.* London: Churchill Livingstone
16 Kennedy, I. (1981) *The Unmasking of Medicine.* London: Allen and Unwin (revised edition, Granada, 1983). The *Journal of Medical Ethics* (1981), **7**, devoted almost all of its December issue to ten critical articles about Kennedy's book, plus a reply from Kennedy, pp. 173–212
17 Taylor, D. (1982) *Medicines, Health and the Poor World.* London (12 Whitehall, SW1A 2DY): Office of Health Economics
18 The Association of the British Pharmaceutical Industry, *Annual Report, 1984–85.* London (12 Whitehall, SW1A 2DY): Office of Health Economics

19 Inglis, B. (1981) *The Diseases of Civilization*. London: Hodder and Stoughton (Granada, 1983)

20 Melville, A. and Johnson, C. (1982) *Cured to Death: the Effect of Prescription Drugs*. London: Secker and Warburg

21 Medawar, C. (1984) *The Wrong Kind of Medicine?* London: Consumers' Association and Hodder and Stoughton

22 Medawar, C. (1984) *Drugs and World Health: An International Consumer Perspective*. London (PO Box 111, London, NW1 8XG): Social Audit

23 Tucker, D. (1984) *The World Health Market: The Future of the Pharmaceutical Industry*. London: Euromonitor Publications

24 Melrose, D. (1982), *Bitter Pills: Medicines and the Third World Poor*. Oxford: Oxfam

25 Haslemere Group (1976), *Who Needs Drug Companies?*, London: Haslemere Group and War on Want

26 Silverman, M. (1977) The epidemiology of drug promotion, *International Journal of Health Services*, **7**, 157–66

27 Greenhalgh, T. (1986) Drug marketing in the Third World: beneath the cosmetic reforms, *Lancet*, **1**, 1318–20

28 Laurance, D.R. (1983), Medicine and the media, *British Medical Journal*, **286**, 218–19, 300–301. See also *Lancet* (1983), 'Opren scandal', **1**, 219–20

29 Melrose, D. (1982) Ref. 24 above, p. 63

30 *Lancet* (1983), Pharmaceutical policies for the Third World – whose responsibility?, **2**, 144

31 Barker, C. (1983), The Mozambique pharmaceutical policy, *Lancet*, **2**, 780–82

32 Eaton, G. and Parish, P. (1976), Sources of drug information used by general practitioners, and general practitioners' views of information about drugs, *Journal of the Royal College of General Practitioners*, Supplement No. 1, **26**, 58–64, and 64–68. See also *Sources of Information for Prescribing Doctors in Britain* (1977). London (12 Whitehall, SW1A 2DY): Office of Health Economics

33 Rawlins, M. D. (1984) Doctors and the drug makers, *Lancet*, **2**, 276–78. See correspondence, pp. 404, 405, 580

34 Veitch, A. (1984) *Guardian*, 28 November

35 Fry, J., Hunt of Fawley, J. H. H., and Pinsent, R. J. F. H. (1983) *A History of the Royal College of General Practitioners*. Lancaster: MTP Press

Chapter 8   Prejudices and irrational practice

1 Hare, E. H. (1962) Masturbatory insanity: the history of an idea, *Journal of Mental Science*, **108**, 1–25

2 Comfort, A. (1967) *The Anxiety Makers*. London: Nelson (Panther, 1968)

3 Anon (1710) *Onania, or the Heinous Sin of Self-Pollution, and All its Frightful Consequences in both sexes, consider'd, with Spiritual and Physical Advice to Those who have already Injur'd themselves by this Abominable Practice*. London: T. Crouch (6th edn, 1722, referred to here)

4 'Then Judah told Onan to sleep with his brother's wife, to do his duty as the husband's brother and raise up issue for his brother. But Onan knew that the

issue would not be his; so whenever he slept with his brother's wife, he spilled his seed on the ground so as not to raise up issue for his brother.' Genesis 38: 8 and 9 (New English Bible). Onan's 'sin' sounds like coitus interruptus, but might have been premature ejaculation or masturbation

5 Tissot, S. A. A. D. (1766) *Onanism: or, A Treatise upon the Disorders produced by Masturbation: or, the Dangerous Effects of Secret and Excessive Venery*, trans. A. Hume. London: J. Pridden

6 ibid. pp. 23–26

7 Hillman, J. (1966) Towards the archetypal model for the masturbation inhibition, *Journal of Analytical Psychology*, **11**, 49–52. Reprinted in Hillman, J. (1975) *Loose Ends: Primary Papers in Archetypal Psychology*. Dallas, Texas: Spring Books

8 The term 'animal' here is derived from the Latin *anima*, meaning breath of life or soul

9 Tissot, S. A. A. D. (1772) *An Essay on Onanism*. Dublin: James Williams. Cited by J. Hillman (1966), ref. 7 above

10 Skultans, V. (1979) *English Madness: Ideas on Insanity, 1580–1890*. London: Routledge and Kegan Paul

11 Rush, B. (1812) *Medical Inquiries and Observations upon the Diseases of the Mind*. Philadelphia: Kimber and Richardson, p. 347

12 Skae, D. (1863), A rational and practical classification of insanity, *Journal of Mental Science*, **9**, 309–19

13 Maudsley, H. (1868), Illustrations of a variety of insanity, *Journal of Mental Science*, **14**, 149–62

14 Hutchinson, J. (1890) On circumcision as preventive of masturbation, *Archives of Surgery (Hutchinson)*, **2**, 267–69

15 Hilton, J. (1863) *On the Influence of Mechanical and Physiological Rest in the Treatment of Accidents and Surgical Diseases, and the Diagnostic Value of Pain*. London: Bell and Daldy, p. 267

16 Hilton, J. (1863) *Rest and Pain*. 6th edn (1950), ed. Walls, E. W., Philipp, E. E. and Atkins, H. J. M. London: G. Bell and Sons, p. 273

17 *Cannabis* Report by the Advisory Committee on Drug Dependence (1968) (The Wootton Report). London: Her Majesty's Stationery Office

18 Mitchell, S. W. (1896) Remarks on the effects of Anhalonium Lewinii (the mescal button), *British Medical Journal*, **2**, 1625–29

19 Ellis, H. (1897) Mescal: a new artificial paradise, *Annual Report of Smithsonian Institution*

20 Campbell, A. M. G., Evans, M., Thomson, J. L. G., and Williams, M. J. (1971) Cerebral atrophy in young cannabis smokers, *Lancet*, **2**, 1219–1224

21 Hastings, J. (ed.) (1910) Circumcision, in *Encyclopaedia of Religion and Ethics*, Vol. 3. Edinburgh: T. and T. Clark (New York: Charles Scribner's Sons), pp. 659–680

22 Gairdner, D. (1949) The fate of the foreskin: a study in circumcision, *British Medical Journal*, **2**, 1433–37

23 Blandy, J. P. (1968) Circumcision, *Hospital Medicine*, **2**, 551–53

24 Masters, W. H. and Johnson, V. E. (1966) *Human Sexual Response*. Boston: Little Brown. London: Churchill. pp. 189–90

25   Gebhard, P. H. and Johnson, A. B. (1979) *The Kinsey Data: Marginal Tabulations of the 1938–63 Interviews conducted by the Institute for Sex Research.* Philadelphia: Saunders, p.127

26   Spock, B. (1965) *Baby and Child Care.* New York: Pocket Books, p. 155. (This book was first published in 1946)

27   Price, W. H. (1963) Gall-bladder dyspepsia, *British Medical Journal,* **2,** 138–41

28   Bakwin, H. (1958) The tonsil-adenoidectomy enigma, *Journal of Pediatrics,* **52,** 339–61

29   Wood, B., Wong, Y. K. and Theodoridis, C. G. (1972) Paediatricians look at children awaiting adenotonsillectomy, *Lancet,* **2,** 645–47

30   Wilson, J. M. G. (1981) Adenotonsillectomy: Scotland is beating England and Wales, *Lancet,* **1,** 895–96

31   Bloor, M. J., Venters, G. A. and Samphier, M. L. (1978) Geographical variation in the incidence of operations on the tonsils and adenoids: an epidemiological and sociological investigation, *Journal of Laryngology and Otology,* **92,** 791–801, 883–95

32   Miller, F. J. W., Court, S. D. M., Walton, W. S. and Knox, E. G. (1960) *Growing Up in Newcastle Upon Tyne: a continuing study of health and illness in young children within their families.* London: Nuffield, Oxford University Press

33   Binning, G. (1950) The influence of the perturbations of childhood life upon the occurrence of appendectomy, *Canadian Medical Association Journal,* **63,** 461–67

34   Tanner, W. E. (1946) *Sir W. Arbuthnot Lane, Bart.: His Life and Work.* London: Baillière, Tindall and Cox, pp. 116–17

35   ibid. p. 117

36   Todd, J. W. (1981) *The State of Medicine: a Critical Review.* Lancaster: MTP Press, Chapter 8 (The Errors of Medicine)

37   Mather, H. G., Pearson, N. G., Read, K. L. Q., *et al.* (1971) Acute myocardial infarction: home and hospital treatment, *British Medical Journal,* **3,** 334–338. Correspondence: **3,** pp. 473, 581–82, 704–05; **4,** p.172

38   Mather, H. G., Morgan, D. C., Pearson, N. G., *et al,* (1976) Myocardial infarction: a comparison between home and hospital care for patients, *British Medical Journal,* **2,** 925–29. Correspondence: p. 1208

39   Rawles, J. M. and Kenmure, A. C. F. (1980) The coronary care controversy, *British Medical Journal,* **281,** 783–86

40   Cochrane, A. L. (1972) *Effectiveness and Efficiency: Random Reflections on Health Services* (Rock Carling Fellowship, 1971). London: Nuffield Provincial Hospitals Trust, p. 53

41   ibid. p. 51

42   Ackner, B., Harris, A. and Oldham, A. J. (1957) Insulin treatment of schizophrenia: a controlled study, *Lancet,* **1,** 607–11

43   Cochrane, A.L. (1972) Ref. 40 above

44   Popper, K.R. (1963) *Conjectures and Refutations: The Growth of Scientific Knowledge.* London: Routledge and Kegan Paul (5th edn. 1974), p.46

45   Discussed in Chapter 1

Chapter 9   Doctors as agents of social control

1   Navarro, V. (1976) *Medicine Under Capitalism*, New York: Prodist; London: Croom Helm. See also A. Reidy (1984) Marxist functionalism in medicine: a critique of the work of Vincente Navarro on health and medicine, *Social Science and Medicine*, **19** No. 9, 897–910

2   Doyal, L. (1979) *The Political Economy of Health*. London: Pluto Press

3   Council for Science and Society (1980) *Childbirth Today: Policy Making in the National Health Service – a Case Study*. London (3 St Andrew's Hill, EC4V 5BY): Council for Science and Society

4   Scully, D. and Bart, P. (1978) A Funny Thing Happened on the Way to the Orifice: Women in Gynecology Textbooks, in *The Cultural Crisis of Modern Medicine*, ed. J. Ehrenreich. New York: Monthly Review Press

5   Donnison, J. (1977) *Midwives and Medical Men: a History of Inter-Professional Rivalries and Women's Rights*. New York: Schocken Books

6   Department of Health and Social Security (1970)*Domiciliary Midwifery and Maternity Bed Needs* (The Peel Report). London: Her Majesty's Stationery Office

7   Office of Population Censuses and Surveys (1985) *Abortion Statistics: Legal Abortions Carried Out under the 1967 Abortion Act in England and Wales, 1984*. Series AB no. 11. London: Her Majesty's Stationery Office

8   Clare, A. (1980) *Psychiatry in Dissent: Controversial Issues in Thought and Practice*, 2nd edn. London: Tavistock, Chapter 7

9   Bridges, P. K. and Bartlett, J. R. (1977) Psychosurgery: yesterday and today, *British Journal of Psychiatry*, **131**, 249–60

10 Bartlett, J., Bridges, P. and Kelly, D. (1981) Contemporary indications for psychosurgery, *British Journal of Psychiatry*, **138**, 507–11

11 Gostin, L. (1979) The merger of incompetency and certification: the illustration of unauthorised medical contact in the psychiatric context, *International Journal of Law and Psychiatry*, **2**, 127–67

12 Szasz, T. (1961) *The Myth of Mental Illness*. New York: Harper and Row. London: Secker and Warburg, 1962. Also Szasz, T. (1974) *Law, Liberty, and Psychiatry: an Inquiry into the Social Uses of Mental Health Services*. New York: Macmillan. London: Routledge and Kegan Paul

13 Szasz, T. (1978) The case against compulsory psychiatric interventions, *Lancet*, **1**, 1035–36. (1985) Psychiatry: rhetoric and reality, *Lancet*, **2**, 711–12

14 Clare, A. (1980) Ref. 8 above, Chapter 8

15 Woods, D. (1978) *Biko*. New York and London: Paddington Press. See also reports from the inquest in *The Times*, 14 November to 24 December 1977; particularly a full-page article by Sir David Napley (Past President of the Law Society), 9 December 1977, p. 10

16 Pollak, L. H. (1978) The Inquest into the Death of Stephen Bantu Biko: a report submitted to the Lawyers Committee for Civil Rights under Law, in M. Arnold (ed.), *Stephen Biko: Black Consciousness in South Africa*. New York: Random House

17 *The Times* (1977) 22 November, p. 8

18 Woods, D. (1978) Ref. 15 above, p. 197

19 *The Times* (1977) 23 November, p. 8

20 Woods, D. (1978) Ref. 15 above, p. 245
21 ibid. p. 255
22 ibid. p. 244
23 ibid. p. 239
24 ibid. p. 199
25 Pollak, L. H. (1978) Ref. 16 above, p. 293
26 Viljoen, C. E. M. (1978) The Steve Biko inquest. *British Medical Journal*, **1**, 239
27 Stover, E. and Nightingale, E. O. (eds) (1985) *The Breaking of Bodies and Minds: Torture, Psychiatric Abuse, and the Health Professions*. New York: W. H. Freeman, p. 109
28 Tobias, P. V. (1980) The South African Medical and Dental Council and the 'Biko doctors', *British Medical Journal*, **2**, 231
29 Shapiro, S. (1980) Medical work against torture: the case of Steve Biko, *New England Journal of Medicine*, **303**, 761
30 Hoffenberg, R. (1984) The Steve Biko case: appeal for funds for court action against South African Medical and Dental Council, *British Medical Journal*, **289**, 1378
31 For later developments see: *British Medical Journal* (1985) **290**, 479; **291**, 1052; *Lancet* (1985) **2**, 136, 1000–1001, 1428; *British Medical Association* (1986) ref. 75 below, p. 12
32 Amnesty International (1984) *Torture in the Eighties*. London: Amnesty International, pp 57–60. More details at the end of this chapter
33 Harris, R. and Paxman, J. (1982) *A Higher Form of Killing: the Secret Story of Gas and Germ Warfare*. London: Chatto and Windus (Triad/Granada, 1983 – references to this edition)
34 Sigmund, E. (1980) *Rage Against the Dying: Campaign against Chemical and Biological Warfare*. London: Pluto Press
35 Murphy, S., Hay, A. and Rose, S. (1984) *No Fire, No Thunder: The Threat of Chemical and Biological Weapons*. London: Pluto Press
36 *Lancet* (1984) Chemical and bacteriological weapons in the 1980s (leading article), **1**, 141–43
37 Harris, R. and Paxman, J (1982) Ref. 33 above, p. 168
38 Webb, H. E., Wetherley-Mein, G., Gordon Smith, C. E. and McMahon, D. (1966) Leukaemia and neoplastic processes treated with Langat and Kyasanur Forest disease viruses: a clinical and laboratory study of 28 patients, *British Medical Journal*, **1**, 258–66
39 Harris, R. and Paxman, J (1982) Ref. 33 above, pp. 76, 140, 152
40 *Unit 731: Did the Emperor Know?* TVS television documentary produced by Peter Williams, transmitted 13 August 1985. Details of the eminent doctors said to have worked at Pinfang were given in *The Mail on Sunday* (London), 11 August 1985
41 Harris, R. and Paxman, J. (1982) Ref. 33 above, p. 141
42 ibid. p. 76
43 Shifrin, A. (1980) *The First Guidebook to Prisons and Concentration Camps in the Soviet Union*. Seewis/GR, Switzerland: Stephanus
44 Bloch, S. and Reddaway, P. (1977) *Russia's Political Hospitals: the Abuse of Psychiatry in the Soviet Union*. London: Gollancz (2nd edn, London: Futura,

1980). New York: Basic Books (1977) under title: *Psychiatric Terror: How Soviet Psychiatry is Used to Suppress Dissent*

45   Bloch, S. and Reddaway, P. (1984) *Soviet Psychiatric Abuse: The Shadow over World Psychiatry*. London: Gollancz

46   Bloch, S. (1981) The Political Misuse of Psychiatry in the Soviet Union, in *Psychiatric Ethics*, ed. S. Bloch and P. Chodoff. Oxford: Oxford University Press

47   Amnesty International (1980) *Prisoners of Conscience in the USSR: Their Treatment and Conditions*, 2nd edn. London: Amnesty International

48   Podrabinek, A. (1980) *Punitive Medicine*. Ann Arbor, Michigan: Karoma

49   Fireside, H. (1979) *Soviet Psychoprisons*. New York: Norton

50   Koryagin, A. (1981) Unwilling patients, *Lancet*, **1**, 821–24

51   Voloshanovich, A. (1982) Soviet Psychiatry, *Medicine and Human Rights*, No. 2, February, London: Amnesty International

52   Fainberg, V. (1975) People listen, but do not hear, *Observer*, 5 January

53   Bloch, S. and Reddaway, P. (1977) Ref. 44 above, pp. 249, 259

54   Snezhnevsky, A.V. (1968) The Symptomatology, Clinical Forms and Nosology of Schizophrenia, in *Modern Perspectives in World Psychiatry*, ed. J. G. Howells. Edinburgh: Oliver and Boyd, pp. 424–47. New York: Brunner/Mazel (1971)

55   Merskey, H. and Shafran, B. (1986) Political hazards in the diagnosis of 'sluggish schizophrenia', *British Journal of Psychiatry*, **148**, 247–56

56   Bloch, S. and Reddaway, P. (1977) ref. 44 above, chapter 8

57   Reich, W. (1985) The World of Soviet Psychiatry. In: Stover and Nightingale (1985) Ref. 27 above, pp. 206–222

58   The dissidents would not necessarily agree that detention in a Special Psychiatric Hospital was preferable to a strict regime labour camp. Political prisoners tended to be kept together in particular camps, their sentence was determinate, and there were regulations concerning their care: none of these conditions applied in the Special Psychiatric Hospitals

59   Gluzman, S. (1982) Fear of freedom: psychological decompensation or existentialist phenomenon?, *American Journal of Psychiatry*, **138**, 575–83 (written in 1970)

60   Bloch, S. and Reddaway, P. (1977) Ref. 44 above, p. 419

61   Koryagin, A. (1981) My cry for help from a Soviet labour camp, *The Times* (London), 13 November. Edited version in *Lancet*, **2**, 1121. See also *Lancet* (1984), **1**, 50

62   Reddaway, P. (1985) Dissident near death in Russian jail, *Observer*, 8 September

63   Bloch, S. and Reddaway, P. (1984) Ref. 45 above

64   Bloch, S. and Reddaway, P. (1977) Ref. 44 above, p. 48

65   McNally, R. T. (1971) *Chaadayev and His Friends: an Intellectual History of Peter Chaadayev and his Russian Contemporaries*. Tallahassee, Florida: The Diplomatic Press

66   Podrabinek, A. (1980) Ref. 48 above, p. 55

67   ibid. pp. 57 et seq

68   Bukovsky, V. (1977) Cited by Bloch and Reddaway (1977) ref. 44 above, p. 201

69   Timerman, J. (1981) *Prisoner Without a Name, Cell Without a Number*. New York: A. A. Knopf. London: Weidenfeld and Nicolson, p. 54
70   Solzhenitsyn, A. (1973) *The Gulag Archipelago, 1, 1918–1956*. New York: Harper and Row. London: Collins/Harvill Press, and Fontana (edition cited here), 1974. p. 208.
71   Mitscherlich, A. and Mielke, F. (1962) *The Death Doctors*. London: Elek, p. 17. (First published as *Medizin Ohne Menschlichkeit*. Heidelberg: Verlag Lambert Schneider, 1949; reissued – Frankfurt: Fischer, 1985. Published in USA as *Doctors of Infamy*. New York: Schuman, 1949). See also Hanauske-Abel, H. M. (1986) From Nazi holocaust to nuclear holocaust: a lesson to learn? *Lancet*, **2**, 172–73
72   ibid. p. 365
73   Amnesty International (1984) Ref. 32 above, pp. 2–3
74   Stover and Nightingale (1985) Ref. 27 above
75   British Medical Association (1986) *The Torture Report: Report of a Working Party of the British Medical Association Investigating the Involvement of Doctors in Torture*. London: British Medical Association
76   de Figueiredo, A. and Steele, J. (1974) Torture films found at police HQ, *Guardian*, 3 May, p. 4.
77   Korovessis, P. (1969) *The Method: A Personal Account of the Tortures in Greece*. London: Allison and Busby 1970, p. 45
78   van Geuns, H. (1984) The Responsibilities of the Medical Profession in connection with Torture. In A. Heijder and H. van Geuns *Professional Codes of Ethics*, 2nd edn. (London: Amnesty International, p. 19). Dr van Geuns discusses the dilemma of doctors who feel that by cooperating with the torturers they might in some way lessen the victim's suffering, and thus be acting in the victim's best interest. Dr van Geuns is emphatic that this view is mistaken, and that any cooperation with the torturers is likely to be used by them to give a false legitimacy to their acts. The BMA shares this view, ref. 75 above
79   See also Sagan, L. A. and Jonsen, A. (1976) Medical ethics and torture, *New England Journal of Medicine*, **294**, 1427–30. Correspondence: **295**, 1018–20
80   Stover and Nightingale (1985) Ref. 27 above, p. 37
81   ibid. p. 13
82   Hawkins, R. and Cohen, J. (1983) Medicine or mutilation?, *World Medicine*, **18**, 24–25
83   Dareer, A. El (1983) *Woman, Why do you Weep? Circumcision and its Consequences*. London: Zed Press
84   Amnesty International (1984) Ref. 32 above, pp. 57–60

Chapter 10   Thinking about illness

1   The term 'illness' is used throughout to refer to what the person experiences, 'disease' to what the doctor diagnoses
2   Helman, C. G. (1984) *Culture, Health and Illness*. Bristol: J. Wright, p. 83.
3   Sigerist, H. E. (1951) *A History of Medicine*, Vol. 1, *Primitive and Archaic Medicine*. New York: Oxford University Press, p. 300
4   Leake, C. D. (1952) *The Old Egyptian Medical Papyri*. Lawrence, Kansas: University of Kansas Press

5   Ebbell, B. (1937) *The Papyrus Ebers*. Copenhagen: Levin and Munksgaard
6   Hussey, E. (1972) *The Presocratics*. London: Duckworth
7   Kirk, G. S., Raven, J. E. and Schofield, M. (1983) *The Presocratic Philosophers*, 2nd edn. Cambridge: Cambridge University Press
8   Burnet, J. (1930) *Early Greek Philosophy*, 4th edn. London: A. and C. Black
9   Guthrie, W. K. C. (1961 and 1965) *A History of Greek Philosophy*, Vol. 1 (1961) *The Earlier Presocratics and the Pythagoreans*; Vol. 2 (1965) *The Presocratic Tradition from Parmenides to Democritus*. Cambridge: Cambridge University Press
10 See Chapter 12 for a diagrammatic representation of humoral theory
11 West, M. L. (1971) *Early Greek Philosophy and the Orient*. Oxford: Clarendon Press. See also Filliozat, J. (1964) *The Classical Doctrine of Indian Medicine: its Origin and its Greek Parallels*. Translated from the original French by D. R. Chanana. New Delhi: Munshiram Manoharlal
12 Kuhn, C. G. (1821–33) *Claudii Galeni, Opera Omnia*. Cnobloch: Leipzig. These run to 22 octavo volumes, in the form of Greek and Latin parallel texts
13 Sarton, G. (1954) *Galen of Pergamon*. Lawrence, Kansas: University of Kansas Press
14 Siegel, R. E. (1968) *Galen's System of Physiology and Medicine: An Analysis of his Doctrines and Observations on Bloodflow, Respiration, Humors and Internal Diseases*.Basel: S. Karger
15 Siegel, R. E. (1970) *Galen on Sense Perception: His Doctrines, Observations, and Experiments on Vision, Hearing, Smell, Taste, Touch and Pain, and their Historical Sources*. Basel: S. Karger
16 Siegel, R. E. (1973) *Galen on Psychology, Psychopathology, and Function and Diseases of the Nervous System: An Analysis of His Doctrines, Observations and Experiments*. Basel: S. Karger
17 Siegel, R. E. (1976) *Galen on the Affected Parts: Translation from the Greek Text with Explanatory Notes*.Basel: S. Karger
18 Duckworth, W. L. H. (trans.) (1962) *Galen on Anatomical Procedures: the Later Books*, ed. M. C. Lyons and B. Towers. Cambridge: Cambridge University Press
19 May, M. T. (1968) *Galen on the Usefulness of the Parts of the Body*, 2 vol. Ithaca, New York: Cornell University Press
20 Brock, A. J. (trans.) (1916) *Galen on the Affected Parts*, Loeb Classical Library. London: Heinemann. New York: G. P. Putnam
21 Brock, A. J. (trans.) (1929) *Greek Medicine: Being Extracts Illustrative of Medical Writers from Hippocrates to Galen*. London: Dent
22 Temkin, O. (1973) *Galenism: Rise and Decline of a Medical Philosophy*. Ithaca: Cornell University Press
23 King. L. S. (1974) The Transformation of Galenism, in *Medicine in Seventeenth Century England*, ed. A. G. Debus. Berkeley: University of California Press
24 Saunders, J. B. de C. M. and O'Malley, C. D. (1950) *The Illustrations for the Works of Andreas Vesalius of Brussels*. New York: Dover, 1973
25 Harvey, W. (1624) . . . *De Motu Cordis* . . . , translated by G. Whitteridge as *An Anatomical Disputation Concerning the Movement of the Heart and Blood in Living Creatures*. Oxford: Blackwell

26 Descartes, R. (1637) *Discourse on Method*, trans. A. Wollaston. Harmonds-worth: Penguin (1960), Part 2, p. 50

27 ibid. Part 3, p. 58

28 ibid. Part 5, p. 79

29 ibid. Part 4, p. 66

30 Kuhn, T. (1970) *The Structure of Scientific Revolutions*, 2nd edn. Chicago: University of Chicago Press, p. 12

31 Vartanian, A. (1960) *La Mettrie's* L'Homme Machine: *A Study in the Origins of an Idea*. Princeton, New Jersey: Princeton University Press

32 Thomson, A. (1981) *Materialism and Society in the Mid-Eighteenth Century: La Mettrie's* Discours Preliminaire. Geneva: Libraire Droz

33 La Mettrie, J. O. de (1747) *Man a Machine*. French text of *L'Homme Machine*, with English translation of the 1748 version by G. C. Bussey (1912). The volume also includes English translations of *Frederick the Great's Eulogy* and *The Natural History of the Soul*. La Salle, Illinois: Open Court Publishing Co., p. 128

34 ibid. p. 141. The translator translated the word *horloge* as 'watch'. I have taken the liberty of substituting the word 'clock'

35 Riese, W. (1953) *The Conception of Disease: its History, its Versions and its Nature*. New York: Philosophical Library, p. 86

36 Noguchi, H. and Moore, J. W. (1913). A demonstration of treponema pallidum in the brain in cases of general paralysis, *Journal of Experimental Medicine*, **17**, 232–38

37 Illich, I. (1976) *Limits to Medicine: Medical Nemesis, the Expropriation of Health*. London: Marion Boyars

38 Parkes, C. M. (1972) *Bereavement: Studies of Grief in Adult Life*. London: Tavistock (Harmondsworth: Penguin)

39 Hinkle, L. E. and Wolff, H. G. (1958) Ecologic investigations of the relationship between illness, life experiences and the social environment, *Annals of Internal Medicine*, **49**, 1373–88

40 Querido, A. (1959) Forecast and follow-up: an investigation into the clinical, social, and mental factors determining the results of hospital treatment, *British Journal of Preventive and Social Medicine*, **13**, 33–49

41 Friedman, M. and Rosenman, R. H. (1959) Association of specific overt behavior pattern with blood and cardiovascular findings, *Journal of the American Medical Association*, **169**, 1286–96

42 Friedman, M. and Rosenman, R. H. (1974) *Type A Behavior and Your Heart*. New York: Knopf. London: Wildwood House

43 Rosenman, R. H., Brand, R. J., Jenkins, C. D., Friedman, M., Straus, R. and Wurm, M. (1975) Coronary artery disease in the Western collaborative group study: final follow-up of 8 years, *Journal of the American Medical Association*, **233**, 872–77

Chapter 11   The doctor's own needs

1 Vaillant, G. E., Sobowale, N. C. and McArthur, C. (1972) Some psychologic vulnerabilities of physicians, *New England Journal of Medicine*, **287**, 372–75

2 Thoroughman, J. C., Pascal, G. R., Jenkins, W. O., Crutcher, J. C. and

Peoples, L. C. (1964) Psychological factors predictive of surgical success in patients with intractable duodenal ulcer: a study of male veterans, *Psychosomatic Medicine*, **26**, 618–24

3   Pascal, G. R. and Thoroughman, J. C. (1967) Psychological studies of surgical intractability in duodenal ulcer patients, *Psychosomatics*, **8**, 11–15

4   McColl, I., Drinkwater, J. E., Hulme-Moir, I. and Donnan, S. P. B. (1971) Prediction of success or failure of gastric surgery, *British Journal of Surgery*, **58**, 768–71

5   The psychological argument (based on Freudian psychology) behind this statement is that the adult still yearns, symbolically, for this kind of unconditional love which is most clearly expressed by feeding at the mother's breast. The deprived infant in adult life expresses this yearning in part by being in a state of constant readiness for a feed which never comes. Thus gastric juice is secreted in anticipation, but since there is no feed, the juices act on the wall of the gut and erode it to produce an ulcer

6   Repression is defined as a psychological process, of which the individual is unaware, by which disturbing ideas and feelings are discreetly removed from consciousness and, as it were, deposited in the unconscious

7   Nichols, K. A. (1984) *Psychological Care in Physical Illness.* London: Croom Helm. Philadelphia: The Charles Press

8   Menzies, I. E. M. (1961) *The Functioning of Social Systems as a Defence against Anxiety: A Report on the Study of the Nursing Service of a General Hospital.* London: Tavistock

9   Bennet, G. (1979) *Patients and their Doctors: the Journey Through Medical Care.* London: Baillière Tindall, pp. 35–40

10 Vere, D. W. (1980) The hospital as a place of pain, *Journal of Medical Ethics*, **6**, 117–19

11 The question of balance and the tension of opposing forces features in Chapter 12

12 Jung, C. G. (1958) *Psychology and Religion: West and East Vol. 11 of The Collected Works.* London: Routledge and Kegan Paul. New York: Bollingen/Pantheon, para. 509

Chapter 12   Early medical alternatives

1   The term 'cosmopolitan' more accurately describes the current world-wide orthodox medical practice often called 'Western', 'modern' or 'scientific'. See F. L. Dunn (1976) Traditional Asian Medicine and Cosmopolitan Medicine as Adaptive Systems, in *Asian Medical Systems: A Comparative Study*, ed. C. Leslie (1976). Berkeley: University of California Press

2   The term 'hermetic' refers in a general way to occult practices dating principally from the time of the Renaissance. They are based on a vision of nature as a whole, and nature as active, animate and psychic, where there can be no meaningful distinction between what we would regard as animate or as inanimate, and all objects are capable of perception and of change. See ref. 33 below; and F. A. Yates (1968) The Hermetic Tradition in Renaissance Science, in *Art, Science, and History in the Renaissance*, ed. C. S. Singleton. Baltimore: Johns Hopkins Press

3 Jung, C. G. (1953) *Psychology and Alchemy* and (1967) *Alchemical Studies*, Vols. 13 and 14 of *The Collected Works*. London: Routledge and Kegan Paul. Princeton, N.J.: Princeton University Press
4 von Franz, M. L. (1980) *Alchemy: an Introduction to the Symbolism and the Psychology*. Toronto: Inner City Books
5 Guthrie, W. K. C. (1965) *A History of Greek Philosophy, Vol. 2, The Presocratic Tradition from Parmenides to Democritus*. Cambridge: Cambridge University Press, p. 471
6 Pagel, W. (1982) *Paracelsus: an Introduction to Philosophical Medicine in the Era of the Renaissance*, 2nd edn. Basel: Karger. See also W. Pagel's article on Paracelsus in *Dictionary of Scientific Biography*, Vol. 10. New York: Charles Scribner's Sons, pp. 304–13
7 Temkin, O. (1952) The elusiveness of Paracelsus, *Bulletin of the History of Medicine*, **26**, 201–17
8 Jung, C. G. (1966) Paracelsus, in *The Spirit in Man, Art and Literature*, Vol. 15 of *The Collected Works*. London: Routledge and Kegan Paul. New York: Bollingen
9 Jung, C. G. (1967) Paracelsus as a Spiritual Phenomenon. In *Alchemical Studies*, Vol. 13 of *The Collected Works*. London: Routledge and Kegan Paul. New York: Bollingen/Pantheon
10 Jacobi, J. (1951) *Paracelsus: Selected Writings*, trans. N. Guterman. London: Routledge and Kegan Paul
11 Stoddart, A. M. (1911) *The Life of Paracelsus*. London: John Murray
12 Debus, A. G. (1977) *The Chemical Philosophy: Paracelsian Science and Medicine in the Sixteenth and Seventeenth Centuries*, Vols 1 and 2. New York: Neale Watson (Science History Publications)
13 *British Medical Journal* (1983), **286**, 65 (1 Jan). Also *The Times*, 16 December 1985
14 Paracelsus, cited by C. G. Jung, ref. 8 above, para. 33
15 ibid. (from *Liber de caducis*), para. 42
16 Debus, A.G. (1977) Ref. 12 above, Vol. 1, Chapter 4
17 Yates, F. A. (1969) *Theatre of the World*. London: Routledge and Kegan Paul
18 Godwin, J. (1979) *Robert Fludd: Hermetic Philosopher and Surveyor of Two Worlds* (with 126 illustrations). London: Thames and Hudson
19 Debus, A. G. (1977) Ref. 12 above, Vol. 1, p. 208
20 Keynes, G. (1966) *The Life of William Harvey*. Oxford: Clarendon Press, p. 320
21 Debus, A. G. (1970) Harvey and Fludd: the irrational factor in the rational science of the seventeenth century, *Journal of the History of Biology*, **3**, 81–105
22 Rosicrucianism: an esoteric Christian sect, probably dating from the early 17th century, claiming secret knowledge from the Egyptian pyramids, Damascus, Plato, Jesus, etc.
23 Pagel, W. (1982) *Joan Baptista van Helmont: Reformer of Science and Medicine*. Cambridge: Cambridge University Press
24 Debus, A. G. (1977) Ref. 12 above, Vol. 2, Chapter 5
25 ibid. p. 546
26 ibid. p. 549
27 Pagel, W. (1982) Ref. 23 above, p. 6

28 ibid. p. 60

29 Debus, A. G. (1977) Ref. 12 above, Vol. 2, p. 341

30 Van Helmont and Fludd were close contemporaries but do not seem to have met. Van Helmont had a low opinion of Fludd, and called him 'a poor doctor and even less of an alchemist, . . . superficially learned [and] of little constancy'. Cited by Debus, A. G. (1977) Ref. 12 above, Vol. 2, p. 296

31 Rattansi, P. M. (1972) Newton's Alchemical Studies, in *Science, Medicine and Society in the Renaissance*, Vol. 2 (of two vol.), ed. A. G. Debus. New York: Science History Publications. London: Heinemann

32 ibid. Quotation taken from Sir David Brewster (1855) *Memoirs of the Life, Writings, & Discoveries of Sir Isaac Newton*. Edinburgh and London: Constable, II, 374–75 (reissued New York, 1965)

33 Westfall, R. S. (1972) Newton and the Hermetic Tradition, in *Science, Medicine and Society in the Renaissance*, Vol. 2 (of two Vols), ed. A. G. Debus. New York: Science History Publications. London: Heinemann

34 McGuire, J. E. and Rattansi, P. M. (1966) Newton and the 'Pipes of Pan', *Notes and Records of the Royal Society of London*, **21**, 108–43

35 Cohen, I. B. (1974) Newton – Alchemy, Prophecy, and Theology. Chronology and History, in Vol. 4, *Dictionary of Scientific Biography*. New York: Charles Scribner's Sons, pp. 81–83

36 Storr, A. (1985) Isaac Newton, *British Medical Journal*, **291**, 1779–84

37 Westfall, R.S. (1972) ref. 33 above, p. 195

38 Keynes, J. M. (1972) Newton, the Man. *In Essays in Biography*, Vol. 10 of *The Collected Writings*. London: Macmillan (St Martin's Press), pp. 363–74

39 Debus, A. G. (1977) Ref. 12 above, Vol. 2, p. 540

40 Debus, A. G. (1982) Scientific truth and occult tradition: the medical world of Ebenezer Sibly (1751–99), *Medical History*, **26**, 259–78

41 Evans, M. (1975) Medicine: Extending the Art of Healing, in *Work Arising from the Life of Rudolf Steiner*, ed. J. Davy. London: Rudolf Steiner Press, pp. 127–50

42 Bott, V. (1978) *Anthroposophical Medicine: Extending the Art of Healing*. London: Rudolf Steiner Press

43 Steiner, R. (1911) *Mystics of the Renaissance*. London: Theosophical Publishing Company (reissued as *Mysticism at the Dawn of the Modern Age*. Englewood, New Jersey: Rudolf Steiner Publications, 1960)

44 British Medical Association (1986) *Alternative Therapy*. Report of the Board of Science and Education. London: British Medical Association

45 British Holistic Medical Association (1986) *Report on the BMA Board of Science Working Party on Alternative Therapy*. London (179 Gloucester Place, NW1 6DX): British Holistic Medical Association

Chapter 13   Harmony and balance in the human system

1 Kirk, G. S., Raven, J. E. and Schofield, M. (1983) *The Presocratic Philosophers*, 2nd edn. Cambridge: Cambridge University Press

2 Hussey, E. (1972) *The Presocratics*. London: Duckworth

3 Burnet, J. (1930) *Early Greek Philosophy*, 4th edn. London: A. and C. Black

4   Guthrie, W. K. C. (1962) *A History of Greek Philosophy*, Vol. 1, *The Earlier Presocratics and the Pythagoreans*; and (1965) Vol. 2, *The Presocratic Tradition from Parmenides to Democritus*. Cambridge: Cambridge University Press

5   Kirk, G. S. (1954) *Heraclitus: The Cosmic Fragments*. Cambridge: Cambridge University Press

6   Marcovich, M. (1967) *Heraclitus: Greek Text with a Short Commentary*. Merida, Venezuela: Los Andes University Press

7   Kahn, C. H. (1979) *The Art and Thought of Heraclitus: An Edition of the Fragments with Translation and Commentary*. Cambridge: Cambridge University Press

8   The numbering of the Heraclitean fragments is according to Diels' classification; and the translations are those of Marcovich (ref. 6 above), unless otherwise indicated

9   Kirk, G. S. (1954) ref. 5 above, p. 5

10   The translation here is as given in Burnet (ref. 3 above p. 136). The fragment is numbered 45 in the classification of Bywaters which he uses

11   Guthrie, W. K. C. (1962) Ref. 4 above, Vol. 1, p. 448

12   Jung, C. G. (1973) *Letters*, Vol. 1, *1906–1950*. London: Routledge and Kegan Paul. New York: Bollingen Foundation/Princeton, p. 116

13   Jung, C. G. (1953) *Two Essays on Analytical Psychology*, Vol. 7 of *The Collected Works*. London: Routledge and Kegan Paul. New York: Bollingen / Pantheon, para. 111. (Jung wrote this passage during the First World War)

14   Sigerist, H. E. (1961) *A History of Medicine*, Vol. 2, *Early Greek, Hindu, and Persian Medicine*. New York: Oxford University Press, pp. 94 et seq

15   Kirk, G. S., Raven, J. E. and Schofield, M. (1983) Ref. 1 above, p. 260

16   Sigerist, H. E. (1961) Ref. 14 above, p. 323

17   Black bile was generally regarded as a toxic substance which could only be destroyed in the spleen. In Mediterranean countries, people are commonly found with enlarged spleens, and probably even more commonly in the ancient world, with malaria one of the prime causes. Any condition involving the discharge of altered blood could be held to be due to black bile; so also any condition in which darkened blood appeared, such as carbuncles, varicose ulcers, and cancer. See Siegel, R. E. (1968) *Galen's System of Physiology and Medicine: An Analysis of his Doctrines and Observations on Bloodflow, Respiration, Humors and Internal Diseases*. Basel: S. Karger, pp. 258–322

18   Sigerist, H. E. (1961) Ref. 14 above, p. 321

19   Lao-Tzu, *Tao Te Ching*, Harmondsworth: Penguin, 1963. The Pinyin spelling – Lao Zi – has been used here for uniformity in this book. See ref. 1 for Chapter 14

20   Filliozat, J. (1964) *The Classical Doctrine of Indian Medicine: its Origins and its Greek Parallels*. Translated from original French by D. R. Chanana. New Delhi: Munshiram Manoharlal, p. 172

21   Majumdar, R. C. (1971) *Medicine* [i.e. Ayurvedic], in *A Concise History of Science in India*, ed. D. M. Bose, S. N. Sen and B. V. Subbarayappa. New Delhi: Indian National Science Academy, p.217

22   West, M. L. (1971) *Early Greek Philosophy and the Orient*. Oxford: Clarendon Press. See also Filliozat, J. (1964) ref. 20 above, pp. 238–79

23 Filliozat, J. (1964) Ref. 20 above
24 Majumdar, R.C. (1971) Ref. 21 above, pp. 213–68
25 Thakkur, C. G., (1974) *Introduction to Ayurveda: Science of Life*, 2nd edn. New York: ASI Publishers Inc
26 Basham, A. L. (1976) The Practice of Medicine in Ancient and Medieval India, in *Asian Medical Systems: A Comparative Study*, ed. C. Leslie (1976). Berkeley: University of California Press
27 Tabor, D. C. (1981) Ripe and unripe: concepts of health and sickness in Ayurvedic medicine, *Social Science and Medicine*, **15B**, 439–55
28 Patterson, T. J. S. (1983) *Science and Medicine in India in Information sources in the History of Science and Medicine*. London: Butterworth Scientific, p. 459
29 Kurup, P. N. V. (1983) *Ayurveda*, in *Traditional Medicine and Health Care Coverage: A Reader for Health Administrators and Practitioners*, ed. R. H. Bannerman, J. Burton and Ch'en Wne-Chieh. Geneva: World Health Organization, pp. 50–60
30 *Caraka-Samhita: Agnivesa's treatise refined and annotated by Caraka and redacted by Drdhabla*, 2 Vols, trans. and ed. by P. V. Sharma (1981 and 1983). Varnasi, India (also Delhi): Chaukhambha Orientalia
31 *Susruta Samhita*, 3 vols, trans. and ed. by K. K. Bhishagratna, 2nd ed. (1963). Varanasi, India: Chowkhamba Sanskrit Series Office
32 Siddiqi, M. Z. (1971) *The Unani Tibb (Greek Medicine) in India*, in *A Concise History of Science in India*, ed. D. M. Bose, S. N. Sen and B. V. Subbarayappa. New Delhi: Indian National Science Academy, pp. 268–73
33 Said, H. M. (1983) *The Unani System of Health and Medicare*, in Bannerman, R. H. *et al.*, ref 29 above
34 Eagle, R. (1980) Your friendly neighbourhood hakim, *World Medicine*, **15** (26 July), 19–22
35 Filliozat, J. (1964) Ref. 20 above, p. 240
36 Leslie, C. (1976) The Ambiguities of Medical Revivalism in Modern India, in *Asian Medical Systems: A Comparative Study*, ed. C. Leslie (1976). Berkeley: University of California Press
37 Thakkur, C.G. (1974) Ref. 25 above, pp. 112–132
38 ibid. p. 2
39 Said, H. M. (1983) Ref. 33 above, p. 62
40 The Ayurvedic and Unani systems have not been described here because to do so would have taken me far from the main line of argument, and the details are not all that relevant here. Also I have felt that the underlying ideas – particularly about the whole – in the Indian medical systems occur also in Chinese thinking, and I have chosen to concentrate on the Chinese. Nevertheless, the Indian systems deserve much closer study by Western scholars, who can deal with the primary sources, than they have hitherto received

Chapter 14   The Dao and Chinese medicine

1 The Pinyin system of romanization of Chinese characters is used throughout as it has been the official form in China since 1979, and it is also phonetically more accurate. However, it is less familiar that the Wade-Giles system, so

that form is given in brackets at the first mention. The titles of books in the reference section are given exactly as published, but Chinese names and words quoted from them are rendered in Pinyin

2 Needham, J. (1956) *Science and Civilisation in China*, Vol. 2, *History of Scientific Thought*. Cambridge: Cambridge University Press, p. 228

3 Lao Tzu (Lao Zi) *Tao te Ching (Dao de Jing), Richard Wilhelm Edition* (1985), translated into English by H.G. Ostwald. London: Arkana/Routledge and Kegan Paul, p. 12

4 Lao Tzu (Lao Zi) *Tao te Ching (Dao de Jing)*. Translated by Gia-Fu Feng and J. English. London: Wildwood. New York: Vintage Books, 1972

5 *Chuang Tzu (Zhuang Zi)* (1926) Translated by H. A. Giles. London: George Allen and Unwin (1980)

6 *I Ching (Yi Jing)*. Translated by R. Wilhelm, 2 vols, London: Routledge and Kegan Paul, 1951

7 Capra, F. (1975) *The Tao of Physics*. London: Wildwood House (London: Fontana, 1976)

8 Lao Tzu, Ref. 4 above, Chapter 40

9 Needham, J. (1956) ref. 2 above, p. 277

10 Lao Tzu, Ref. 4 above, Chapter 48

11 ibid. Chapter 56

12 ibid. Chapter 73

13 Porkert, M. (1979) Chinese Medicine: a Traditional Healing Science, in *Ways to Health: Holistic Approaches to Ancient and Contemporary Medicine*, ed. D. S. Sobel. New York: Harcourt Brace Jovanovich, pp. 150–51

14 Porkert, M. (1974) *The Theoretical Foundations of Chinese Medicine: Systems of Correspondence*. Cambridge, Mass.: MIT Press

15 Needham, J. (1956) Ref. 2 above. General reference

16 Kaptchuk, T. J. (1983) *Chinese Medicine: The Web that has no Weaver*. London: Rider

17 Jung, C. G. (1966) Richard Wilhelm: In Memoriam, in *The Spirit in Man, Art, and Literature*, Vol. 15 of *The Collected Works*, London: Routledge and Kegan Paul. New York: Bollingen/Pantheon, para. 81

18 Jung, C. G. (1952) Synchronicity: An Acausal Connecting Principle, in *The Structure and Dynamics of the Psyche*, Vol. 8 of *The Collected Works*. London: Routledge and Kegan Paul. New York: Bollingen/Pantheon. For writings by Jung on Chinese modes of thinking, see Wilhelm, R. and Jung, C. G. (1935) *The Secret of the Golden Flower: a Chinese Book of Life*. London: Kegan Paul, Trench, Trubner and Co. Commentary by C. G. Jung also (retranslated) in *Alchemical Studies*, Vol. 13 (1967) of *The Collected Works*. London: Routledge and Kegan Paul. Princeton, N. J.: Princeton University Press. Also Jung, C. G. (1949) Foreword to the *I Ching*, ref. 6 above, p. ii. It also appears in *Psychology and Religion: West and East*, Vol. 11 (1958) of *The Collected Works*. London: Routledge and Kegan Paul. New York: Bollingen/Pantheon, paras 968–69

19 Needham, J. (1956) Ref. 2 above, p. 279

20 ibid. p. 280

21 ibid. pp. 280–81

22 ibid. p. 288, citing the French sinologist Marcel Granet

23 ibid. p. 287
24 *Chuang Tzu*, Ref. 5 above, Chapter 2, p. 36. Quotation taken from Needham, J. (1956) Ref. 2 above, p. 52
25 Porkert, M. (1974) Ref. 14 above, p.1
26 Needham, J. (1956) Ref. 2 above, p. 294 et seq.
27 Porkert, M. (1974) Ref. 14 above, p. 9
28 Kaptchuk, T. J. (1983) Ref. 16 above, pp. 8 et seq.
29 Bennett, S. J. (1978) Chinese science: theory and practice, *Philosophy East and West*, **28**, 439–53
30 The term 'Evolutive Phase' is one of Porkert's, and he uses it for two reasons. First, he says, the Chinese words *wu xing (wu hsing)* do not translate as 'five elements', even though that has been the standard translation hitherto, and it has led to a misunderstanding of the concept. *Xing* really means 'passing through', and the term 'evolutive phase'. Secondly, the system is not describing the composition of the world (usually imagined in the West as static) but qualities of energy (which are constantly changing). Porkert, M. (1974) Ref. 14 above, p. 45
31 Needham, J. (1956) Ref. 2 above, p. 266
32 ibid. p. 262
33 Kaptchuk, T. J. (1983) Ref. 16 above, p. 352
34 Lock, M. M. (1980) *East Asian Medicine in Urban Japan*. Berkeley: University of California Press p. 64
35 ibid. p. 15
36 ibid. General reference
37 See also Otsuka, Y. (1976) Chinese Traditional Medicine in Japan, in *Asian Medical Systems: A Comparative Study*, ed. C. Leslie (1976). Berkeley: University of California Press
38 In Taiwan there is a similar mixing of traditional Chinese (East Asian) medicine with cosmopolitan medicine. See Kleinmann, A. (1980) *Patients and Healers in the Context of Culture: an Exploration of the Borderland between Anthropology, Medicine, and Psychiatry*. Berkeley: University of California Press. Also, Croizier, R. C. (1968) *Traditional Medicine in Modern China: Science, Nationalism and the Tensions of Cultural Change*. Cambridge, Mass.: Harvard University Press
39 Lock, M. M. (1980) Ref. 34 above, p. 113
40 The traditional art of pulse diagnosis in which twelve distinct pulses are identified by palpation (three superficial and three deep at each wrist), is regarded sceptically by Western doctors. However, pulsograph tracings of these do seem to support the contentions of the Chinese practitioners. See G. T. Lewith (1982) *Acupuncture: Its Place in Western Medical Science*. Wellingborough, Northamptonshire: Thorsons, p. 26
41 Lock, M. M. (1980) Ref. 34 above, p. 114
42 German was used on the 'cosmopolitan' part of the form, because, according to Margaret Lock, 'the major Western source of influence on Japanese medicine was Germany' (p. 114). The *first* Western influence in Japan, however, was Portuguese in the sixteenth century
43 Lock, M. M. (1980) Ref. 34 above, p. 127
44 ibid. p. 128

45 ibid. p. 134
46 ibid. p. 77
47 ibid. p. 80

Chapter 15   The wounded healer

1 Morris, J. (1976) *Radio Times*, 22 October
2 That is, Ulysses, or *Ulixes*, derived from the Greek: *oulos* wound, and *ischion* thigh. This is according to Robert Graves (1955) *The Greek Myths*, Vol. 2. Harmondsworth: Penguin, p. 369
3 Wilson, E. (1941) *The Wound and the Bow: Seven Studies in Literature*. Cambridge, Mass.: Houghton Mifflin Company. London: Secker and Warburg (London: Methuen, 1961)
4 Heracles had been poisoned by a garment smeared with the blood of Nessus, a centaur, whom he had killed some time before for making advances to his wife, Deianira. As Nessus was dying, he had given Deianira some of his blood, saying it was a love-potion, and later Deianira had sent it to Heracles to try to win back his affection, but the blood killed him
5 Homer, *The Iliad*, Book 2, line 718 (Harmondsworth: Penguin edn, p.58)
6 Jung says that Chryse represented the anima (the unconscious feminine principle) which had risen up in revenge against Philoctetes for rejecting the unconscious. In *Symbols of Transformation* (1958), Vol. 5 of *The Collected Works*. London: Routledge and Kegan Paul. New York: Bollingen/ Pantheon, para. 450
7 Kerenyi, C. (1959) *Asklepios: Archetypal Image of the Physician's Existence*. New York: Pantheon, p.7
8 Deuteronomy 32: 39
9 Edelstein, E. J. and L. (1945) *Asclepius: A Collection and Interpretation of the Testimonies*, 2 Vols. Baltimore: Johns Hopkins Press, Vol. 1, para. 458 (p. 263). Galen had a right subphrenic abscess which he developed at the age of twenty-eight while he was still living at Pergamon, then one of the principal centres for the Asclepians
10 Edelstein, L. (1967) The Hippocratic Oath: Text, Translation and Interpretation, in *Ancient Medicine: Selected Papers of Ludwig Edelstein*, ed. O. and C. L. Temkin. Baltimore: Johns Hopkins Press, pp. 3–63
11 Edelstein, E.J. and L. (1945) Ref. 9 above. General reference
12 Meier, C.A. (1967) *Ancient Incubation and Modern Psychotherapy*. Evanston: Northwestern University Press
13 Eliade, M. (1964) *Shamanism: Archaic Techniques of Ecstasy*. London: Routledge and Kegan Paul
14 Harner, M. (1980) *The Way of the Shaman: a Guide to Power and Healing*. New York: Harper and Row
15 Halifax, J. (1982) *Shaman: the Wounded Healer* (with 131 illustrations). London: Thames and Hudson
16 Hultkrantz, A. (1985) The shaman and the medicine-man, *Social Science and Medicine*, **20**, No. 5, 511–15
17 Lewis, I. M. (1971) *Ecstatic Religion: An Anthropological Study of Spirit Possession and Shamanism*. Harmondsworth: Penguin, p. 192

18   Matthew 4: 1,2
19   Vanstone, W. H. (1982) *The Stature of Waiting*. London: Darton, Longman and Todd, Chapter 2
20   ibid. pp. 30, 35
21   1 Peter 2: 24
22   2 Corinthians 12: 9,10
23   The term 'archetype' is imprecise and is used in various ways, in modern times notably by Jung. See Jung, C. G. (1964) *Civilization in Transition*, Vol. 10 of *The Collected Works*. London: Routledge and Kegan Paul. New York: Bollingen/Pantheon, para. 847. See also Stevens, A. (1982) *Archetype: A Natural History of the Self*. London: Routledge and Kegan Paul. And Guggenbühl-Craig, A. (1971) ref. 25 below
24   Jung, C. G. (1960) *The Structure and Dynamics of the Psyche*, Vol. 8 of *The Collected Works*. London: Routledge and Kegan Paul. New York: Bollingen/Pantheon, para. 198
25   Guggenbühl-Craig, A. (1971) *Power in the Helping Professions*. Dallas: Spring Publications
26   Cousins, N. (1979) *Anatomy of an Illness as Perceived by the Patient: Reflections on Healing and Regeneration*. New York: W. W. Norton, p. 69
27   Jung, C. G. (1954) *The Practice of Psychotherapy*, Vol. 16, *The Collected Works*. London: Routledge and Kegan Paul. New York: Bollingen/Pantheon, para. 163
28   Adler, G. (1984) Regarding the wounded healer, *British Journal of Holistic Medicine*, **1**, 131–32
29   Jung, C. G. (1954) Ref. 27 above, para. 422
30   Zigmond, D. (1984) Physician heal thyself: the paradox of the wounded healer, *British Journal of Holistic Medicine*, **1**, 63–71

Chapter 16   The whole, health and systems

 1   Hillman, J. (1975) *Re-Visioning Psychology*. New York: Harper and Row
 2   Russell, B. (1912) *The Problems of Philosophy*. London: Williams and Norgate (Home University Library), p. 249
 3   Heisenberg, W. (1958) *Physics and Philosophy: The Revolution in Modern Science*. London: Allen and Unwin, 1959. New York: Harper and Row, 1962, pp. 96 and 173
 4   Niels Bohr's coat of arms shown on BBC Television 'Everyman' programme, featuring Fritjof Capra, 26 January 1986
 5   Krishnamurti, J. (1954) *The First and Last Freedom*. London: Victor Gollancz, Chapter 15, 'The thinker and the thought'
 6   Bohm, D. (1980) *Wholeness and the Implicate Order*. London: Routledge and Kegan Paul (reprinted with corrections 1981), p. 11
 7   ibid. p. 48
 8   ibid. p. 64
 9   ibid. p. 39
10   ibid. p. 177
11   ibid. p. xiv

12 Capra, F. (1975) *The Tao of Physics.* Berkeley: Shambala. London: Wildwood and Fontana

13 Capra, F. (1982) *The Turning Point: Science, Society, and the Rising Culture.* London: Wildwood House

14 Lovelock, J. E. (1979) *Gaia: A New Look at Life on Earth.* Oxford and New York: Oxford University Press

15 Jantsch, E. (1980) *The Self-Organizing Universe: Scientific and Human Implications of the Emerging Paradigm of Evolution.* Oxford and New York: Pergamon

16 An exception to this, among philosophers, was Leibniz, who also interested himself in Chinese thought. See Needham, J. (1956) *Science and Civilisation in China*, Vol. 2. Cambridge: Cambridge University Press, pp. 340–45

17 Heisenberg, W. (1958) Ref. 3 above, p. 96

18 Smuts, J. C. (1926) *Holism and Evolution.* London: Macmillan

19 ibid. p. 100

20 ibid. p. 109

21 ibid. p. 101

22 Weiss, P. A. (1969) The Living System, in *Beyond Reductionism: New Perspectives in the Life Sciences*, ed. A. Koestler and J. R. Smythies. Boston: Beacon Press. London: Hutchinson, pp. 47 and 55

23 In Jung's words: 'the unconscious [is] the only available source of religious experience. This is certainly not to say that what we call the unconscious is identical with God or is set up in his place. It is simply the medium from which religious experience seems to flow. As to what the further cause of such experience may be, the answer to this lies beyond the range of human knowledge. Knowledge of God is a transcendental problem.' Jung, C. G. (1956) The Undiscovered Self, in *Civilization in Transition* (1964), Vol. 10 of *The Collected Works*. London: Routledge and Kegan Paul. New York: Bollingen/Pantheon, para. 565

24 Ziegler, A. (1983) *Archetypal Medicine* (original title in German: *Morbismus*). Dallas: Spring Books

25 Needham, J. (1956) ref. 16 above, p. 476

26 Lock. M. M. (1980) *East Asian Medicine in Urban Japan.* Berkeley: University of California Press, p.77

27 Simonton, O. C., Matthews-Simonton, S. and Creighton, J.L. (1978) *Getting Well Again.* Los Angeles: J. P. Tarcher (New York: Bantam Books, 1980). See also *Lancet* editorial (1985) Emotion and immunity, **2**, 133–34

28 Pearce, I. (1983) *The Gate of Healing.* Jersey: Neville Spearman

29 Beishon, J. and Peters, G. (1976) *Systems Behaviour*, 2nd edn London: Harper and Row (Open University)

30 Bertalanffy, L. von (1968) *General System Theory.* New York: Brazillier. London: Allen Lane

31 Laszlo, E. (1972a) *The Systems View of the World: theNatural Philosophy of the New Developments in the Sciences.* New York: George Brazillier. Oxford: Blackwell, Chapter 2

32 Laszlo. E. (1972b) *Introduction to Systems Philosophy: Toward a New Paradigm of Contemporary Thought.* New York: Gordon and Breach

33 Laszlo, E. (1972a) Ref. 31 above, p. 23

34 This schema is modified from H. Brody and D. S. Sobel A Systems View of Health and Disease, in *Ways to Health: Holistic Approaches to Ancient and Contemporary Medicine* (1979), ed. D. S. Sobel. New York: Harcourt Brace Jovanovich. The original idea of a hierarchy of systems is usually attributed to George Engel (1977) The need for a new medical medical model: a challenge for biomedicine, *Science*, **196**, 129–36; and, more importantly, (1980) The clinical application of the biopsychosocial model, *American Journal of Psychiatry*, **137**, 535–44. Ervin Laszlo (1972b) Ref. 32 above, describes something similar, p. 29

35 Weiss, P. A. (1969) Ref. 22 above, p. 13

36 Houk, J. C. (1980) Homeostasis and Control Principles, in *Medical Physiology*, Vol. 1, ed. V. B. Mountcastle. St Louis: C. V. Mosby

37 Bernard, C. (1878) Extract from *Leçons sur les phénomènes de la vie communs aux animaux at aux végétaux*, in *Selected Readings in the History of Physiology*, trans. and ed. by J.F. Fulton (1930). Springfield, Ill.: C. C. Thomas, pp. 307–09

38 Cannon, W.B. (1929) Organization for physiological homeostasis, *Physiological Reviews*, **9**, 399–431

39 This is the Uroborus (or Ouroboros), a Gnostic and alchemical symbol of continuity and unity in all things. The serpent devouring its own tail symbolizes destruction and nourishment at the same time, and so represents the interplay of opposites

40 Bernard, C. (1865) *An Introduction to the Study of Experimental Medicine*, trans. H. C. Green (1927). New York: Dover, 1957 (Also London: Constable) p. 88

41 ibid. p. 89

42 ibid. Foreword

Chapter 17 Personal reorientations

1 Kerenyi, C. (1959) *Asklepios: Archetypal Image of the Physician's Existence*. New York: Pantheon, p.7

2 Alma Ata Declaration (made at Alma-Ata, Kazakhstan, USSR, 12 September 1978). See Horder, J. (1983) *British Medical Journal*, **286**, 191–94

3 Ziegler, A. (1983) *Archetypal Medicine* (original title in German edition: *Morbismus*). Dallas: Spring Books. Quotations here taken from an interview with Ann Shearer, *Guardian*, 23 April 1986

4 Bennet, G. (1983) *Beyond Endurance: Survival at the Extremes*. London: Secker and Warburg. New York: St Martin's Press, mainly chapters 8 and 9

5 See references in Chapter 7, mainly refs. 6 to 12

6 Sanford, J. A. (1982) *Ministry Burnout*. London: Arthur James (1984), p. 104

7 Eliot, T. S. (1944) *Four Quartets*, East Coker, III. London: Faber and Faber

8 Dante. *The Inferno*. Temple Classics translation (1900). London: J. M. Dent

Chapter 18 Partnership and participation

1 References to this topic in Chapter 2

2 References in Chapter 1, mainly nos 16–21

3   Sanford, J. A. (1982) *Ministry Burnout*. London: Arthur James (1984)
4   General Medical Council (1985) *Professional Conduct and Discipline: Fitness to Practise*. London: General Medical Council, p. 7
5   ibid. p. 30
6   The Association of Surgeons of Great Britain and Ireland evolved a scheme in 1982 whereby surgeons whose competence to practise was in doubt could be reported confidentially and then discreetly investigated. For doctors, in Britain, seeking personal help there is the National Counselling and Welfare Service for Sick Doctors, 7 Marylebone Road, London, NW1 5HH; tel. (during office hours) 01–580–3160. The network of support in the United States is much more extensive: see Schreiber, S. C. and Doyle, B. D. (eds) (1983) *The Impaired Physician*. New York and London: Plenum, Appendix A
7   The words 'feeling' and 'feelings' crop up frequently in this section and may need some explanation. 'Feeling' can refer to straightforward displays of feeling, or emotion, as in an outburst of distress or anger. It has a broader meaning when contrasted with thinking: that is, the feeling and empathic functions as opposed to the thinking, rational and intellectual functions. Many people who mainly employ their rational and intellectual functions (such as doctors) have difficulty with their feeling functions. It is as though these functions are less well developed, and the person concerned is liable to be less comfortable and assured in situations where feelings are prominent in the interaction. The doctor with poorly developed feeling functions can become uneasy when patients show distress or when personal relationships (which are all about feeling) enter into the medical dialogue. This is not to say that such people are not capable of deep feeling – far from it – merely that they are less confident and comfortable where feelings are concerned, as opposed to ideas or factual information
8   2 Corinthians 12: 9, 10
9   Reedy, B. L. (1978) *The New Health Practitioners in America: a Comparative Study*. London: Pitman (for King's Fund)
10   Bowling, A. (1981) *Delegation in General Practice: a Study of Doctors and Nurses*. London: Tavistock
11   In the United States, in addition to Nurse Practitioners, who are registered nurses with special extra training, there are Physician's Assistants. These are mostly men who have previously been medical technicians or members of the medical corps in the armed forces. They have training and duties comparable with those of the nurse practitioners but they are employed directly by physicians (as opposed to working in health organizations), and they identify with the physicians. See Reedy, B. L. (1978) ref. 8 above
12   Allibone, A. (1981) It does work, *British Medical Journal*, **283**, 1581–82
13   Hart, J. T. (1985) Practice nurses: an underused resource, *British Medical Journal*, **290**, 1162–63
14   Hayes, T. M. and Harries, J. (1984) Randomised controlled trial of routine hospital clinic care versus routine general practitioner care for type II diabetes, *British Medical Journal*, **289**, 728–30
15   Speight, A. N. P. (1978) Is childhood asthma being underdiagnosed and undertreated?, *British Medical Journal*, **2**, 331–32

16 Fox, S. (1984) Hippocrates unbound, *Journal of the American Medical Association*, **251**, 490–94

17 General Medical Council (1985) Ref. 4 above, p. 11

18 Marks, I. (1985) Controlled trial of psychiatric nurse therapists in primary care, *British Medical Journal*, **290**, 1181–84

19 Some doctors may think I am presenting the health professionals as flawless people, but, of course, nurses, social workers, complementary and alternative practitioners and others can be authoritarian, dogmatic and prejudiced like anyone else. In this book about doctors I have not discussed these other workers except insofar as they can enhance the overall quality of medical care

20 Paine, T. (1983) Survey of patient participation groups in the United Kingdom: Parts 1 and 2, *British Medical Journal*, **286**, 768–72, 847–49

21 Mann, R. H. (1985) Why patient participation groups stop functioning: general practitioners' viewpoint, *British Medical Journal*, **290**, 209–11

22 Sand, P. (1978) Patient Participation Groups: an Analysis of Consumer Participation in General Practice. Unpublished thesis for MSc in social research, University of Surrey. Summary in Pritchard, P. (1981), ref. 23 below, pp. 17–19

23 Pritchard, P. (ed.) (1981) *Patient Participation in General Practice*, Occasional Paper 17. London: Royal College of General Practitioners

24 Patient Participation – More or Less?, a debate by several authors, in *Common Dilemmas in Family Medicine*, ed. J. Fry (1983). Lancaster: MTP Press, pp. 229–69

25 Pritchard, P. (1983) Patient Participation, in *Doctor-Patient Communication*, ed. D. Pendleton and J. Hasler. London: Academic Press

26 McEwen, J., Martini, C. J. M. and Wilkins, N. (1983) *Participation in Health*. London: Croom Helm

27 Bates, E. (1983) *Health System and Public Scrutiny: Australia, Britain, and the United States*. London: Croom Helm. New York: St Martin's Press

28 Maxwell, R. and Weaver, N. (eds) (1984) *Public Participation in Health: Towards a Clearer View*. London: King Edward's Hospital Fund for London

29 Wilson, A. T. M. (1977) Patient participation in a primary care unit, *British Medical Journal*, **1**, 398

30 Wilson, A. (1981) In Aberdare, *British Medical Journal*, **282**, 1284–86

31 Graffey, J. P. (1981) Patient participation in primary health care. In P. Pritchard (1981) ref. 23 above, pp. 23–26

32 An important early attempt at participation occurred at the Pioneer Health Centre at Peckham (south London), and ran for nine years in the 1930s and 40s. See *Lancet* (1986), **1**, 422–23

33 *Journal of the Royal College of General Practitioners* (1974) Patient power, Editorial, **24**, 1–3

34 Levin, L. S. (1976) The layperson as the primary health care practitioner, *Public Health Records*, **91**, 206–10

35 Shearer, A. (1983) The patient revolution in Kentish Town, *Self Health* (Journal of the College of Health), **1** (No. 1), 7–9

36 Nottinghamshire County Council (1984) *Mansfield Community Health Project*. Nottingham: Social Services Department, 20 pages. (This is a description of one community project)

37 Gunn, A. D. G. (1984) Self Help, *British Medical Journal*, **288**, 1024
38 Robinson, D. (1978) Self-help groups, *British Journal of Hospital Medicine*, **20**, 306–11
39 National Association of Health Authorities (in England and Wales) (1985) *Index of Consumer Relations in the NHS*. NAHA, Garth House, 47 Edgbaston Park Road, Birmingham B15 2RS. (Descriptions of 93 surveys into consumer attitudes towards all aspects of health care)
40 College of Health. For their journal, see ref. 35 above

Index